Dermatology

Editors

DARIO D'OVIDIO
DOMENICO SANTORO

VETERINARY CLINICS
OF NORTH AMERICA:
EXOTIC ANIMAL PRACTICE

www.vetexotic.theclinics.com

Consulting Editor
JÖRG MAYER

May 2023 • Volume 26 • Number 2

ELSEVIER

1600 John F. Kennedy Boulevard • Suite 1800 • Philadelphia, Pennsylvania, 19103-2899
http://www.vetexotic.theclinics.com

VETERINARY CLINICS OF NORTH AMERICA: EXOTIC ANIMAL PRACTICE Volume 26, Number 2
May 2023 ISSN 1094-9194, ISBN-13: 978-0-323-93991-1

Editor: Stacy Eastman
Developmental Editor: Axell Ivan Jade M. Purificacion

Veterinary Clinics of North America: Exotic Animal Practice (ISSN 1094-9194) is published in January, May, and September by Elsevier, Inc., 360 Park Avenue South, New York, NY 10010-1710. Subscription prices are $305.00 per year for US individuals, $614.00 per year for US institutions, $100.00 per year for US students and residents, $355.00 per year for Canadian individuals, $739.00 per year for Canadian institutions, $370.00 per year for international individuals, $739.00 per year for international institutions, $100.00 per year Canadian students/residents, and $165.00 per year for international students/residents. To receive student/resident rate, orders must be accompanied by name of affiliated institution, date of term, and the *signature* of program/residency coordinator on institution letterhead. Orders will be billed at individual rate until proof of status is received. Foreign air speed delivery is included in all *Clinics* subscription prices. All prices are subject to change without notice. **POSTMASTER:** Send address changes to *Veterinary Clinics of North America: Exotic Animal Practice*, Elsevier Health Sciences Division, Subscription Customer Service, 3251 Riverport Lane, Maryland Heights, MO 63043. **Customer Service: Telephone: 1-800-654-2452** (U.S. and Canada); **1-314-447-8871** (outside U.S. and Canada). **Fax: 1-314-447-8029. E-mail: journalscustomerservice-usa@elsevier.com (for print support); journalsonlinesupport-usa@elsevier.com (for online support).**

Reprints. For copies of 100 or more of articles in this publication, please contact the Commercial Reprints Department, Elsevier Inc., 360 Park Avenue South, New York, New York 10010-1710. Tel.: 212-633-3874; Fax: 212-633-3820; E-mail: reprints@elsevier.com.

Veterinary Clinics of North America: Exotic Animal Practice is covered in *MEDLINE/PubMed (Index Medicus).*

Contributors

CONSULTING EDITOR

JÖRG MAYER, Dr med vet, Msc
Diplomate, American Board of Veterinary Practitioners (Exotic Companion Mammals); Diplomate, European College of Zoological Medicine (Small Mammals); Diplomate, American College of Zoological Medicine; Associate Professor of Zoological Medicine, Department of Small Animal Medicine and Surgery, University of Georgia College of Veterinary Medicine, Athens, Georgia, USA

EDITORS

DARIO d'OVIDIO, DVM, MS, SpecPACS, PhD
Diplomate, European College of Zoological Medicine (Small Mammals); Private Practitioner, Arzano, Naples, Italy; Anicura Clinica Veterinaria Malpensa, Samarate, Italy

DOMENICO SANTORO, DVM, DrSc, MS, PhD
Diplomate, European College of Veterinary Dermatology; Diplomate, American College of Veterinary Dermatology; Diplomate, American College of Veterinary Microbiologists; Department of Small Animal Clinical Sciences, College of Veterinary Medicine, University of Florida, Gainesville, Florida, USA

AUTHORS

TARIQ ABOU-ZAHR, BVSc, CertAVP(ZooMed), MRCVS
Diplomate, European College of Zoological Medicine (Avian); Valley Exotics, Vet Partner's Practices Ltd T/A Valley Vets, Gwaelod-Y-Garth, Cardiff, United Kingdom

GRACIELA AGUILAR, DVM
Department of Veterinary Clinical Sciences, Louisiana State University, School of Veterinary Medicine, Baton Rouge, Louisiana, USA

NORIN CHAI, DVM, MSc, PhD
Diplomate, European College of Zoological Medicine (Zoo Health Management); Yaboumba, Paris, France

DARIO d'OVIDIO, DVM, MS, SpecPACS, PhD
Diplomate, European College of Zoological Medicine (Small Mammals); Private Practitioner, Arzano, Naples, Italy; Anicura Clinica Veterinaria Malpensa, Samarate, Italy

GRAYSON A. DOSS, DVM
Diplomate, American College of Zoological Medicine; Department of Surgical Sciences, School of Veterinary Medicine, University of Wisconsin-Madison, Madison, Wisconsin, USA

DAVID ESHAR, DVM
Diplomate, American Board of Veterinary Practitioners (Exotic Companion Mammal); Diplomate, European College of Zoological Medicine (Small Mammal, Zoo Health Management); Department of Clinical Sciences, College of Veterinary Medicine, Kansas State University, Manhattan, Kansas, USA

METTE LOUISE HALCK, DVM
Master of Exotic Companion and Hobby Animal Medicine, AniCura Københavns Dyrehospital, Denmark

MARK A. MITCHELL, DVM, MS, PhD
Diplomate, European College of Zoological Medicine (Herpetology); Department of Veterinary Clinical Sciences, Louisiana State University, School of Veterinary Medicine, Baton Rouge, Louisiana, USA

MARIALETIZIA PALOMBA, Biol, PhD
Department of Ecological and Biological Sciences, University of Tuscia, Largo dell'Università sn, Viterbo, Italy

MARCIA RAQUEL PEGORARO DE MACEDO, Biol, PhD
Department of Integrative Marine Ecology, Stazione Zoologica Anton Dohrn, Naples, Italy

ENDRE SÓS, DVM, PhD
Diplomate, European College of Zoological Medicine (Zoo Health Management); Budapest Zoo and Botanical Garden, Hungary

VIKTÓRIA SÓS-KOROKNAI, DVM, PhD
Budapest Zoo and Botanical Garden, Hungary

DOMENICO SANTORO, DVM, DrSc, MS, PhD
Diplomate, European College of Veterinary Dermatology; Diplomate, American College of Veterinary Dermatology; Diplomate, American College of Veterinary Microbiologists; Department of Small Animal Clinical Sciences, College of Veterinary Medicine, University of Florida, Gainesville, Florida, USA

MARIO SANTORO, DVM, MSc, PhD
Diplomate, European College of Zoological Medicine (Wildlife Population Health); Department of Integrative Marine Ecology, Stazione Zoologica Anton Dohrn, Naples, Italy

JASMINE SARVI, DVM
Department of Clinical Sciences, College of Veterinary Medicine, Kansas State University, Manhattan, Kansas, USA

NICO J. SCHOEMAKER, DVM, PhD
Diplomate, European College of Zoological Medicine (Small Mammal, Avian); Department of Clinical Sciences, Faculty of Veterinary Medicine, Utrecht University, the Netherlands

YVONNE R.A. VAN ZEELAND, DVM, MVR, PhD
Diplomate, European College of Zoological Medicine (Avian, Small Mammal); Department of Clinical Sciences, Faculty of Veterinary Medicine, Utrecht University, the Netherlands

STEPHEN D. WHITE, DVM
Diplomate, American College of Veterinary Dermatology; Distinguished Professor, Chief of Service, Dermatology, Department of Veterinary, Medicine and Epidemiology, School of Veterinary Medicine, University of California, Davis, Davis, California, USA

Contents

Dermatologic disorders are some of the most common conditions affecting exotic companion mammals. This article provides a clinical approach of the conditions presenting with alopecia, pruritus, scaling/crusting, erosion/ulceration, and nodules in order to select and interpret the appropriate diagnostic tests to achieve a diagnosis for a successful treatment.

Dermatologic conditions are common in avian practice and can be caused by a huge array of potential disorders, ranging from infectious diseases, ectoparasites, metabolic disorders, nutritional deficiencies, and management deficits. The skin is the largest organ in the body and has the potential to lead to significant discomfort and welfare compromise when pathology is present. Some conditions may be relatively pathognomonic based on gross findings, whereas others may require a full diagnostic workup to investigate. Getting to the bottom of skin lesions and disorders often involves identification and correction of the underlying cause, rather than just treating the lesions present in the integument.

The majority of rabbit skin disease presentations can be divided into pruritus, alopecia, scaling, and nodules. Some disease will have more than one of these clinical signs. Ectoparasites, bacterial and fungal infections, and neoplasia account for most of the causes seen. Diagnostic tests include skin scraping and cytology, microbial culture, and biopsy. Therapy is dependent on cause. In addition to discussing the various causes and their treatments, important clinical care points are noted.

Skin diseases commonly affect pet ferrets, with neoplastic, endocrine, and parasitic diseases being the most common. This review includes clinical presentation, diagnostic workup, and treatment of diseases with a dermatologic presentation in ferrets.

The article deals with the primary aspects of how to maintain healthy integument in zoo mammals and in particular why husbandry-related health problems can occur in general in a zoologic setting. While working with these species we are often faced with diagnostic challenges, which may include a general approach (often requiring anesthesia or medical training), lack of "normal" references, and difficulties, especially if the cutaneous signs are not a primary ailment, but a manifestation of a generalized disease (eg, immune-suppression). The different etiologies of skin problems are discussed with clinical examples.

Elasmobranch fishes comprise sharks and sawfish (infraclass Selachii) and rays, skates, and stingrays (infraclass Batoidea). Many elasmobranch species are popular fish exhibited in zoos and public aquariums. They may serve as hosts for a great variety of parasites. Among these, parasitic copepods are commonly known to cause serious damage to their hosts. The Pandaridae (Milne Edwards, 1840) (Siphonostomatoida; Burmeister, 1835) comprises copepod ectoparasites of fish (primarily of sharks), whose taxonomic information is conflicting, and data on biology, ecology, biogeography, phylogeny, and pathogenesis remain incomplete or poor known.

Integumentary disorders caused by zoonotic agents are very common in exotic companion mammals. This article provides an understanding of the main zoonotic dermatoses including parasitic, fungal, bacterial, and viral diseases to provide the most updated information on their epidemiology, diagnosis, reported clinical signs, and therapies in cohabitant people.

VETERINARY CLINICS OF NORTH AMERICA: EXOTIC ANIMAL PRACTICE

FORTHCOMING ISSUES

September 2023
Critical Care
Lily Parkinson, *Editor*

January 2024
Exotic Animal Nutrition
Amanda Ardente, *Editor*

May 2024
Pediatrics
João Lemos Brandão and Peter M. DiGeronimo, *Editors*

RECENT ISSUES

January 2023
Pain Management
David Sanchez-Migallon Guzman, *Editor*

September 2022
Exotic Animal Clinical Pathology
J. Jill Heatley and Karen E. Russell, *Editors*

May 2022
Cardiology
Michael Pees, *Editor*

SERIES OF RELATED INTEREST

Veterinary Clinics: Small Animal Practice
https://www.vetsmall.theclinics.com/
Advances in Small Animal Care
https://www.advancesinsmallanimalcare.com

THE CLINICS ARE NOW AVAILABLE ONLINE!
Access your subscription at:
www.theclinics.com

Preface

(Exotic Animal) Dermatology

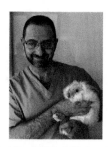 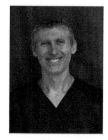

Dario d'Ovidio, DVM, MS, SpecPACS, PhD   Domenico Santoro, DVM, DrSc, MS, PhD
Editors

Due to the increase in popularity of exotic animals as pets in households as well as their recognized importance on the entire ecosystem, zoologic medicine has made significant advances in the past decades. Consequently, all areas of this field have developed considerably. Dermatologic disorders are some of the most common problems affecting companion animals (eg, dogs, cats, horses), and exotic animals are not the exception. This issue of the *Veterinary Clinics of North America: Exotic Animal Practice* brings, in separate articles, up-to-date information on bird, rabbit, ferret, rodent, reptile, amphibian, four-toed hedgehog, zoo mammal, and fish dermatology. For the first time, we are proposing a problem-oriented approach in exotic animals to help diagnose dermatologic conditions based on the predominance of their main clinical sign, such as alopecia, pruritus, scaling/crusting, erosion/ulceration, and nodular lesions. The information presented in the articles included in this issue highlights the impressive progress made in this field of veterinary medicine over the last 20 years, with numerous scientific articles and case reports documenting newly diagnosed dermatologic diseases, new diagnostic methods as well as evaluation of new treatment modalities for different types of exotic animal species. Finally, an overview of the main zoonotic dermatoses, including parasitic, fungal, bacterial, and viral diseases, is provided to gather the most updated information on their epidemiology, diagnosis, and treatment.

We would like to thank all the authors for their valuable contribution to this issue, and we hope that clinicians will find the information presented here applicable and clinically useful. Also, we would like to acknowledge and dedicate this issue of *Veterinary Clinics of North America: Exotic Animal Practice* to our friend and colleague, Dr Dunbar Gram. Dunbar was an exceptional human being and an enthusiastic and kind friend. He made teaching the new generation of veterinarians and current veterinary practitioners his professional mission. In addition, Dunbar worked very closely with the zoo medicine service at the University of Florida for the past decade, managing dermatologic

Vet Clin Exot Anim 26 (2023) ix–x
https://doi.org/10.1016/j.cvex.2023.02.001
1094-9194/23/© 2023 Published by Elsevier Inc.

conditions in a variety of animals, including bats, large ruminants, elephants, and other exotic and zoo animals. He will always be remembered and missed by all the people that had the pleasure and honor to meet him.

Dario d'Ovidio, DVM, MS, SpecPACS, PhD
Private Practitioner
Via Colombo 118
Arzano, NA 80022, Italy

Domenico Santoro, DVM, DrSc, MS, PhD
Department of Small Animal Clinical Sciences
College of Veterinary Medicine
University of Florida
2015 Southwest 16th Avenue
Gainesville, FL 32610, USA

E-mail addresses:
dariodovidio@yahoo.it (D. d'Ovidio)
dsantoro@ufl.edu (D. Santoro)

Problem-Oriented Approach in Exotic Companion Mammals

Dario d'Ovidio, MS, SpecPACS, PhD, Dip.ECZM (Small Mammals)[a,b,*],
Stephen White, DVM, DACVD[c],
Domenico Santoro, DVM, DrSc, MS, PhD, Dip.ECVD, Dip.ACVD, Dip.ACVM[d]

KEYWORDS

- Exotic companion mammals • Dermatology • Skin disease • Management • Rabbit
- Rodents • Ferrets

KEY POINTS

- Dermatologic disorders are extremely common in exotic companion mammals (ECMs).
- The problem-oriented approach (POA) is a rational method to manage clinical cases in human as well as veterinary patients.
- The POA can help the development of evidence-based dermatology in ECM practice.

INTRODUCTION

Exotic companion mammals (ECMs; eg, rabbits, rodents, ferrets) are becoming increasingly popular as house pets. Skin disorders are some of the most common diseases affecting these species. They can be either infectious (eg, viral, bacterial, parasitic, and fungal) or noninfectious (eg, endocrine, neoplastic, and allergic) in origin and can be characterized by several clinical signs such as alopecia, pruritus, scaling/crusting, erosion/ulceration, and nodules. Dermatologic diseases in exotic pets are currently approached by class/species of animals (eg, reptiles, avian, small mammals) and/or primary etiologic agents (eg, viruses, bacteria, fungi, parasites).[1] The problem-oriented approach (POA) is a rational step-wise method to manage clinical cases in human as well as veterinary patients emphasizing the patient's problems (clinical signs caused by patient's disease), which influence the clinical reasoning that the clinician uses to achieve the diagnosis.[2,3] This approach begins with gathering all the information (history and clinical): step 1: Database collection: following to create a problem list

[a] Private Practitioner, Via C. Colombo 118, Arzano, Naples 80022, Italy; [b] Anicura Clinica Veterinaria Malpensa, Samarate, Italy; [c] Dermatology, School of Veterinary Medicine, University of California, 2108 Tupper Hall, One Shields Avenue, Davis, CA 95616, USA; [d] Department of Small Animal Clinical Sciences, College of Veterinary Medicine, University of Florida, 2015 Southwest 16th Avenue, Gainesville, FL 32610, USA
* Corresponding author. Private Practitioner, Via C. Colombo 118, Arzano, Naples 80022, Italy.
E-mail address: dariodovidio@yahoo.it

Vet Clin Exot Anim 26 (2023) 309–326
https://doi.org/10.1016/j.cvex.2023.01.003
1094-9194/23/© 2023 Elsevier Inc. All rights reserved.

including all the clinical signs, presenting complaints, and diagnostic findings that the clinician has identified is formulated and step 2: Problem identification: this list is refined overtime. After identification of the problems, a plan including diagnostic tests, therapy, and client/owner education is developed (step 3: Plan formulation). In the final step, progress notes containing new or additional data and their assessments, collected from the initial and all subsequent plans, are written and used to take the appropriate decisions and improve the medical action (step 4: Assessment and follow-up).[2]

Alopecia

The main causes of hair loss are listed in **Tables 1** and **2**.

Several physiologic or behavioral factors may affect the evaluation of hair loss in ECMs. These may include gender and reproductive status, age and time of onset, husbandry conditions, and pattern of alopecia. Hair pulling, generally from the abdomen, occurs in pregnant does (rabbits) before giving birth or in case of false pregnancy in order to prepare a nest.[4] A seasonal hair loss is normal during moulting (or shedding), which occurs generally in young rabbits at around puberty (5–6 months) and twice yearly (spring and fall) in adult animals.[4] In client-owned pets, the moulting season may occur in different times of the year, depending on the temperature in the household. Partial rather than total alopecia can be seen during the moulting. On the contrary, during specific medical conditions, different patterns of alopecia may occur in rabbits. The most common patterns include focal, multifocal, patchy, diffuse, and symmetric alopecia. Some conditions may start with focal or multifocal alopecia, but they can progress to diffuse or generalized alopecia.

In intact ferrets of both sexes, a bilateral symmetric alopecia involving the tail and the perianal area may be seen during the breeding season, from March to August (in the northern hemisphere).[5,6] With the exception of this seasonal alopecia, a complete work-up should be performed to identify the reason for the hair loss.

Non-pruritic hair loss in guinea pigs can be frequently seen in late pregnancy or during lactation due to hormonal changes.[7] Improper handling may cause fur slip in chinchillas that may release a patch of hair due to defensive behavior.[8] Rodents trying to escape from the cage may develop alopecia of the muzzle or face without other cutaneous signs.[9]

Clinical presentation

The presence, features, and distribution of lesions can help guide the clinician to formulate a list of differential diagnoses.

- Patchy alopecic, non-pruritic lesions on the head (ear, eyes, chin), limbs (feet and nail beds), or generalized distribution, sometimes with crusting and erythema, are seen in rabbits with dermatophytosis.[4,10,11] In ferrets, dermatophytosis is characterized by annular alopecia, associated with scaling, crusting, erythema, and papules.[6,12]
- The concurrent presence of seborrhea sicca, otitis externa, crusts of the face, head, and neck, and extensive alopecia should alert the clinician to search for *Demodex* mite infestation in rabbits although rare.[4,13]
- The presence of alopecic areas with broken hairs all over the body (self-barbering) or even on the head of animals housed with (dominant) cage-mates is commonly suggestive of barbering. Rarely barbering may be associated with actual self-inflicted wounds. Lesions can be diagnosed on observation or via trichogram.[4,14,15]
- Generalized alopecia in rabbits presented with paradoxic hyperexia, weight loss, and cardiac abnormalities (atrial fibrillation and dilatation) may be suggestive of Idiopathic hyperthyroidism.[16]

Table 1
Dermatologic diseases causing alopecia, pruritus, scales/crusts, erosion/ulcer, and nodule in exotic companion mammals

Clinical Sign	Definition	Main Conditions	Species Affected
Alopecia	Partial (hypotrichosis) or complete loss of hair	Barbering, improper husbandry	ECM
		Fur slip/fur chewing	Chinchillas, other ECM
		Dermatophytosis	ECM
		Endocrinopathies	Ferrets, other ECM
		Neoplasia	ECM
		Demodex infestation (see **Table 2**)	Rabbits/rodents
Pruritus	Uncomfortable sensation associated with the urge of scratch, rub, chew, or pull	Ectoparasites	ECM
		Pinworms	Rabbits/rodents
		Bacterial infections	ECM
		Endocrinopathies	Ferrets, other ECM
		Neoplasia	ECM
		Idiopathic ulcerative dermatitis	Mice
Scales/crusts	Scale: Accumulation of loose corneocytes Crust: Dried accumulation of cells, blood, and exudate	Ectoparasites	ECM
		Bacterial infections (rabbit syphilis)	Rabbit
		Sebaceous adenitis	Rabbit
		Viral diseases (distemper, poxvirus infection)	Ferrets, guinea pigs, other ECM
		Dermatophytosis	Ferrets and rodents
		Neoplasia (epitheliotropic lymphoma)	Ferrets and guinea pigs
		Other conditions (pemphigus foliaceus-like, erythema multiforme)	Ferrets
Erosion/ulcer	Erosion: Loss of epidermis up to the basement membrane Ulcer: Loss of epidermis affecting the basement membrane	Ulcerative pododermatitis	ECM
		Bacterial infections (necrobacillosis)	ECM
		Neoplasia (epitheliotropic lymphoma)	ECM
		Idiopathic ulcerative dermatitis	Mice
		Bacterial ulcerative dermatitis	Rats
Nodule	Circumscribed, raised, cell-filled, firm lesion >1 cm	Parasitic nodules (see **Table 2**)	ECM
		Viral nodules (myxomatosis, Shope fibroma/papilloma)	Rabbits
		Mycotic nodules	Ferrets
		Neoplasia	Guinea pigs, other ECM

- A diffuse generalized alopecia, associated with erythema, erosions, crusts, and plaques may be seen in ferrets with cutaneous lymphoma.[6,17,18]
- Neutered/spayed ferrets affected with adrenal gland disease may show a symmetric, bilateral, not-well-demarcated (in more than 33% of cases) alopecia beginning on the tail, rump, or flanks and progressing to the trunk, dorsum, and ventrum.[6,19–21]

Table 2
Parasites causing dermatologic disorders in exotic companion mammals

Causative Agent	Main Clinical Sign	Species Affected
Ectoparasites		
Mites and Gamasids		
Demodex spp.	Alopecia/scales/pruritus (rare)	Hamsters/prairie dogs/hedgehogs other ECM (rare)
C. parasitovorax, L. gibbus, Chirodiscoides caviae, P. cuniculi, O. cynotis, Sarcoptes scabiei, T. caviae, N. cati, C. tripilis, Caparinia erinacei, Chorioptes, Myocoptes	Pruritus/scales/crusts/erosion/ulcer	Rabbits/guinea pigs/hedgehogs
Gamasids (*O bacoti*)	Pruritus/alopecia	ECM
Myobia musculi, Myocoptes musculinus, Radfordia affinis, Radfordia ensifera	Pruritus/ulcer	Rats/mice
Fleas		
Spilopsyllus cuniculi, Cediopsylla simplex, Odontopsyllus multispinosus, Echidnophaga gallinacea, Hoplopsyllus spp, *Ceratophyllus sciorum, Ceratophyllus gallinae, Pulex irritans, Nosopsylla* spp., *Archeopsylla erinacei, Ctenocephalides* spp.	Pruritus/scales/crusts	ECM
Ticks		
Haemaphysalis, Ixodes spp., *Rhipicephalus* spp., *Otobius* spp., *Dermacentor* spp., *Amblyomma* spp., *Boophilus* spp.	Pruritus	ECM
Lice		
H. ventricosus, Gliricola porcelli, Gyropus ovalis, Polyplax serrata, Polyplax spinulosa	Pruritus	Rabbits/rodents
Insects		
Cuterebra, Lucilia, Calliphora, H. bovis	Nodule	ECM
Endoparasites		
Pinworms (*P. ambiguus*)	Pruritus	Rabbits
Tapeworms (*Coenurus serialis*)	Nodule	Rabbits

- A focal or diffuse not-well-demarcated alopecia (generalized form) and less commonly a pruritic, crusting pododermatitis (localized form), can be seen in ferrets affected with sarcoptic mange.[6,22]
- A not-well-demarcated alopecia, associated with comedones, skin discoloration, erythema, and brown ceruminous debris in the ferrets' external ear canal, is associated with *Demodex* infestation.[5,6,23]
- Nutritional deficiencies, poor hygiene, and improper bedding material may cause hair loss in the ventrum in guinea pigs.[7,24,25]

- Guinea pigs affected with follicular ovarian cysts may show a bilateral, symmetric, well-demarcated alopecia in up to 60% of cases.[26,27] Similarly, a well-demarcated symmetric alopecia associated with adrenal disease can be seen in hamsters.[28]
- A clean, alopecic area, where the hair has been pulled out, can be seen in chinchillas with fur slip.[8,29]
- Alopecia and short hair only on the dorsum, lumbar area, tail, and flanks can be seen in chinchillas affected with fur chewing (**Fig. 1**). This behavioral disorder can occur in chinchillas of any age from continual stressful conditions (eg, small cage, lack of enrichment or exercise wheels, and presence of dominant cage mates) or in older animals with dental disorders.[8,30,31]
- Alopecia associated with scaling and/or erythema can be seen in hamster affected with demodicosis (**Fig. 2**).[32]

Pruritus

Diseases causing pruritus in ECM can have an infectious, hormonal, or environmental origin (see **Tables 1** and **2**).

Pruritus in rabbits, rodents, and hedgehogs is caused mainly by infectious parasitic diseases, whereas in ferrets, it is more commonly associated with adrenal disease rather than ectoparasites (eg, fleas or mites).[4,6,21,32–47] Parasitic dermatoses are commonly caused by mites and less commonly fleas, lice, and ticks (see **Table 2**). Internal parasites (eg, pinworms) may also cause perianal pruritus in rabbits.[4] The development of new spines in young hedgehogs may be associated with pruritus.[43] A thorough history can give important information on husbandry conditions, direct or indirect contact with infected pets as well as current and previous antiparasitic treatments.

Clinical presentation

Dealing with a pruritic ECM can be challenging to the veterinarian and frustrating for the owner who is concerned with the risk of contagion to other pets or people.

- A unilateral or bilateral, intensely pruritic otitis with thick crusts extending from the proximal to the external ear pinna, with lesions occasionally located around the face or at the genital area, is frequently associated with *Psoroptes cuniculi* infection in rabbits.[4,10,48,49]
- Alopecic, erythematous, severely pruritic, crusted lesions at the nose, mouth, ears, limbs, and less frequently genitals are commonly caused by *Sarcoptes scabiei* infection (**Fig. 3**).[4,45,48]

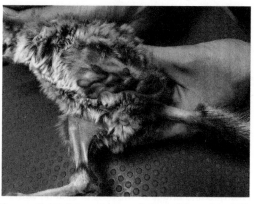

Fig. 1. Alopecia of the medial tights and base of the tail in a chinchilla with fur chewing.

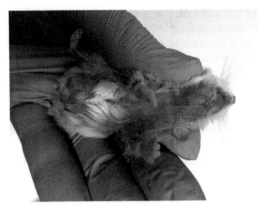

Fig. 2. Diffuse alopecia and erythema in a hamster affected with demodicosis.

- A moderate to severe pruritus, associated with erythema and excoriations, less frequently with crusts on head and trunk can be seen in case of infestation by fleas, ticks, and mites. Owing to their size, these parasites and/or their excrements (fleas) can be commonly seen at naked eye.[4,10,40,48]
- Perianal pruritus caused by the rabbit pinworm (*Passalurus ambiguus*) eggs can be the only dermatologic sign found in cases of pinworm infestation.[4,10]
- Contact or allergic dermatitis may be suspected in ECM showing pruritic behavior once alternate causes have been ruled out.[4,50]
- Ferrets affected with ear mite infestation may present for head shaking, ear scratching, periaural excoriations, and crusting (otitis externa) as well as presence of dark ear exudate filling the ear canal.[6,51] Similarly, otic debris and otic pruritus may be seen in African hedgehogs infested by ear mites (*Notoedres cati*).[43]
- Ferrets with mild reactions to vaccines may show pruritus and skin erythema.[44]
- Chronic pruritus, along with diffuse alopecia, erythema, erosions, crusts, and ulcerated plaques, may be seen in ferrets affected with epitheliotropic lymphoma.[17]
- Intense pruritus, alopecia, scales, crusts, and hyperkeratosis, potentially associated with pruritic behavior in cohabitant humans, are typically seen in guinea pigs with *Trixacarus caviae* infestation.[5,24,25,34]

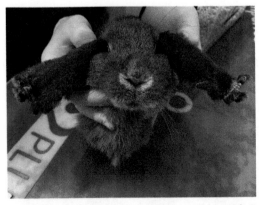

Fig. 3. Crusts on ears margins and bridge of the nose in a rabbit with *S. scabiei* var. *cuniculi* infection.

- Pruritus, erythema, and poorly demarcated dorsal alopecia on the neck and midline can be seen in ECM affected with *Ornithonyssus bacoti* infestation.[39,40]
- Greasy fur and self-inflicted ulcerations may occur in rats/mice with heavy mite infestation (see **Tables 1** and **2**).[5,42]

Scaling/Crusting

The diseases more commonly causing scaling/crusting of the skin and the mucocutaneous junctions are listed in **Tables 1** and **2**.

These conditions can be pruritic (fur mite infestation) or non-pruritic (treponematosis, sebaceous adenitis) and can be associated with systemic or organ-specific signs (eg, metritis, abortion, neonatal death in the case of treponematosis).[4]

Clinical presentation

The presence of lesions in specific areas of the body and the presence of concurrent signs in cohabitant pets or owners should help narrow the list of differential diagnoses.

- Facial (nose, eyelids, and muzzle) crusts and proliferative lesions as well as around the perineum are commonly associated with treponematosis.[4,29,48]
- A diffuse scaling/crusting (neck, shoulder, dorsum, ventral areas) associated with papular eruptions in owners is commonly associated with fur mite infestation (cheyletiellosis, leporacariasis).[20,35,37]
- A papular-crusted dermatitis involving the tail, ventrum, or medial thighs of ferrets may be seen in case of flea infestation.[5,6]
- Otitis externa with excoriations and crusting can be seen in ferrets affected with ear mites.[5,6,51]
- Ferrets affected with sarcoptic mange may develop a crusting pododermatitis.[5,6,51]
- A generalized orange-tinged dermatitis, along with diarrhea and mucopurulent nasal and ocular discharges leading to crusts on the facial area and foot pads, or rarely pruritus, generalized erythema and scaling, can be seen in ferrets affected with canine distemper.[5,52–54]
- A sudden onset of crusting and erythema on the ventral inguinal area can be seen in ferrets with epitheliotropic lymphoma; similarly, guinea pigs affected by epitheliotropic T-cell lymphoma may show well-demarcated alopecia, erythema, severe scaling, and lichenification of the front and rear limbs and the ventral region.[5,6,17,55]
- Crusting around the face (eyes, mouth, chin) as well as foot pads and prepuce can be seen in ferrets with pemphigus foliaceus-like skin disease.[5,56]
- See alopecia for clinical signs of cutaneous lymphoma
- Scaling, patchy alopecia with crusty edges on the face (eyes, nose, and ears), feet, and dorsum are frequently seen in guinea pigs affected with dermatophytosis.[57–59]
- Crusty, erythematous areas with excoriations can be seen in case of ectoparasitic infestations (lice, mites), particularly in case of mange by *T. caviae.*[5,25,60]
- Crusts and pustules around the muzzle and nose that can progress to necrosis can be seen in guinea pigs affected by poxvirus infection (**Fig. 4**).[5,20]
- Alopecia, erythema, scaling, and crusting over the face, head, neck, and tail may occur in mice with ringworm (*Trichophyton mentagrophytes* infection).[5,42]
- A chronic exfoliative dermatitis and patchy alopecia can be seen in rabbits with sebaceous adenitis (**Fig. 5**A, B).[61]
- Severe crusting progressing to lichenification can be seen in African hedgehogs affected with *Caparinia tripilis* mite dermatitis (**Fig. 6**).[46]

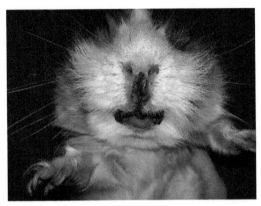

Fig. 4. Crusting ulcerated lesions around the lips and nose in a guinea pig affected with poxvirus infection.

Erosion/Ulceration

The diseases more commonly causing erosion/ulceration of the skin and the mucocutaneous junctions are listed in **Tables 1** and **2**.

Erosive and ulcerative conditions are particularly common in mice and rats.[42] In rabbits, most of the erosive/ulcerative diseases cause systemic signs such as pain (hocks) leading to lameness and reluctance to move, lethargy, fever, and anorexia (necrobacillosis).[4] Hematological abnormalities such as neutrophilia may be associated with tissue inflammation and necrosis as well as nonregenerative anemia associated with advanced stage pododermatitis and osteomyelitis.[62]

Clinical presentation
Specific conditions may be found in specific areas such as limbs and perianal/genital area.

- Granulomatous ulcerative lesions affecting the tarsal/metatarsal skin or less frequently the carpal/metacarpal skin are associated with pododermatitis.[4,63–65]
- Perianal ulcers are suggestive of perianal dermatitis or necrobacillosis (*Fusobacterium necrophorum*).[4,5,29,48]

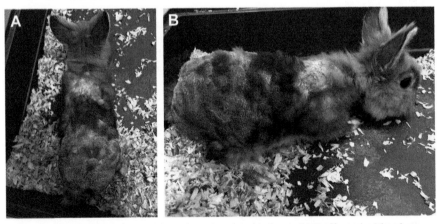

Fig. 5. (*A, B*) Exfoliative dermatitis and patchy alopecia in a rabbit affected with sebaceous adenitis.

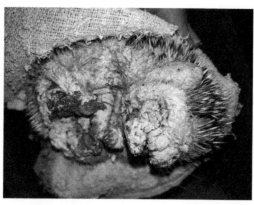

Fig. 6. Severe crusting and lichenification of the ventral skin and limbs in an African hedgehog with *C. tripilis* mite dermatitis.

- Ferrets affected with pyoderma may present skin erosions, ulcerative dermatitis, crusts, and erythematous macules.[66]
- See alopecia for clinical signs of cutaneous lymphoma
- Black laboratory mice (C57BL/6 strain) as well as pet mice can be affected with the idiopathic ulcerative dermatitis characterized by excoriations and ulcerative lesions on the thorax and head, eventually progressing to severe dermatitis.[42,67]
- Rats affected by pruritus associated with fur mite infestation or viral sialodacryoadenitis may develop a secondary bacterial ulcerative dermatitis caused by *Staphylococcus aureus*.[5,42]
- Guinea pigs may develop ulcerative pododermatitis of the palmar or plantar surfaces of the feet. The initial erythematous lesions may progress to granulomatous swellings that, in severe cases, may eventually lead to bacterial invasion of the underlying anatomic structures (eg, tendons, joints, and bone).[5,63]

Nodular Lesions

Diseases causing skin and subcutaneous nodules can have an infectious or noninfectious origin (see **Tables 1** and **2**).

Affected animals may show clinical signs associated with systemic involvement (eg, fever, lethargy, dyspnea, and secondary bacterial infections) in case of systemic diseases (eg, myxomatosis) or organ-specific signs in cases of neoplasms. However, in most of the cases, the skin/subcutaneous nodules do not affect the rabbit's general conditions and only cause a localized problem (eg, non-metastasized tumors, parasitic nodules).[4,50]

Benign or malignant skin neoplasms represent the most frequent cause of nodular lesions in ferrets.[5,6] Rare causes of nodules in ferrets include abscesses caused by *Actinomyces* spp. or infections due to *Blastomyces* spp., *Histoplasma* spp., and *Coccidioidomycosis* spp.[6,68,69]

Benign or malignant tumors are frequently seen in guinea pigs, mice, and rats (particularly in inbred strains used in the laboratory), whereas they are uncommon in chinchillas (<3% prevalence) and degus.[8,31,41,70]

Clinical presentation

Specific conditions may be found in specific body regions such as limbs and perianal/genital area.

- Skin nodules on the head and genital area associated with ocular edema and blepharo-conjunctivitis (subacute form) are highly suggestive of rabbit myxomatosis.[71,72]
- Soft-tissue swellings, around the head, over the limbs, and perianal region can be associated with rabbit Shope fibromatosis, whereas horn-like lesions around ears, eyelids, neck, and shoulders can be seen in case of rabbit Shope papillomatosis.[71,72]
- Integumentary tumors of any origin may appear as solitary or multiple, well-circumscribed or infiltrative, intradermal or subcutaneous masses, sometimes pigmented occurring anywhere on the body. They can enlarge and may become ulcerated.[18,70,73,74]
- Parasitic nodules (eg, *Cuterebra* spp. and *Hypoderma bovis*) may generally resemble abscesses and are fluctuant nodules closed or fistulated, sometime painful.[4,6,75]
- Ferrets affected with skin tumors may present nodular (or plaque-like) lesions on the head, trunk, limbs, or preputial gland.[6] Main tumors reported include mast cell tumors, basal cell tumors, sebaceous adenomas/epitheliomas, squamous cell carcinoma, adenocarcinoma, and cutaneous (nonepitheliotropic) lymphoma.[6,73]
- Ferrets affected by fungal infections with dermatologic involvement (eg, blasto-mycosis, histoplasmosis, and coccidioidomycosis) may present with subcutaneous nodules.[6,20,29,68,69]
- *Actinomyces* spp., an anaerobic bacterium, may cause nodular lesions in the cervical area, so-called "lumpy jaw."[76]
- Trichofolliculomas are the most common tumor of guinea pigs. They appear as large, solitary masses most common along the back and flanks that can ulcerate and discharge a sebaceous exudate (**Fig. 7**).[18,70]
- Fibroadenomas occur anywhere along the mammary chain and represent the most common subcutaneous tumor in the rat. There is no gender predisposition.[8,70]
- All ECM may have various skin tumors anywhere on the body (**Figs. 8** and **9**).[18,70]

Diagnostic Tests

A detailed general history including the pet's signalment, lifestyle, health management, and general health condition will help identify husbandry-related conditions

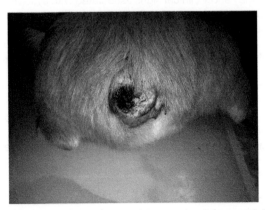

Fig. 7. Trichofolliculoma in a guinea pig appearing as a nodule containing keratinous and hemorrhagic material.

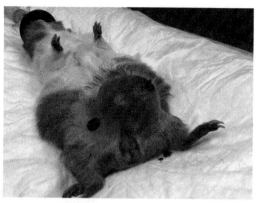

Fig. 8. Mammary carcinoma in a female guinea pig.

(eg, nutritional deficiencies) as well as behavioral dermatopathies (eg, barbering). Diagnosis of infectious or endocrine conditions is based on results of several dermatologic tests.

- Diagnosis of ectoparasite infestation can be done by several methods. Microscopic identification of mites or their eggs on hair plucking, combing, or brushing (fur mites and gamasids) as well as by adhesive tape test or superficial skin scraping is generally easily done in case of nonburrowing mites (eg, *P. cuniculi*, *Otodectes cynotis*, *Cheyletiella parasitovorax*, *Leporacarus gibbus*), and lice (eg, *Haemodipsus ventricosus*, *Gliricola porcelli*, and *Gyropus ovalis*) from hairs, ear

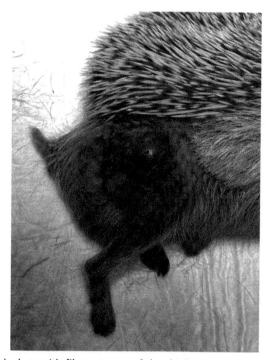

Fig. 9. African hedgehog with fibrosarcoma of the thigh.

crusts, or debris.[4,35–37,40,42,45,60,77] A deep skin scrape is needed to identify burrowing mites or their eggs such as by *S. scabiei, T. caviae, N. cati,* and *Demodex* spp.[10,42] However, due to the poor sensitivity of skin scraping, identification can be challenging.[5,6] Macroscopic and microscopic identification of ticks, fleas, lice, and their excrements is generally easily done particularly in animals with a clean haircoat. Identification of gamasids (*O. bacoti*) can be performed at light microscopy after harvesting the parasites on the host skin or from the environment (eg, cage).[40] Fecal examination, perianal acetate tape test, and molecular methods (polymerase chain reaction [PCR]) can be used to detect pinworm (*P. ambiguus*) infection, particularly when fecal sampling is performed in the afternoon and evening hours.[78] Parasitologic evaluation of tapeworm cysts is needed to identify parasitic nodules.[79]

- Identification of the bacterial causative agent should be performed by bacterial culture and sensitivity testing as well as PCR. Microscopic visualization of skin scrapings (dark-field microscopy), serology (to detect the human syphilis agent), and PCR may be used to detect *Treponema paraluisleporidarum*. Samples from exudative lesions as well as infected wounds should be submitted for bacterial culture and sensitivity testing in all cases to identify the causative agents.[4,5,8] An anaerobic culture is needed to confirm the diagnosis of rabbit necrobacillosis, as *F. necrophorum* is a gram-negative anaerobic bacterium.[4,5,29,48] Bacterial culture and sensitivity is required to identify the causative agents of ulcerative dermatitis.[42]

- Diagnosis of dermatophytosis caused by *T. mentagrophytes, Trichophyton benhamiae, Trichophyton porcellae, Microsporum canis,* and *Microsporum gypseum* is based on clinical signs, ultraviolet light (Wood's lamp) (only for 50% of *Microsporum* spp.), results of cytologic examination, dermatophyte culture, and PCR (**Fig. 10**).[57,59]

Microscopic observation of affected hairs (trichogram) differentiates normal broken hairs (barbering) from those with abnormalities caused by infectious agents (eg, parasites or fungi). Potassium hydroxide 10% or lactophenol cotton blue can be added to the collected material enables in order to clearly identify fungal arthrospores or hyphae.[4] Serology may be used to detect *Trichophyton* spp. in rabbits through an indirect enzyme-linked immunosorbent assay (ELISA).[80,81] However, fungal cultures (dermatophyte test medium and Sabouraud's dextrose agar plates) represent the most used tests to identify dermatophytes.[82] Molecular methods (eg, PCR) can also

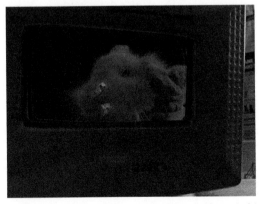

Fig. 10. Wood's lamp test in a rabbit affected with dermatophytosis (ringworm).

be used to reliably and accurately identify fungal pathogens before treatment as ancillary or sole test for the diagnosis of dermatophytosis.

- Cytologic evaluation of fine-needle aspirates may provide preliminary information on mycotic nodules and cutaneous masses. In addition, cytologic evaluation can help identify bacterial rods in case of rabbit *F. bacterium* infection.[18,42,70,73,74,83]
- Viral diseases can be detected through several tests. Diagnosis of canine distemper in ferrets relies on serologic (fluorescent antibody labeling) or molecular (PCR) testing performed on blood or respiratory samples (eg, conjunctival and tonsillar), respectively.[52,54] Intracytoplasmic or rarely intranuclear inclusion bodies may be detected in the respiratory system, skin, brain, and urinary bladder.[52,54] Rabbit myxoma virus isolation can be performed through ELISA and PCR.[71] Histopathologic examination as well as virus isolation from skin lesions can diagnose rabbit myxomatosis, Shope fibromatosis, and papillomatosis and guinea pig poxvirus infection.[29,71,72]
- Histopathologic and immunohistochemical evaluation of skin biopsy samples provides a definitive diagnosis in cases of suspect neoplasms or autoimmune conditions (eg, pemphigus foliaceus-like skin disease and erythema multiforme) and may achieve a histologic diagnosis of rabbit syphilis (through silver staining) as well as ferret pyoderma (eg, periphery of the ulcerative lesions).[6,18,56,66,70,73,74,84] In addition, the use of staining with periodic acid-Schiff, Gridley, or Gomori's methenamine silver stain can be used to identify fungal elements on a histopathological sample.[4] Histopathologic examination of skin samples is necessary to diagnose murine idiopathic ulcerative dermatitis.[85]
- Finally, radiography, ultrasonography, computed-tomography, MRI, blood work (complete blood count to detect hyperestrogenism-secondary pancytopenia, plasma biochemical analysis), and a hormonal panel including androstenedione, estradiol, and 17α-hydroxyprogesterone may detect endocrine disorders (eg, hyperadrenocorticism/hyperandrogenism, thyroid disorders, or follicular ovarian cysts).[6,21] In ECM affected by pododermatitis, besides dermatologic tests, further diagnostic procedures (eg, imaging of the hocks) may be performed to stage/grade the condition (eg, evaluate underlying bone and joint involvement) and better plan a therapeutic approach.[63]

SUMMARY

ECM can be affected by many dermatologic diseases presenting with variable or multiple clinical signs. An approach to these conditions based on the predominance of their main clinical sign (eg, alopecia, pruritus, scaling/crusting, erosion/ulceration, and nodular lesions) should be encouraged as it can help rule out the most likely differential diagnosis and eventually achieve a final diagnosis.

CLINICS CARE POINTS

- In the northern hemisphere, a breeding season alopecia involving the tail and the perianal area is commonly seen in ferrets from March to August.
- Skin neoplasms are the most common differentials for nodular lesions in ferrets.
- Trichogram is the fastest diagnostic test to differentiate normal broken hairs (barbering) from abnormal hair caused by follicular dysplasia or by infectious agents (eg, parasites or fungi).

- Exotic companion mammals affected with ulcerative dermatitis of the palmar or plantar surfaces of the feet should be promptly treated to avoid bacterial invasion of the underlying anatomic structures (eg, tendons, joints, and bone).
- Fibroadenomas are the most common subcutaneous neoplasia present in the rat and may occur anywhere along the mammary chain.

DISCLOSURE

The authors have nothing to disclose.

REFERENCES

1. Palmeiro BS, Roberts H. Clinical approach to dermatologic disease in exotic animals. Vet Clin North Am Exot Anim Pract 2013;16:523–77.
2. Lorenz MD. The Problem-Oriented Approach. In: Lorenz MD, Neer TM, DeMars P, editors. Small animal medical diagnosis. Ames, IA: Blackwell Publishing; 2013. p. 3–12.
3. Maddison J. Encouraging a problem-based approach to diagnosis. Veterinary Record [Internet]. 2014 [i-ii pp.]. Available at: http://veterinaryrecord.bmj.com/content/175/3/i.
4. Varga M, Paterson S. Dermatologic diseases of rabbits. In: Quesenberry KE, Orcutt CJ, Mans C, et al, editors. Ferrets, rabbits and rodents clinical medicine and surgery. 4th edition. St Louis, MO: Elsevier Saunders; 2021. p. 220–32.
5. de Matos R, Kalivoda K. Dermatoses of exotic small mammals. In: Scott DW, Miller WH, Griffin CE, editors. Muller & Kirk's small animal dermatology. 7th edition. St Louis: Elsevier; 2013. p. 844–87.
6. d'Ovidio D, Santoro D. Dermatologic diseases of ferrets. In: Quesenberry KE, Orcutt CJ, Mans C, et al, editors. Ferrets, rabbits and rodents clinical medicine and surgery. 4th edition. St Louis, MO: Elsevier Saunders; 2021. p. 109–16.
7. Meredith A, Johnson-Delaney CA. Guinea pigs. In: Meredith A, Johnson-Delaney CA, editors. BSAVA manual of exotic pets: a foundation manual. 5th edition. Quedgeley: British Small Animal Veterinary Association; 2010. p. 52–64.
8. Mans C, Donnelly TM. Chinchillas. In: Quesenberry KE, Orcutt CJ, Mans C, et al, editors. Ferrets, rabbits and rodents clinical medicine and surgery. 4th edition. St Louis, MO: Elsevier Saunders; 2021. p. 298–322.
9. Miwa Y, Mayer J. Hamsters and Gerbils. In: Quesenberry KE, Orcutt CJ, Mans C, et al, editors. Ferrets, rabbits and rodents clinical medicine and surgery. 4th edition. St Louis, MO: Elsevier Saunders; 2021. p. 368–84.
10. White SD, Bourdeau P, Meredith A. Dermatologic problems of rabbits. Semin Avian Exot Pet Med 2002;11(3):141–50.
11. Kramer A, Muller RS, Hein J. Environmental factors, clinical signs, therapy and zoonotic risk of rabbits with dermatophytosis. Tierarztl Prax Ausg K Kleintiere Heimtiere 2012;40:425–31.
12. Meredith A. Ferret dermatoses, In: Keeble E. and Meredith A., BSAVA manual of rodents and ferrets. Gloucester, 2009, British Small Animal Veterinary Association, Gloucester, England, 269.
13. Harvey RG. *Demodex cuniculi* in dwarf rabbits (*Oryctolagus cuniculus*). J Small Anim Pract 1990;31:204–7.
14. Reinhardt V. Hair pulling: a review. Lab Anim 2005;39(4):361–9.

15. Tynes VV. Behavioral dermatopathies in small mammals. Vet Clin North Am Exot Anim Pract 2013;16:801–20.

16. Di Geronimo P, Brandao J. Updates on Thyroid Disease in Rabbits and Guinea Pigs. Vet Clin Exot Anim 2020;23:373–81.

17. Rosenbaum MR, Affolter VK, Usborne AL, et al. Cutaneous epitheliotropic lymphoma in a ferret. J Am Vet Med Assoc 1996;209:1441–4.

18. Kanfer S, Reavill DR. Cutaneous neoplasia in ferrets, rabbits, and guinea pigs. Vet Clin Exot Anim Pract 2013;16:579–98.

19. Scott DW, Gould WJ, Cayatte SM, et al. Figurate erythema resembling erythema annulare centrifugum in a ferret with adrenocortical adenocarcinoma-associated alopecia. Vet Dermatol 1994;5:111–5.

20. Scott DW, Miller WH, Griffin CE. Dermatoses of pet rodents, rabbits and ferrets. In: Scott DW, Miller WH, Griffin CE, editors. Small animal dermatology. 6th ed. Philadelphia: WB Saunders; 2001. p. 1417.

21. Schoemaker NJ, van Zeeland YRA. Endocrine diseases of ferrets. In: Quesenberry KE, Orcutt CJ, Mans C, et al, editors. Ferrets, rabbits and rodents clinical medicine and surgery. 4th edition. St Louis, MO: Elsevier Saunders; 2021. p. 77–91.

22. Patterson MM, Fox JG, Eberhard ML. Parasitic diseases. In: Fox JG, Marini RP, editors. Biology and diseases of the ferret. 3rd edition. Ames (IA): John Wiley & Sons; 2014. p. 566.

23. Noli C, van der Horst HH, Willemse T. Demodicosis in ferrets (*Mustela putorius furo*). Vet Q 1996;18:28–31.

24. White SD, Guzman DS, Paul-Murphy J, et al. Skin diseases in companion guinea pigs (*Cavia porcellus*): a retrospective study of 293 cases seen at the Veterinary Medical Teaching Hospital, University of California at Davis (1990-2015). Vet Dermatol 2016;27:395, e100.

25. Pignon C, Mayer J. Guinea pigs. In: Quesenberry KE, Orcutt CJ, Mans C, et al, editors. Ferrets, rabbits and rodents clinical medicine and surgery. 4th edition. St Louis, MO: Elsevier Saunders; 2021. p. 270–97.

26. Beregi A, Zorn S, Felkai F. Ultrasonic diagnosis of ovarian cysts in ten guinea pigs. Vet Radiol Ultrasound 1999;40(1):74–6.

27. Bean AD. Ovarian cysts in the guinea pig (*Cavia porcellus*). Vet Clin North Am Exot Anim Pract 2013;16(3):757–76.

28. Bauck LB, Orr JP, Lawrence KH. Hyperadrenocorticism in three teddy bear hamsters. Can Vet J 1984;25:247–50.

29. Meredith A. Dermatology of mammals. In: Patterson S, editor. Skin diseases of exotic pets. Oxford: Blackwell Science; 2006. p. 173–324.

30. Jekl V, Hauptman K, Knotek Z. Quantitative and qualitative assessments of intraoral lesions in 180 small herbivorous mammals. Vet Rec 2008;162:442–9.

31. Jekl V. Degus. In: Quesenberry KE, Orcutt CJ, Mans C, et al, editors. Ferrets, rabbits and rodents clinical medicine and surgery. 4th edition. St Louis, MO: Elsevier Saunders; 2021. p. 323–33.

32. White SD, Bourdeau PJ, Brement T, et al. Companion hamsters with cutaneous lesions; a retrospective study of 102 cases at two university veterinary teaching hospitals (1985–2018). Vet Dermatol 2019a;30:243, e74.

33. d'Ovidio D, Santoro D. Orodental diseases and dermatological disorders are highly associated in pet rabbits: a case-control study. Vet Dermatol 2013;24(5):531, e125.

34. Singh SK, Dimri U, Ahmed QS, et al. Efficacy of doramectin in *Trixacarus caviae* infestation in guinea pig (*Cavia porcellus*). J Parasit Dis 2013;37(1):148–50.

35. d'Ovidio D, Santoro D. *Leporacarus gibbus* infestation in client-owned rabbits and their owner. Vet Dermatol 2014;25(1):46, e17.

36. d'Ovidio D, Santoro D. Prevalence of fur mites (*Chirodiscoides caviae*) in pet guinea pigs (*Cavia porcellus*) in southern Italy. Vet Dermatol 2014;25(2):135-7, e37-e38.

37. d'Ovidio D, Noviello E. Corner Diagnostico Animali Esotici Rivista ufficiale della SCIVAC 2015;29:65-7.

38. Mayer J, Marini RP, Fox JG. Biology and diseases of ferrets. In: Fox JG, Andersen LC, Otto GM, et al, editors. Laboratory animal medicine. 3rd edition. Boston: Academic Press; 2015. p. 577–616.

39. d'Ovidio D, Noviello E, Santoro D. Tropical rat mite (*Ornithonyssus bacoti*) infestation in pet Syrian hamsters (*Mesocricetus auratus*) and their owner. Vet Dermatol 2017;28(2):256-7.

40. d'Ovidio D, Noviello E, Santoro D. Prevalence and zoonotic risk of tropical rat mite (*Ornithonyssus bacoti*) in exotic companion mammals in southern Italy. Vet Dermatol 2018;29(6):522, e174.

41. White SD, Bourdeau PJ, Brément T, et al. Companion rats (*Rattus norvegicus*) with cutaneous lesions: a retrospective study of 470 cases at two university veterinary teaching hospitals (1985-2018). Vet Dermatol 2019b;30(3):237, e72.

42. Frohlich J. Rats and Mice. In: Quesenberry KE, Orcutt CJ, Mans C, et al, editors. Ferrets, rabbits and rodents clinical medicine and surgery. 4th edition. St Louis, MO: Elsevier Saunders; 2021. p. 345–67.

43. Doss GA, Carpenter JW. African Pigmy Hedgehogs. In: Quesenberry KE, Orcutt CJ, Mans C, et al, editors. Ferrets, rabbits and rodents clinical medicine and surgery. 4th edition. St Louis, MO: Elsevier Saunders; 2021. p. 401–15.

44. Quesenberry C, de Matos J. Basic Approach to Veterinary Care of Ferrets. In: Quesenberry KE, Orcutt CJ, Mans C, et al, editors. Ferrets, rabbits and rodents clinical medicine and surgery. 4th edition. St Louis, MO: Elsevier Saunders; 2021. p. 13–26.

45. d'Ovidio D, Santoro D. Efficacy of Fluralaner in the Treatment of Sarcoptic Mange (*Sarcoptes scabiei*) in 12 Pet Rabbits. Top Companion Anim Med 2021;43: 100528.

46. d'Ovidio D, Santoro M, Santoro D. A clinical retrospective study of *Caparinia tripilis* (*Psoroptidae*) mite dermatitis in pet African pygmy hedgehogs (*Ateletrix albiventris*) in southern Italy. Vet Dermatol 2021;32(5):434, e115.

47. d'Ovidio D, Santoro D. Efficacy of a spot-on combination of fluralaner plus moxidectin (Bravecto® Plus) against naturally acquired *Sarcoptes scabiei* infestation in 10 pet rabbits: retrospective case series. Vet Dermatol 2022;34(1):3–6.

48. Jenkins JR. Skin disorders of the rabbit. Vet Clin North Am Exot Anim Pract 2001; 4(2):543–63.

49. Bulliot C, Mentre V, Marignac G, et al. A case of atypical psoroptic mange in a domestic rabbit. J Exot Pet Med 2013;22:400–4.

50. Harcourt-Brown F. Skin diseases. In: Harcourt-Brown F, editor. Textbook of rabbit medicine. Oxford: Butterworth Heinemann; 2002. p. 224–48.

51. Rosenthal KL. Ferrets. Vet Clin North Am Exot Anim Pract 1994;24:1.

52. Fox JG, Pearson RC, Gorham JR. Viral diseases. In: Fox JG, editor. Biology and diseases of the ferret. 2nd edition. Baltimore: Lippincott Williams and Wilkins; 1998. p. 335–74.

53. Zehnder AM, Hawkins MG, Koski MA, et al. An unusual presentation of canine distemper virus infection in a domestic ferret (*Mustela putorius furo*). Vet Dermatol 2008;19(4):232–8.

54. Perpinan D. Respiratory Diseases of Ferrets. In: Quesenberry KE, Orcutt CJ, Mans C, et al, editors. Ferrets, rabbits and rodents clinical medicine and surgery. 4th edition. St Louis, MO: Elsevier Saunders; 2021. p. 71–6.
55. Martorell J, Such R, Fondevila D, et al. Cutaneous Epitheliotropic T-cell Lymphoma with Systemic Spread in a Guinea Pig (*Cavia porcellus*). J Ex Pet Med 2011;20(4):313–7.
56. Eckerman-Ross C. Pemphigus foliaceus-like skin disease in a ferret. Exot DVM 2007;9:5.
57. Vangeel I, Pasmans F, Vanrobaeys M, et al. Prevalence of dermatophytes in asymptomatic guinea pigs and rabbits. Vet Rec 2000;146:440–1.
58. Hoppman E, Barron WH. Ferret and Rabbit Dermatology. J Exot Pet Med 2007;4: 225–37.
59. d'Ovidio D, Grable SL, Ferrara M, et al. Prevalence of dermatophytes and other superficial fungal organisms in asymptomatic guinea pigs in Southern Italy. J Small Anim Pract 2014c;55(7):355–8.
60. Nath AJ. Treatment and control of *Trixacarus caviae* infestation in a conventional guinea pig (*Cavia porcellus*) breeding colony. J Parasit Dis 2016;40(4):1213–6.
61. Jassies-van der Lee A, van Zeeland Y, Kik M, et al. Successful treatment of sebaceous adenitis in a rabbit with ciclosporin and triglycerides. Vet Dermatol 2009; 20(1):67–71.
62. Moore DM, Zimmerman K, Smith SA. Hematological assessment in pet rabbits: blood sample collection and blood cell identification. Vet Clin Exot Anim 2015; 18:9–19.
63. Bumblefoot Blair J. A Comparison of Clinical Presentation and Treatment of Pododermatitis in Rabbits, Rodents, and Birds. Vet Clin Exot Anim 2013;16(3):715–35.
64. Snook TS, White SD, Hawkins MG, et al. Skin diseases in pet rabbits: a retrospective study of 334 cases seen at the University of California at Davis, USA (1984-2004). Vet Dermatol 2013;24(6):613–7, e148.
65. Mancinelli E, Keeble E, Richardson J, et al. Husbandry risk factors associated with hock pododermatitis in UK pet rabbits (*Oryctolagus cuniculus*). Vet Rec 2014;174(17):429.
66. King WW, Lemarié SL, Veazey RS, et al. Superficial spreading pyoderma and ulcerative dermatitis in a ferret. Vet Dermatol 1996;7:43–7.
67. Lejnieks DV. Treatment of Ulcerative Dermatitis in Mice (*Mus musculus*) with Gabapentin: 14 cases 2011-2019. J Exot Pet Med 2022;41:54–61.
68. Lenhard A. Blastomycosis in a ferret. J Am Vet Med Ass 1985;186:70.
69. DuVal-Hudelson KA. Coccidioidomycosis in Three European Ferrets. J Zoo Wild Med 1990;21:353–7.
70. Hocker SE, Eshar D, Wounda RM. Rodent Oncology: Diseases, Diagnostics, and Therapeutics. Vet Clin Exot Anim 2017;20:111–34.
71. Kerr PJ, Donnelly TM. Viral Infections of Rabbits. Vet Clin Exot Anim 2013;16: 437–68.
72. Meredith AL. Viral skin diseases of the rabbit. Vet Clin North Am Exot Anim Pract 2013;16(3):705–14.
73. Schoemaker NJ. Ferret Oncology: Diseases, Diagnostics, and Therapeutics. Vet Clin North Am Exot Anim Pract 2017;20(1):183–208.
74. van Zeeland Y. Rabbit Oncology: Diseases, Diagnostics, and Therapeutics. Vet Clin North Am Exot Anim Pract 2017;20(1):135–82.
75. Collins S, Cotton R. Subcutaneous arthropod larva consistent with *Cuterebra* sp. in a rabbit. J Exot Pet Med 2021;37:16–7.

76. Swennes AG, Fox JG. Bacterial and mycoplasmal diseases. In: Fox JG, Marini RP, editors. Biology and diseases of the ferret. 3rd Edition. Ames (IA): John Wiley & Sons; 2014. p. 519.

77. Fehr M, Koestlinger S. Ectoparasites in Small Exotic Mammals. Vet Clin Exot Anim 2013;16:611–57.

78. Rinaldi L, Russo T, Schioppi M, et al. *Passalurus ambiguus*: new insights into copromicroscopic diagnosis and circadian rhythm of egg excretion. Parasitol Res 2007;101(3):557–61.

79. Fountain K. *Coenurus serialis* in a pet rabbit. Vet Rec 2000;147:340.

80. Zrimsek P, Kos J, Pinter L, et al. Detection by ELISA of the humoral immune response in rabbits naturally infected with *Trichophyton mentagrophytes*. Vet Microbiol 1999;70(1–2):77–86.

81. Zrimsek P, Kos J, Pinter L, et al. Serum-specific antibodies in rabbits naturally infected with *Trichophyton mentagrophytes*. Med Mycol 2003;41(4):321–9.

82. Overgaauw PAM, Avermaete KHAV, Mertens CARM, et al. Prevalence and zoonotic risks of *Trichophyton mentagrophytes* and *Cheyletiella* spp. in guinea pigs and rabbits in Dutch pet shops. Vet Microbiol 2017;205:106–9.

83. Garner M. Cytologic Diagnosis of Diseases of Rabbits, Guinea Pigs, and Rodents. Vet Clin Exot Anim 2007;10:25–49.

84. Fisher P. Erythema multiforme in a ferret (*Mustela putorius furo*). Vet Clin North Am Exot Anim Pract 2013;16:599–609.

85. Kastenmayer RJ, Fain MA, Perdue KA. A retrospective study of idiopathic ulcerative dermatitis in mice with a C57BL/6 back- ground. J Am Assoc Lab Anim Sci 2006;45:8–12.

Avian Dermatology

Tariq Abou-Zahr, BVSc, CertAVP(ZooMed), DipECZM(Avian), MRCVS

KEYWORDS

- Feather destructive behavior • Pododermatitis • Bumblefoot • Knemidocoptes
- Pyoderma • Folliculitis • SCUD • Dermatitis

KEY POINTS

- Dermatologic abnormalities may result from primary skin disease or may occur secondary to systemic disorders.
- Infectious causes of skin diseases are common, including ectoparasitic, bacterial, fungal, and viral causes.
- To assess the skin itself, skin biopsy with histology is a useful diagnostic modality. The use of paired biopsies from affected and unaffected regions for comparison is often recommended.
- Chronic dermatitis often occurs secondary to auto-mutilation, potentially an extreme manifestation of feather destructive behavior in psittacine birds
- Pododermatitis is often manageable, but treatment is futile without addressing the underlying cause(s).
- The main disorders of the uropygial gland are impaction, infection, and neoplasia and it is possible to surgically remove the gland if there is no response to medical treatment.
- Birds may suffer from several cutaneous neoplastic processes. Squamous cell carcinomas are particularly common and surgical resection is the treatment of choice.

INTRODUCTION

As with traditional companion animals, disorders of the integument form an important part of avian veterinary practice. The skin, the largest organ in the body, primarily acts as an environmental barrier, but also has many other roles, for example, vitamin D production, temperature regulation, adnexal production, and immune regulation.[1] Primary skin disorders as well as conditions that manifest in the skin as a result of more systemic processes, both infectious and noninfectious, are seen commonly in a range of avian species and especially in psittacine birds. In a great number of cases, the clinician will need to look beyond just the skin of the bird and consider its behavioral, nutritional, management, and systemic status to resolve clinical dermatologic presentations.[1,2]

Valley Exotics, Vet Partner's Practices Ltd T/A Valley Vets, Unit 2C Gwaelod-Y-Garth Industrial Estate, Gwaelod-Y-Garth, Cardiff, CF15 9AA, UK
E-mail address: ta9797@my.bristol.ac.uk

Vet Clin Exot Anim 26 (2023) 327–346
https://doi.org/10.1016/j.cvex.2022.12.001
1094-9194/23/Crown Copyright © 2022 Published by Elsevier Inc. All rights reserved.
vetexotic.theclinics.com

Anatomy and Physiology

The avian skin is considerably thinner than that of mammals.[3] The only exception is the skin of the beak and the scales of the legs, which are greatly thickened to resist mechanical stress.[3,4] As in mammals, an epidermis, dermis, and subcutaneous layer exists. In feathered areas, the epidermis is only around 10 cells thick and consists of an outer keratinized epithelium (*stratum corneum*), an intermediate transitional layer, and a deeper *stratum germinativum*, which produces new cells to replace those that are lost at the surface.[3,4] The dermis is also very thin and is composed of superficial and deep layers. The deep layer of the dermis contains the smooth muscle of the feathers and non-feathered skin (apteria) which are interconnected by elastic tendons. It also contains the feather follicles, onto which the feather muscles attach.[3] The subcutaneous layer contains fat, which is particularly abundant in waterfowl and penguins and in many migratory birds, where it acts as an energy reserve. It also contains subcutaneous muscles that attach to the underlying bone or skeletal muscle and regulate skin tension.[3]

Feathers are made of keratin. Their structure consists of a main, hollow shaft (the rachis) which ends in the quill or calamus. The calamus anchors the feather into the follicle. The feather vane exists on both sides of the rachis and is composed of barbs, from which hooked barbules emanate and interlock with the barbules of the adjacent barb, leading to the vane acting as a single membrane.[4,5] Birds usually molt once or twice a year, whereby feathers are lost and new feathers grow to replace them (**Fig. 1**). Molting occurs in a bilaterally symmetric fashion, normally after the breeding

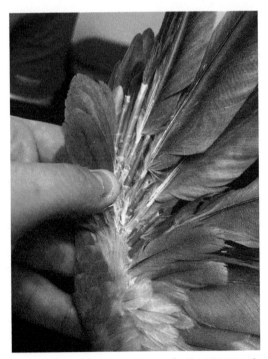

Fig. 1. During the process of moulting, new "blood feathers" grow through with vascular supply into the calamus, such as in this African gray parrot (*Psittacus erithacus erithacus*), visible as a blue or red coloration (depending on the color of the feather). As the feather matures, the vascular supply regresses.

season. Thyroid hormones, sex hormones and prolactin are all believed to affect the molt, although more research is needed to understand its precise physiologic control.[6] It is thought that in particular, falling levels of prolactin and rising T_3 and T_4 levels are important initiating factors for molting.[1,7] Some species of bird undergo a "catastrophic molt," where all the feathers are replaced at once, for example, in penguins.[1]

There are seven main feather types, contour, semiplume, down, powder down, hypopenna, filoplume, and bristle feathers.[3] Contour feathers include body feathers and flight feathers. Flight feathers include the remiges (the primary and secondary flight feathers of the wings) and retrices (tail feathers). Semiplumes have a wholly fluffy vane and a rachis which is longer than the longest barb. They have a function in thermal insulation and buoyancy in aquatic birds. Down feathers are also insulative and are entirely fluffy. Hypopennae are also called "after feathers" and are usually very small, but in ratites, they are almost as long as the main rachis, giving the appearance of a "double feather."[8] Powder down feathers grow continuously in dense tracts and disintegrate, shedding powder, which supplements the uropygial secretions, to aid in maintaining and waterproofing the feathers.[9] Filoplumes exist close to each contour feather and have many nerve endings in their follicles. These serve a proprioceptive function, to ensure feathers are in an optimum position. Bristles are largely devoid of barbs and have a tactile function, like a cat's whiskers.[3] Feather color may manifest as a result of pigments or because of feather structure. Pigments include carotenoids, melanins, and porphyrins. Some birds (for example flamingos) derive feather pigments from their diet. Parrots synthesize all of their red and yellow pigments from scratch. Melanocytes in the skin and feathers produce melanins, whereas psittacin pigments are usually produced in the liver. The microscopic feather structure may alter refraction and reflection of light, leading to changes in the color of the feathers. In psittacines, blue coloration is usually structural.[3,10]

Birds have a single gland associated with the skin—the uropygial gland, or preen gland, located at the base of the tail. The remainder of the skin is devoid of glands, although epidermal cells may secrete a lipoid sebaceous material.[1] The uropygial gland is a bilobed holocrine tubuloalveolar gland, which is generally pair shaped and features a "nipple-like" papilla, into which ducts from the different lobes empty.[4] The uropygial section, which is oily, is spread over the feathers during preening and helps keep the feathers, beak, and scales supple and waterproof. The gland therefore is usually particularly large in waterfowl. Some species of birds, including ratites, pigeons, and Amazon parrots do not have a uropygial gland.[3,4]

EXAMINATION AND DIAGNOSTIC INVESTIGATION OF THE SKIN

An external examination of the skin and feathers is a fundamental part of the physical examination of the avian patient. The skin may vary from grossly normal, to severely inflamed or necrotic. Feather disease may be observed with or without skin pathology. The distribution of skin and feather lesions and the presence of ulcers, plaques or exudates may assist the clinician in reaching a diagnosis.[4] Although most of the contour feathers and the skin associated with the head and legs may be examined before any restraint, examination of the flight feathers and most of the skin of the body will require hands-on physical examination. For a thorough examination of the skin and to facilitate the parting of feather tracts etc., general anesthesia is usually indicated. In many species of birds, inhalational anesthesia with a volatile gaseous agent such as isoflurane is the preferred means of facilitating a detailed physical examination.[11] A complete dermatologic examination includes examination of the skin around the eyes, beak, nares and ear openings, as well as over the whole body, including the axillae and inguinal regions, the rhamphotheca, the scales of the pelvic limbs and the claws. Abnormally colored feathers, feather dystrophy, regions of feather loss, the presence of any skin scurf, distinct skin lesions or dermatitis, and the presence of any visible ectoparasites should be noted. "Fret marks" also known as "stress bars" or "fault bars" may be seen along the length of the vane and rachis on some feathers. These indicate that at that point while the feather was developing, the bird was stressed or malnourished.[12]

A full diagnostic workup to include hematology and biochemistry analysis and survey radiographs is usually indicated initially, where there is evidence of potential systemic causes of skin and feather abnormalities, including feather destructive behavior. Infectious disease testing for conditions such as dermatophytosis, chlamydiosis, psittacine beak and feather disease, and polyoma virus is also often indicated, depending on the clinical signs.[1,13]

Potentially the most useful direct means of assessing the skin itself is with skin biopsy and histologic analysis. In many cases and especially in cases of feather-destructive behavior, paired biopsies are indicated. A full-thickness skin biopsy is collected to include a feather follicle from a region of the body affected by a skin or feather abnormality, as well as one from an unaffected region.[14,15] The biopsy site for the "unaffected" region should be an area of the body that is inaccessible to the bird, such as the back of the neck. Comparison of these paired biopsies has proven essential for determining whether there is inflammatory skin disease present, as accessible lesions will often be inflamed as a result of attention from the bird's beak or nails.[14]

Common Disorders of the Skin

Congenital and genetic disorders

Feather cysts may be observed in all species, but Norwich and crested canaries seem to have an underlying genetic predisposition.[3] Feather cysts present as oval or elongated swellings of a feather follicle. The cyst contains a yellowish or cream, layered, dry material. In some cases, there may be secondary infection. Where cysts are not thought to be heritable, they may also be caused by infection, trauma, or any condition which interferes with the normal growth of the feather.[1,3] Surgical removal of the cyst is normally necessary for resolution and is usually curative. The use of microsurgical instruments and radiosurgery is useful to help ensure the complete removal of the feather follicle.[16,17]

Feather duster syndrome, also known as "chrysanthemum disease," is seen in budgerigars, where birds have continuously grown, dystrophic contour feathers. No treatment is available.[18] There is evidence that there is an underlying genetic basis for this disease.[19]

Lutino cockatiels often have a region on their crown which is devoid of feathers; this is a mutation-related genetic trait.[20]

ECTOPARASITES

Knemidocoptes mites cause "scaly face" (*Knemidocoptes pilae*) and "scaly leg" (*Knemidocoptes mutans*). Severe hyperkeratosis and acanthosis of the cere and legs are observed, with thickening, flaking, and gross irregularity of the skin. Budgerigars, canaries and domestic chickens are most frequently presented, but several species may potentially be affected (**Fig. 2**). The mites may be found in all layers of the stratum corneum and are usually readily observed on skin scrapings.[3] Treatment with ivermectin and fipronil have been described, with ivermectin resulting in a quicker resolution of clinical signs in one study.[21] In severe cases of "scaly face," there may be secondary

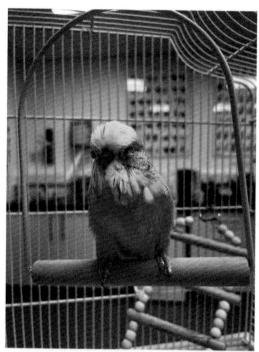

Fig. 2. Hyperkeratotic proliferative lesions around the eye in a budgerigar (*Melopsittacus undulatus*), typical of *Knemidocoptes pilae* (scaley face mite) infection.

deformities of the beak.[22] In severe cases of "scaly leg" there may be secondary necrosis of the digits.[23]

The poultry red mite (*Dermanyssus gallinae*) and the northern fowl mite (*Ornithonyssus sylviarum*) may occasionally be found on cage birds and both are especially common in domestic fowl. The northern fowl mite lives on the bird and can be seen during the day, whereas the red mite usually only feeds on the birds at night and lives in the birds' environment during the day.[3] Mites cause inflammation in the skin and can lead to noticeable proliferation of the epidermis.[3] Feather mites from the family Analgoidea may affect various avian species and lead to feather damage. The same is true of quill mites, which invade the calamus. To confirm their presence, the calamus must be split lengthwise. Maceration in a 10% potassium hydroxide solution will break down keratin while leaving chitin in the exoskeleton of mites undamaged and can be used to help detect mites from deeper scrapings, or from inside feather material.[24,25]

Ivermectin is an effective treatment for most of mite infestations in birds. In the case of red mites in poultry (*Dermanyssus*), the use of oral fluralaner (Exzolt, Intervet International B.V., The Netherlands; Bravecto, Merck, USA) is fast becoming the treatment of choice, as it seems both effective and safe. The Exzolt preparation is licensed for use in chickens for the treatment of red mites at a dose of 0.5 mg/kg, administered twice, 7 days apart.[23] It has also shown promise in the treatment of *O sylviarum* and *Allopsoroptoides galli* too. It remains to be seen how effective this may be as a treatment for birds other than poultry and for other species of ectoparasites.[23]

Lice may occasionally be seen and are especially common in columbiformes, galliformes, and wild birds. They are rarely pathogenic and unless there is a very severe burden, there are not usually any gross lesions to appreciate.[3]

Fungal Skin Disease

Several fungal organisms have been associated with skin disease in birds, including *Microsporum gypseum*, *Trichophyton* spp., *Aspergillus* spp., *Mucor* spp., and *Candida* sp. Dermatophytosis seems to be much less common in birds than in mammals, potentially as a result of their usually higher body temperatures, as many species have inhibited growth at 40°C.[26] When present, swelling of feather follicles, reddening of the skin, hyperkeratosis, and skin crusts may all be observed. Occasionally, *Malassezia*-like yeasts may be seen causing dermatitis lesions in birds (especially in passerines), with lichenification, erythema, and pruritus potentially leading to auto-mutilation.[3]

In poultry, dermatophytosis is frequently referred to as "favus." Most commonly, unfeathered areas of the body are affected, such as the comb and wattles and the skin of the head. Diagnosis is via demonstration of septate hyphae from lesions, alongside histologic lesions. Because of the species of dermatophytosis generally affecting birds, dermatophytes of birds do not fluoresce under ultraviolet light. Treatment is with antifungal drugs and a variety have been used, including topical enilconazole and miconazole and systemic itraconazole.[27]

Folliculitis and Pyoderma

This may take the form of dermatitis (pyoderma), or may be confined to the feather follicle, leading to folliculitis.[3,28,29]

In folliculitis, *Staphylococcus* spp. are reported to be the most commonly associated bacteria. Swelling of the follicle with erythema is seen grossly, potentially with hyperkeratosis, crusting, and perifollicular swelling, potentially with abnormal coloration of the feather[3,28] (**Fig. 3**). An affected feather may be pulled aseptically, opened. and the pulp cytologically examined to look for evidence of infectious agents. In the case of bacterial folliculitis, treatment based on the results of culture and sensitivity testing is recommended. In the case of fungal folliculitis (such as those caused by *Trichophyton* sp., *M gypseum*, *Aspergillus* sp. or *Candida sp.*, treatment with antifungal medications is indicated and often, treatment courses of at least 3 weeks are needed to clear an infection.[28]

Polyfolliculitis is a particular skin presentation often observed in small psittacines, such as budgerigars and most notoriously, lovebirds (*Agapornis* spp.). This is different to the typical folliculitis described above and is recognized as multiple feathers growing from the same follicle. The feathers of the dorsal neck and tail are most commonly affected. The condition results in pruritus and feather-destructive behavior is a common sequel. The cause is unknown, but an instigating viral infection may play a role. Secondary bacterial infection may be seen.[28]

In backyard poultry, a cutaneous form of Marek's disease is associated with reddened enlargement of feather follicles. Transmission is via feather follicle dander and asymptomatic carrier birds may shed the virus for life. Biopsy and histologic examination are recommended to assist with diagnosis. There is no cure for Marek's disease and the virus (gallid herpes virus 2, GaHV-2) can survive for years in the environment and is largely regarded as ubiquitous.[28]

Bacterial dermatitis (pyoderma) is usually observed as generalized erythema with crust formation and often ulceration.[3] Secondary infections often follow skin trauma, which may occur in the first place as a result of automutilation—an extreme manifestation of feather-destructive behavior in psittacines[2,3,14] (**Fig. 4**). Superficial Chronic Ulcerative Dermatitis (SCUD) is a syndrome recognized frequently in psittacine birds in practice. In a retrospective study by the author looking at 11 cases, African gray parrots were overrepresented.[29] Fungal cultures from SCUD lesions were negative in all

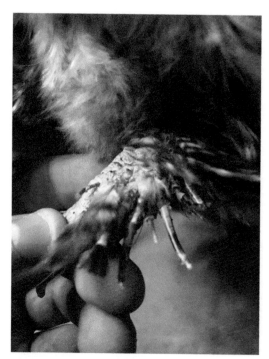

Fig. 3. Folliculitis with severe erythema observed on the foot of a domestic fowl (*Gallus gallus domesticus*).

cases and *Enterobacter cloacae*, followed by *Escherichia coli* and *Staphylococcus aureus* were the most common bacterial organisms cultured from lesions. In all cases, an underlying cause of behavioral automutilation with secondary infection was suspected to be the cause.[30,31] Treatment of bacterial dermatitis lesions involves prevention of the patient from causing further trauma. A collar around the bird's neck is usually needed in the short term (**Fig. 5**). Several weeks of antimicrobial therapy based on culture and sensitivity results from lesions is likely to be needed. Topical antiseptic preparations such as silver sulfadiazine and systemic nonsteroidal anti-inflammatory drugs (NSAIDs) such as meloxicam are also valuable. In the study mentioned looking

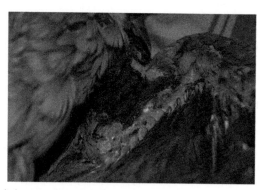

Fig. 4. A superficial chronic ulcerative dermatitis (SCUD) lesion in the axillary region of an African gray parrot (*Psittacus erithacus erithacus*).

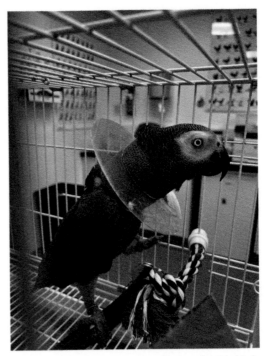

Fig. 5. A neck collar can be made to prevent interference by the bird with skin lesions, to facilitate healing. In this African gray parrot (*Psittacus erithacus erithacus*), a piece of foam pipe lagging is used in combination with a round plastic disk. This is not a suitable solution for preventing long -term feather destructive behavior but is suitable for short-term use where there are dermatitis lesions or wounds.

at SCUD, median time to resolution was 2 months, but took up to 21 months in one case. When lesions affect a region under constant tension, such as the propatagium, the use of radiographic film, sutured in place and replaced regularly, to temporarily reduce movement and stretching and to facilitate healing has proven very useful. In cases where self-mutilation is the cause of dermatitis lesions, addressing the underlying behavioral, environmental, and medical causes is paramount to minimize the risk of recurrence of lesions.[30]

Mycobacterial infections of the skin are seen in birds and may be localized, or an indication of systemic mycobacteriosis. Typically, granulomas are seen, either individual or multiple, which may be nonpainful and non-pruritic, or they may resemble abscesses caused by other bacteria. Several species of Mycobacterium can cause cutaneous disease in birds, including *M avium*, *M genavense*, and *M tuberculosis*.[3] There are zoonotic concerns and treatment is challenging. Successful treatment usually requires a combination of antibiotics, which are administered for a year or longer.[32]

Pododermatitis

Pododermatitis (bumblefoot) is another example of a usually bacterial skin condition that is common in avian medicine. Birds of prey (especially falcons) and waterfowl seem predisposed to it. It is also commonly seen in psittacines, particularly in budgerigars (**Fig. 6**). Broadly, the underlying causes include nutritional deficiencies (in particular, hypovitaminosis A), obesity, poor hygiene, inappropriate perching surfaces, and

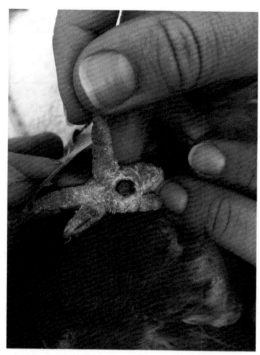

Fig. 6. A grade 3/5 pododermatitis lesion in a galah cockatoo (*Eolophus roseicapilla*), with a central scab and a necrotic core.

too much time spent by the bird on its feet, due to reduced time spent flying or swimming. It may often occur secondary to trauma—particularly where the bird subsequently has reduced weight bearing on one leg and bears more weight than necessary on the contralateral pelvic limb. It is a very common complication following surgical amputation of pelvic limbs in avian medicine. Dermatitis and cellulitis can progress if it is left untreated and lead to deep-seated infections and plantar abscess formation.[3,33]

Pododermatitis lesions are often graded. Different grading systems exist, one that is frequently used is that suggested by Oaks, 1993.[33] Broadly, classification and suggestions for treatment are as per **Table 1**.

Bumblefoot surgery aims to remove all caseous, nonviable, and necrotic tissue. The central Crust is removed followed by the necrotic core and any pus, which is typically inspissated and solid, rather than liquid. Necrotic tissue is debrided, taking care not to damage the tendons of the foot. The presence of viscous liquid during surgery can indicate synovial of tendon sheath involvement. Samples from the cavity should be taken for culture and sensitivity testing. Sterile cotton swabs, bone curettes, and flushing with sterile saline can all be used to remove all infected material. Antibiotic-impregnated polymethylmethacrylate (PMMA) beads can be placed inside the wound cavity to reduce the risk of recurrence of infection. In some cases, repeated surgeries may be needed for clinical resolution. The wound in the plantar aspect of the foot is sutured following surgery to reduce dead space and oppose skin edges. Donut-type bandages are used widely in the treatment of bumblefoot, particularly following surgery, as they take the weight off the sole of the foot while allowing monitoring of the wound and application of topical preparations if needed.[33]

Table 1
A grading system for pododermatitis, including the characteristics for each grade and the suggested approach to treatment

Grade	Characteristics of the Plantar Aspect of the Foot	Treatment
1	Erythema and atrophy of the callused skin	Topical preparations, husbandry improvements, use of NSAIDs
2	Hyperkeratosis, early skin necrosis, discoloration, and small crusts/mild swelling	Topical preparations, husbandry improvements, use of NSAIDs, bandages, Antimicrobials
3	A hyperkeratotic/necrotic core penetrating the skin. Inflammation of the subcutaneous tissues with distinct swelling and the presence of a caseous abscess	Topical preparations, husbandry improvements, use of NSAIDs, bandages, Antimicrobials. Surgery needed to debride the abscess and necrotic core.
4	Involving the tendon sheaths and tendons leading to ascending infection to the intertarsal joint	Topical preparations, husbandry improvements, use of NSAIDs, bandages, Antimicrobials. Surgery needed to debride the abscess and necrotic core. Antibiotic impregnated PMMA beads. Guarded prognosis.
5	Affecting the bone (osteolysis/osteomyelitis) or septic arthritis of the tarsometatarsal and interphalangeal joints	As above, with aggressive and protracted treatment. However, with severe osteomyelitis and if osteolysis is present, the prognosis is grave. Euthanasia should be considered in most of the cases on welfare grounds.

Abbreviations: NSAIDs, nonsteroidal anti-inflammatory drugs; PMMA, polymethylmethacrylate.

Correction of husbandry deficiencies is incredibly important in the treatment of pododermatitis. Ensuring adequate vitamin-A provision and in the case of obese birds, weight loss, are both potentially important steps. Using appropriate perches is incredibly important to reduce the risk of pododermatitis development. Ideal perches are nonabrasive and allow weight to be bored on slightly different parts of the feet. For caged birds, the use of abrasive sandpaper or cement perches is not recommended. Natural wooden branches rather than uniform dowels are often the most appropriate way forward. Perches should be cleaned regularly with a nontoxic, nonirritant, broad-spectrum disinfectant. In the case of waterfowl, hard surfaces such as concrete yards should be replaced with soft material, such as fine sand, or grass. Importantly, waterfowl should be allowed the opportunity to access water, as they have evolved to do, which naturally takes the pressure off the pelvic limbs.[33] In the case of falcons, stress results in immunosuppression, which can predispose to infectious processes such as pododermatitis developing. Ensuring that hard, smooth perching surfaces are avoided is important as these favor keratin buildup, inadequate desquamation, and pressure ischemia.[34] The use of AstroTurf on perching surfaces has proven useful in the prevention of pododermatitis developing.[33] Sharp overgrown talons can facilitate accidental puncture and introduction of microbial organisms into the foot[34] (**Fig. 7**).

Viral skin disease
Papillomavirus has been uncommonly reported in several bird species and causes papillomatous skin lesions. In finches, lesions seem most common on the feet. In

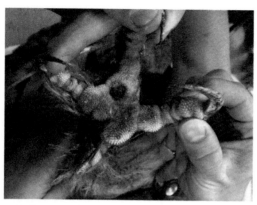

Fig. 7. A grade 3/5 pododermatitis lesion in a Eurasian eagle owl (*Bubo bubo*), with a central scab and a necrotic core.

canaries, they are reportedly most common at the commissure of the beak. In African gray parrots, lesions are reported to occur most commonly around the face.[3,35,36]

Polyomavirus is seen commonly, particularly in psittacines.[37] Budgerigars are often affected, with the condition being termed "French moult" by bird keepers.[38] Feather dystrophy is prevalent in affected young birds and the hallmark presentation is the fledging of young birds with primary flight feathers and/or tail feathers either being totally absent, or having thick feather sheaths, with potential hemorrhage into their calamus. Owing to the absence of flight feathers, these young birds have difficulties flying and are often called "runners" by breeders. Young budgerigars affected with psittacine beak and feather disease virus (PBFDV), caused by a circovirus, may also present in a similar way and many affected birds are infected with both viruses concurrently.[37] Polyoma virus also affects larger psittacines, where it rarely causes feather dystrophy, but often causes skin and subcutaneous hemorrhages. Polyomavirus can be challenging to diagnose due to a short viremia and inconsistent shedding of the virus, which means false negative polymerase chain reaction tests are reasonably common.[1,3,30]

Poxvirus infection may present with dermatologic signs. It is particularly commonly seen in chickens, ostriches, and canaries.[39] In the "dry" or cutaneous form, pox virus causes proliferative nodules and pustules, which may ulcerate. Most often these are confined to the head and feet, but in severe infections, nodules may be seen elsewhere. Providing the "wet" or septicemic forms of pox are not present, lesions may often resolve of their own accord after 2 to 4 weeks.[3]

Psittacine herpes virus is another example of a virus that can lead to the formation of proliferative lesions on the pelvic limbs, or mucocutaneous papillomas of the oral cavity and eye.[3,32]

Finally, PBFDV (psittacine beak and feather disease virus), caused by a circovirus is seen very commonly in psittacine birds.[40] The disease is enzootic in Australia and is transmitted by oral ingestion or inhalation of infected feather dust. Australian and old-world parrots are particularly predisposed, although new-world species may also be affected, albeit less commonly. In the acute form of the disease, which typically occurs in younger birds, death is common within 2 weeks as a result of severe immunosuppression and hepatic necrosis.[41] In the chronic form of the disease, which is generally seen in 8 month—3-year-old birds, dystrophic feathers replace the existing ones when the bird goes through its first molt. Powder-down feathers are often the first affected, commonly leading to a "shiny" beak. With time, feathers may be markedly dystrophic, and birds are observed to have severe feather loss (**Fig. 8**). Birds eventually succumb to secondary infections; however, the course of the chronic form of the disease may take several years.[41]

Allergic skin disease

This has been reported, but it is not common, or well-documented.[42] Clinical signs include pruritus, feather loss, feather-destructive behavior, and erythema. Skin biopsies can be used to determine the type and level of inflammation; however, histology is not definitive for allergic skin disease at the present time, due to low numbers of cases with follow up information. Treatment is predominantly with anti-inflammatories.[1,3] Intradermal allergy testing is possible in birds, although it presents difficulties due to the lack of information regarding antigen dosages in most species, availability of fresh allergens, and the availability of only a small area of skin for testing.[1,43]

Disorders of the uropygial gland

Impaction, infection, and neoplasia of the gland are all observed. This is a potential cause of feather-destructive behavior and the gland should be examined as part of the physical examination, to ensure that it is not distended and that there is normal oily secretion exuding from its papilla when the tip is wiped with a finger. Impaction of the gland usually happens secondary to hypovitaminosis A. Vitamin A supplementation along with hot, moist compressing of the gland and gentle expression of the contents may ultimately lead to resolution without the need for surgery (**Fig. 9**). In very severe cases of impaction, the gland has been known to rupture. Excision of

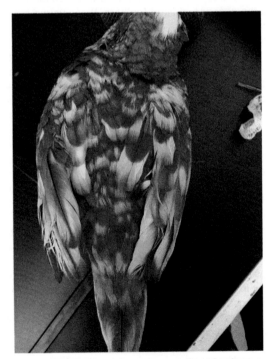

Fig. 8. Abnormally colored feathers, such as these yellow feathers on a normally green colored bird, such as this Blue-fronted Amazon parrot (*Amazona aestiva*) can indicate infection with PBFDV.

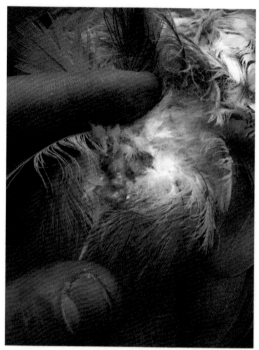

Fig. 9. A preen gland abscess in an African gray parrot (*Psittacus erithacus erithacus*). Note the purulent exudate coming from the uropygial duct.

the gland should be considered in cases where impaction is unresponsive to medical management, where it persistently recurs, where it has ruptured or where a tumor is present.[43,44] Uropygial gland tumors are typically adenomas or carcinomas and gross differentiation is difficult.[3]

Otitis
Otitis externa is reported uncommonly and may be associated with an extension of generalized skin disease. Self-trauma as a result of scratching the ears is common, which may lead to secondary hemorrhage and inflammation. In cases of otitis externa in birds, exudates are often seen coming from the external ear openings. Potential causes include bacterial (eg, *Corynebacterium kroppenstedtii*) and fungal infections (eg, *Aspergillus sp.*), or ectoparasites (eg, *Knemidocoptes pilae*).[45–48] Taking samples from the ear canal for cytology and culture is recommended initially. Occasionally carcinomas may be observed within the ear canal.[3]

Neoplasia
Several neoplastic conditions of the skin may be seen in avian practice. One of the most common cutaneous neoplasms is the squamous cell carcinoma.[49] These are typically infiltrative, growing slowly and often becoming large. They may arise anywhere on the skin or uropygial gland[3] (**Fig. 10**). A retrospective study looking at 87 birds with cutaneous or oral squamous cell carcinomas found that surgical excision was the only treatment approach associated with complete or partial response and increased survival time.[50] Basal cell tumors can present as solitary nodules, or they may arise in feather cysts and are benign, but often quite locally expansile lesions.[51] They have sometimes been termed "feather folliculomas." Basal cell carcinomas are

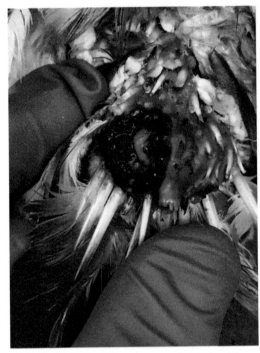

Fig. 10. A squamous cell carcinoma affecting the uropygial gland in an African Gray Parrot (*Psittacus erithacus erithacus*).

rare, although seem to have a high propensity for metastasis.[3,52] Keratoacanthomas are seen sporadically, involving the beak and claws. Although benign, they can cause severe local structural and mechanical problems.[53]

Lipomas are common and are seen especially frequently in budgerigars. Liposarcomas are rare.[54] Fibrosarcomas again are relatively common.[3] In one case, a fibrosarcoma in a blue and gold macaw was treated with a combination of intratumoral cisplatin and radiotherapy, following initial surgical debulking. The bird was in remission for 29 months.[55]

Melanomas have been diagnosed several times in psittacines. They are malignant, usually brown-black masses that most frequently affect the face. Mast cell tumors have occasionally been observed in chickens and owls. There are very sparing reports of their occurrence in psittacines.[56]

Xanthomas are very common, especially in budgerigars and cockatiels.[57,58] They are variably sized masses, frequently occurring on the wing, sternopubic region and keel, and even the conjunctiva.[57] They are formed by accumulations of lipid-containing macrophages. Surgical resection is indicated when the movement or function of the bird is compromised, or when the masses are becoming damaged or ulcerated. It has been speculated that trauma, high-fat diets, and derangements in lipid metabolism may all predispose to xanthomatosis.[1,3]

Hypovitaminosis A

Vitamin A deficiencies are especially common in psittacines, which leads to squamous metaplasia of epithelial surfaces. Scaling of the skin, hyperkeratosis, rhinitis, blepharitis, white plaques in the oral cavity, blunted choannal papillae and sublingual swellings may all be observed (**Fig. 11**). Treatment is with improvement of the diet and supplementation of vitamin A, taking care not to induce hypervitaminosis A (which can lead to bone abnormalities, conjunctivitis, enteritis, fatty liver and kidneys, and deficiencies of other fat-soluble vitamins).[1,59]

Endocrinopathies

Hypothyroidism is a rare disorder that has been associated with decreased molting events, alopecia, abnormally colored feathers and hyperkeratosis. Birds may be prone to obesity. Although a TSH stimulation test is needed for a definitive diagnosis in the antemortem case, no avian TSH assay is commercially available. In the research setting where this test is possible, there is a two- to four-fold increase in T_4 levels when TSH is administered. As in domestic animals, a low baseline T_4 is not necessarily diagnostic for hypothyroidism.[1,3]

Hepatic disease

The liver controls keratin metabolism. It is also responsible for synthesizing feather pigments in many bird species. Birds with hepatic disease may frequently be observed to have poor quality, or dystrophic feathers. Abnormally colored feathers are also frequently observed. Rapid overgrowth of the beak and nails is another common integumentary consequence of liver disease.[1]

Feather Destructive Behavior

Feather destructive behavior, FDB, (self-inflicted) is such a complex topic, that it is virtually a subject in its own right[60] (**Fig. 12**). This is a huge problem of captive

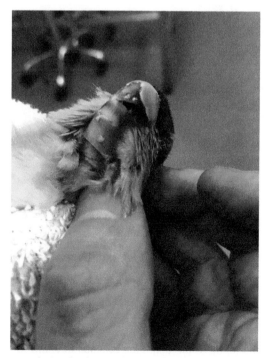

Fig. 11. Squamous metaplasia of submandibular salivary glands and conjunctivitis are both common findings with hypovitaminosis A, as seen in this red-fronted kakariki (*Cyanoramphus novazelandiae*).

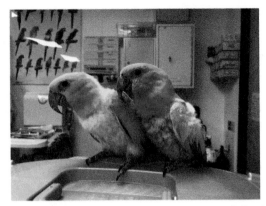

Fig. 12. Some species are more predisposed to feather destructive behavior than others. The Queen of Bavaria (*Guaruba guarouba*) is an example of a species that seems particularly predisposed.

psittacines, which may be multifactorial and is often difficult to solve.[60] In severe cases, it may progress to include automutilation of the skin. Causes of FDB include medical issues, such as liver disease, kidney disease, heavy metal toxicosis, hypocalcemia, infectious disease, inappropriate nutrition, etc.[60,61] Often, the problem stems from environmental or behavioral issues. A reduced amount of time spent foraging

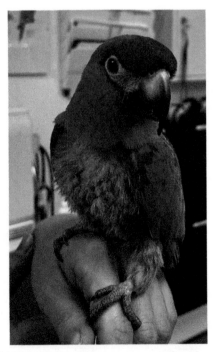

Fig. 13. The breast and inside of the thighs are common locations for feather destructive behavior, such as in this Hahn's macaw (*Diopsittaca nobilis*). Note that the plumage on the head is absolutely normal, reflecting the fact that the bird cannot reach this area with its beak. This can help distinguish FDB from other causes of feather loss.

for food in captivity (the main past time of parrots in the wild), a segregation from members of their own species, a lack of stimulation and enrichment, and a stressful environment are all possible underlying issues.[62] Other possible instigating factors may include wing trimming (which results in a sharp end of the transected rachis which may irritate the bird), the presence of environmental irritants, and a lack of opportunities for bathing. This disorder is considered a compulsive or stereotypical behavior by some and in many cases, even once the initiating cause is resolved, the behavior may continue on a long-term basis[1,60] (**Fig. 13**). A diagnostic workup to exclude medical causes, of which there are many, to include hematology and biochemistry analysis, infectious disease screening and diagnostic imaging should ideally be performed in all cases.[60,63]

CLINICS CARE POINTS

- Skin biopsies and infectious disease tests may get right to the heart of what's likely to be causing many dermatological disorders. However as skin disease often occurs secondarily to systemic or behavioural disorders, do not neglect to consider the history, blood work and diagnostic imaging findings when working up a case.

- Ensure the expectations of the client are realistic, as some disorders, for example feather destructive behaviour, may never fully resolve and similarly with chronic skin and feather disease, permanent scarring of the skin, or failure of feathers to regrow may result.

- In the case of pododermatitis, a common pitfall is to treat the clinical lesions, without thoroughly investigating all of the potential underlying causes. Failure to address the cause will result in recurrence and often fairly quickly.

- Never underestimate the welfare compromises that can result from skin disease and, in addition to addressing the skin disease, ensure that you prescribe suitable analgesia where applicable. This will also potentially minimise interference with uncomfortable lesions by the patient.

- Do not be tempted to approach avian skin disease in the same way that you may other domestic species. Treatment with steroid medications is fraught with danger in birds, which are very sensitive to the immusuppressive effects and while skin disease as a result of hypersensitivity disorders can occur in birds, it is described relatively infrequently, unlike in more traditional pet species.

DISCLOSURE

The author has nothing to disclose.

REFERENCES

1. Perry S, Sander S, Mitchell M. Integumentary System. In: Mitchell MA, Tully Jr TH, editors. Current therapy in exotic pet practice. 1st edition. Missouri: Elsevier; 2016. p. 17–75.
2. Gill JH. Avian skin diseases. Vet Clin North Am: Exot Anim Pract 2001;4(2): 463–92.
3. King AS, McLelland J. Integument. In: Birds their structure and function. 2nd edition. Bath: Bailliere Tindall; 1984. p. 23–42.
4. Schmidt RE, Reavill DR, Phalen DN. Integument. In: Pathology of pet and aviary birds. 2nd edition. New Jersey: John Wiley & Sons, Inc; 2003. p. 237–62.
5. Prum RO. Development and evolutionary origin of feathers. J Exp Zoolog 1999; 285(4):291–306.

6. Dawson A. Avian molting. In: Scanes C, editor. Sturkie's avian physiology. Massachusetts: Academic Press; 2015. p. 907–17.

7. Dawson A, Perrins CM, Sharp PJ, et al. The involvement of prolactin in avian molt: the effects of gender and breeding success on the timing of molt in Mute swans (Cygnus olor). Gen Comp Endocrinol 2009;161(2):267–70.

8. Smith DA. Palaeognathae: Apterygiformes, Casuariiformes, Rheiformes, Struthioniformes; Tinamiformes. In: Terio KA, McAloose D, Leger JS, editors. Pathology of wildlife and zoo animals. Academic Press; 2018. p. 635–51.

9. Menon GK, Menon J. Avian epidermal lipids: functional considerations and relationship to feathering. Am Zoologist 2000;40(4):540–52.

10. Tinbergen J, Wilts BD, Stavenga DG. Spectral tuning of Amazon parrot feather coloration by psittacofulvin pigments and spongy structures. J Exp Biol 2013; 216(23):4358–64.

11. Koski MA. Dermatologic diseases in psittacine birds: an investigational approach. Semin Avian Exot Pet Med 2002, July;11(3):105–24.

12. Murphy ME, Miller BT, King JR. A structural comparison of fault bars with feather defects known to be nutritionally induced. Can J Zoolog 1989;67(5):1311–7.

13. Langlois I. Medical causes of feather damaging behavior. Vet Clin Exot Anim Pract 2021;24(1):119–52.

14. Garner MM, Clubb SL, Mitchell MA, et al. Feather-picking psittacines: histopathology and species trends. Vet Pathol 2008;45(3):401–8.

15. Clubb SL, Garner MM, Cray C. Detection of Inflammatory Skin Disease in Psittacine Birds Using Paired Skin Biopsies. Monterey, California: Proceedings of the Annual Conference of the AAV; 2002. p. 193–4.

16. Özsemir, KG., & Demir, A. Multiple feather cysts and surgical resection with radio cautery in a canary. Journal of Istanbul Veterinary Sciences, 2019, 57–57.

17. Harrison GJ. Microsurgical procedure for feather cyst removal in a citron-crested cockatoo (Cacatua sulphurea citrinocristata). J Avian Med Surg 2003;17(2): 86–90.

18. van Zeeland YR. Plumage Disorders In Birds. In: Proceedings of the 8th World Congress of Veterinary Dermatology, Bordeaux, France, 2016, 415-420.

19. Baker JR. Survey of feather diseases of exhibition budgerigars in the United Kingdom. Vet Rec 1996;139(24):590–4.

20. Kubiak M. Feather plucking in parrots. Practice 2015;37(2):87–95.

21. Akhtar S, Durrani UF, Mahmood AK, et al. Comparative efficacy of ivermectin and fipronil spot on against Knemidocoptes pilae in budgerigars. Indian J Anim Res 2021;55(1):105–8.

22. Elbal P, Alarcón M, Salido VJC, et al. Severe beak deformity in Melopsittacus undulatus caused by Knemidocoptes pilae. Turkish J Vet Anim Sci 2014;38(3): 344–6.

23. Soares NM, Tucci EC, Perdoncini G, et al. Efficacy of fluralaner (Exzolt®) for the treatment of natural Allopsoroptoides galli infestations in laying hens. Poult Sci 2022;101(10):102099.

24. Morishita TY, Johnson G, Johnson G, et al. Scaly-leg mite infestation associated with digit necrosis in bantam chickens (Gallus domesticus). J Avian Med Surg 2005;19(3):230–3.

25. Schuster RK. Skin and Feather Examination. In: Avian Medicine. 3rd edition. Missouri: Elsevier; 2015. p. 121–2.

26. Pugh GJF, Evans MD. Keratinophilic fungi associated with birds: II. Physiological studies. Trans Br Mycol Soc 1970;54(2):241–50.

27. Wernery U. Infectious Diseases. In: Samour J, editor. Avian medicine. 3rd edition. Missouri: Elsevier; 2016. p. 434–521.

28. Lennox A. Dermatological Diseases. In: Greenacre CB, Morishita TR, editors. Backyard poultry medicine and surgery A guide for veterinary practitioners. 1st edition. Massachusetts: John Wiley & Sons Inc.; 2015. p. 160–8.

29. Abou-Zahr T, Carrasco DC, Shimizu N, et al. Superficial chronic ulcerative dermatitis (SCUD) in psittacine birds: Review of 11 cases (2008-2016). J Avian Med Surg 2018;32(1):25–33.

30. van Zeeland YR, Schoemaker NJ. Plumage disorders in psittacine birds-part 1: feather abnormalities. Eur J Companion Anim Pract 2014;24(1):34–47.

31. Wellehan JFX Jr, Lierz M, Phalen D, et al. Infectious Disease. In: Speer B, editor. Current therapy in avian medicine and surgery. 1st edition. Missouri: Elsevier; 2016. p. 22–106.

32. Zsivanovits P, Monks D. Management Related Conditions. In: Samour J, editor. Avian medicine. 3rd edition. Missouri: Elsevier; 2016. p. 260–93.

33. Oaks JL. Immune and inflammatory responses in falcon staphylococcal pododermatitis. In: Redig PT, Cooper JE, Remple JD, et al, editors. Raptor biomedicine. Minneapolis, MN: University of Minnesota Press; 1993. p. 72–87.

34. O'Banion K, Jacobson ER, Sundberg JP. Molecular cloning and partial characterization of a parrot papillomavirus. Intervirology 1992;33(2):91–6.

35. Tachezy R, Rector A, Havelkova M, et al. Avian papillomaviruses: the parrot Psittacus erithacus papillomavirus (PePV) genome has a unique organization of the early protein region and is phylogenetically related to the chaffinch papillomavirus. BMC Microbiol 2002;2(1):1–9.

36. Johne R, Müller H. Avian polyomavirus in wild birds: genome analysis of isolates from Falconiformes and Psittaciformes. Arch Virol 1998;143(8):1501–12.

37. Rott O, Kröger M, Müller H, et al. The genome of budgerigar fledgling disease virus, an avian polyomavirus. Virology 1988;165(1):74–86.

38. Raidal SR, Sarker S, Peters A. Review of psittacine beak and feather disease and its effect on Australian endangered species. Aust Vet J 2015;93(12):466–70.

39. Lüschow D, Hoffmann T, Hafez HM. Differentiation of avian poxvirus strains on the basis of nucleotide sequences of 4b gene fragment. Avian Dis 2004;48(3): 453–62.

40. Fogell DJ, Martin RO, Groombridge JJ. Beak and feather disease virus in wild and captive parrots: an analysis of geographic and taxonomic distribution and methodological trends. Arch Virol 2016;161(8):2059–74.

41. Doneley RJT. Acute Beak and Feather Disease in juvenile African Grey parrots-an uncommon presentation of a common disease. Aust Vet J 2003;81(4):206–7.

42. Freeman N, Tuyttens FA, Johnson A, et al. Remedying contact dermatitis in broiler chickens with novel flooring treatments. Animals 2020;10(10):1761.

43. Colombini S, Foil CS, Hosgood G, et al. Intradermal skin testing in Hispaniolan parrots (Amazona ventralis). Vet Dermatol 2000;11(4):271–6.

44. Remple JD, Al-Ashbal AA. Raptor Bumblefoot: Another Look at Histology & Pathogenesis. In: Redig PT, Cooper JE, Remple D, Hunter B, editors. Raptor biomedicine. 1st edition. Minnesota: Chiron Publications; 1993. p. 92–8.

45. Martel A, Haesebrouck F, Hellebuyck T, et al. Treatment of otitis externa associated with Corynebacterium kroppenstedtii in a peach-faced lovebird (Agapornis roseicollis) with an acetic and boric acid commercial solution. J Avian Med Surg 2009;23(2):141–4.

46. Schiavon E, Piccirillo A, Baruchello M, et al. Ceruminous otitis in native chicken breeders belonging to Robusta Lionata breed [Veneto]. Ital J Anim Sci (Italy) 2006;1594–4077.

47. Rival, F. Auricular diseases in birds. In: Proceedings of the 8th European AAV conference, 2005, Arles, France, 333-339.

48. Montesinos A. Systemic Diseases. In: Samour J, editor. Avian medicine. 3rd edition. Missouri: Elsevier; 2016. p. 359–433.

49. Bennett RA, Harrison GJ. Soft Tissue Surgery. In: Avian medicine: principles and application. 1st edition. Florida: Wingers Publishing Inc; 1994. p. 1096–136.

50. Zehnder AM, Swift LA, Sundaram A, et al. Clinical features, treatment, and outcomes of cutaneous and oral squamous cell carcinoma in avian species. J Am Vet Med Assoc 2018;252(3):309–15.

51. Tell LA, Woods L, Mathews KG. Basal cell carcinoma in a blue-fronted Amazon parrot (Amazona aestiva). Avian Dis 1997;41(3):755–9.

52. Reavill DR. Tumors of pet birds. Vet Clin Exot Anim Pract 2004;7(3):537–60.

53. Doukaki C, Papaioannou N, Huynh M. Beak keratoacanthomas in two budgerigars (Melopsittacus undulatus) with Knemidocoptes spp. infection. J Exot Pet Med 2021;36:80–3.

54. De Voe RS, Trogdon M, Flammer K. Preliminary assessment of the effect of diet and L-carnitine supplementation on lipoma size and bodyweight in budgerigars (Melopsittacus undulatus). J Avian Med Surg 2004;18(1):12–8.

55. Riddell C, Cribb PH. Fibrosarcoma in an African grey parrot (Psittacus erithacus). Avian Dis 1983;27(2):549–55.

56. Guthrie AL, Gonzalez-Angulo C, Wigle WL, et al. Radiation therapy of a malignant melanoma in a thick-billed parrot (Rhynchopsitta pachyrhyncha). J Avian Med Surg 2010;24(4):299–307.

57. Souza MJ, Johnstone-McLean NS, Ward D, et al. Conjunctival xanthoma in a blue and gold macaw (Ara ararauna). Vet Ophthalmol 2009;12(1):53–5.

58. Lipar M, Horvatek D, Prukner-Radovčić E, et al. Subcutaneous xanthoma in a cockatiel (Nymphicus hollandicus)-a case report. Veterinarski arhiv 2011;81(4):535–43.

59. Bailey T. Biochemistry Analyses. In: Samour J, editor. Avian medicine. 3rd edition. Missouri: Elsevier; 2016. p. 100–12.

60. van Zeeland YRA, Friedman SG, Bergman L. Behavior. In: Speer B, editor. Current therapy in avian medicine and surgery. 1st edition. Missouri: Elsevier; 2016. p. 177–251.

61. Fluck A, Enderlein D, Piepenbring A, et al. Correlation of avian bornavirus-specific antibodies and viral ribonucleic acid shedding with neurological signs and feather-damaging behaviour in psittacine birds. Vet Rec 2019;184(15):476.

62. Jayson SL, Williams DL, Wood JL. Prevalence and risk factors of feather plucking in African grey parrots (Psittacus erithacus erithacus and Psittacus erithacus timneh) and cockatoos (Cacatua spp.). J Exot Pet Med 2014;23(3):250–7.

63. Owen DJ, Lane JM. High levels of corticosterone in feather-plucking parrots (Psittacus erithacus). Vet Rec 2006;158(23):804.

Rabbit Dermatology

Stephen D. White, DVM, DACVD

KEYWORDS

- Dermatology • Rabbit • *Psoroptes cuniculi* • *Treponema paraluiscuniculi*

KEY POINTS

- Ectoparasites are the most common reason for pruritus in rabbits.
- Do not use fipronil in rabbits due to the possibility of toxicity.
- The serologic tests used to diagnose syphilis in humans can be used to diagnose rabbit treponematosis.
- Domestic rabbits, which are Old World rabbits, are very susceptible to myxomatosis.

INTRODUCTION

A report from a university veterinary teaching hospital indicated that almost one-third of all rabbits examined had evidence of skin disease.[1] Skin disorders in rabbits can manifest in the form of pruritus, alopecia without pruritus, scaling or nodules, and these are the most common reasons owners seek veterinary care for their pet rabbits. Combinations of one or more of these clinical presentations may be observed in an individual.

PRURITUS

Causes for pruritic skin disorders usually include ectoparasites (most common[2]) or environment (contact, bedding). Pruritus is not always present in the examination room and can be elicited by scraping or rubbing the rabbit's skin.

Parasites: *Psoroptes cuniculi*, *Ctenocephalides* spp., *Spilopsyllus cuniculi*, *Sarcoptes scabiei*, *Ornithonyssus bacoti*, lice.

Various degrees of pruritus will be associated with the dermatoses caused by these parasites. Skin lesions in those cases are often the result of self-inflicted trauma and secondary infections and may include excoriation, exudation, crusting, and alopecia. Some of these are important to discuss in greater detail:

P cuniculi (rabbit ear mite): This parasite causes otitis externa and rarely otitis media that can result in neurologic signs.[3,4] Rabbits will present with head shaking, pruritus of ears, and head and/or ear dropping (this may be the initial sign). Pinna and canals

Department of Veterinary, Medicine and Epidemiology, School of Veterinary Medicine, University of California, 2108 Tupper Hall, One Shields Avenue, Davis, CA 95616, USA
E-mail address: sdwhite@ucdavis.edu

Vet Clin Exot Anim 26 (2023) 347–357
https://doi.org/10.1016/j.cvex.2022.12.002
1094-9194/23/© 2022 Elsevier Inc. All rights reserved.

will be erythematous and will have a thick crust, which is often red-brown in color (**Fig. 1**). Other parts of the body may be rarely affected. Attempting to remove these crusts is quite painful and should be avoided. Use systemic parasiticides as discussed below.

O bacoti has been documented in rabbits, although its infestation is often without clinical signs.[5] The author is aware of one rabbit with *O bacoti* that exhibited pruritus.

Sarcoptic mange has also been reported in pet rabbits and especially in rabbit colonies.[6–9]

Lice are usually seen in small numbers in rabbits. Large numbers may indicate an infestation with another skin parasite, or an underlying systemic disease.

Fleas: Domestic rabbits are often exposed to the flea *Ctenocephalides* spp. when they share the household with a dog or cat.[3,4] In pet rabbits housed outside or exposed to wild rabbits, various flea species may be found including the rabbit flea *S cuniculi*. Infestations of *S cuniculi* are common in rabbit colonies. The life cycle of this flea is controlled by the hormonal cycle of the host, which explains the sudden proliferation seen on pregnant does and young rabbits.[10] *S cuniculi* is also important as a vector for myxomatosis. *S cuniculi* most often bites on the pinnae and face and may also bite cats and dogs. Pruritus is variable in flea infestation in rabbits but may be severe.

Diagnoses of these parasitic disorders can be confirmed by finding the parasites on multiple skin scrapings (mites) or by visualization of fleas or their excrements. The use of scalpel blades for skin scraping is to be avoided. Medical grade spatulas are safe and easy-to-use instruments to perform the scrapings.

Treatment of Epidermal Mites, Fleas, and Lice

Ivermectin 0.2 to 0.4 mg/kg q 2 weeks for 2 to 3 treatments PO or SQ. In rabbits, ivermectin also has been used to treat *Cheyletiella* infestations in doses ranging from 0.2 to 2.1 mg/kg SQ q11 days × 3 or 0.6 to 2.7 mg/kg PO q10 days × 3.[11]

Selamectin (Revolution, Zoetis, Parsipanny, NJ) has been reported as safe and effective in rabbits for the treatment of ear mites when used at the dosage of 6 or 18 mg/kg twice, 28 days apart.[12] It has also been shown to be effective against *Cheyletiella* at 6.2 to 20.0 mg/kg q2-4 weeks × 1-3[11] as well as at one dose of 12 mg/kg.[13]

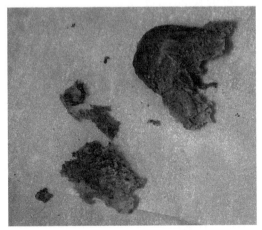

Fig. 1. Brown debris from ear of a 2-year-old female rabbit with otitis externa due to *P cuniculi*.

Selamectin should also be effective in treating lice but dosages have not been well researched. *Selamectin* has also been shown to be effective and safe in treating rabbits with *Ctenocephalides felis*.[14]

Imidacloprid/moxidectin (Advocate, Advantage Multi; Elanco, Greenfield, IN) has also been shown to be effective for ear mites applied 3 times, 30 days apart,[15] as well as effective against *O bacoti*.[5] A single subcutaneous dose of *eprinomectin* at 200 or 300 μg/kg was able to eliminate *P cuniculi* infection in rabbits,[16] although topical protocols with this drug have not been as effective.[17]

Imidacloprid (Advantage, Elanco) should be effective in treating lice (but not mite) infestation; however, again, dosages have not been well researched. *Imidacloprid* is also a topical adulticide, and it has been shown to be safe and effective in flea control in rabbits, and is licensed for this purpose in the United Kingdom.[4]

Fluralaner (Bravecto, Merck Animal Health, Rahway, NJ) One report showed successful treatment of *P cuniculi* in 15 rabbits with one oral dose of fluralaner at 25 mg/kg.[18] Two other articles reported the successful treatment of *S scabiei* in companion rabbits with oral fluralaner at the same dose.[19,20] Presumably fluralaner would also be effective against fleas.

Do *not* use *fipronil* (Frontline/Frontline Plus, Boehringer Ingelheim Animal Health USA Inc., Duluth, GA) in rabbits because its use has been associated with fatalities.[3,21]

Environmental causes of pruritus such as contact and bedding are not often seen at the author's practice because most cases have already tried changing the bedding. However, the veterinarian should determine if the pet is exposed to any harsh chemicals, particularly in the cleaning of its cage: an example would be a cage disinfected in bleach but not thoroughly washed before placing the rabbit back in it. In addition, there are anecdotal reports of certain wood shavings (especially cedar) causing contact pruritus or irritation.

ALOPECIA WITHOUT PRURITUS

Causes of this clinical presentation include dermatophytes, shedding, and barbering.

Dermatophytes

Dermatophytes are variable in their frequency in rabbits; in one study, only 2 of 334 were diagnosed with dermatophyte infection.[1] The usual dermatophyte species affecting rabbits are *Trichophyton mentagrophytes, Microsporum canis, and Microsporum gypseum*. *T mentagrophytes* is the most common in laboratory colonies, pet shops, and so forth but *M canis* may be more common in house pets.[22] Clinical signs besides alopecia may include scales, crusts, and erythema (**Fig. 2**).

Diagnosis: Fungal culture (most accurate), polymerase chain reaction, direct examination of hair (trichogram), or scales mounted in 10% KOH or mineral oil (often nondiagnostic) and/or Wood's lamp. Fluorescence of the latter test was positive in 8 of 29 rabbits with culture-verified dermatophytosis, although only one had *M canis*, the other 7 cultures were identified as *T mentagrophytes*; this finding needs to be further investigated because, traditionally, only *M canis* is capable of fluorescing.[22,23]

Treatment of dermatophytosis

Itraconazole 5 to 10 mg/kg daily, for 1 month, although the drug is probably safe for up to 3 months.[3,4,24]

Griseofulvin 15 to 25 mg/kg PO for 4 weeks. Avoid its use in pregnant animals (teratogenic).

Lime sulfur topical 1:32 dilution with water 2 to 3 times weekly—can be used as a sole treatment or adjunctive.

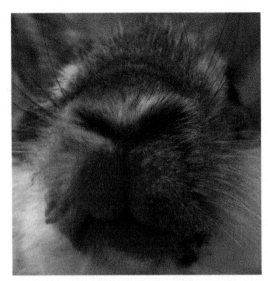

Fig. 2. A 5-year-old castrated male rabbit with dermatophytosis (*T mentagrophytes*).

Enilconazole (Imaverol, Elanco—not available in United States) 2 times weekly is effective; however, rabbits are frequent groomers, and thus may ingest too much of the medication.

Clipping is not recommended due to difficulties and stress. The environment should be disinfected by discarding bedding and first washing off all organic matter from cages and any other surfaces. The cages should then be washed in either lime sulfur, dilute bleach (1:10 with water), enilconazole or an accelerated hydrogen peroxide product; the first 2 may be irritating to owners and animals, so should always be washed thoroughly. Disinfection has been discussed recently in more detail.[23]

Shedding/Barbering

Rabbits especially may shed hair normally in uneven patterns, giving the owner and the clinician the impression that there is a pathologic process. The major differential in those cases is dermatophytosis, which should be ruled out with a fungal culture. Conspecifics may barber each other. The doe may self-pluck hairs as a nesting behavior.

Scaling and crusting

Causes of scaling and crusting dermatoses include *Cheyletiella* spp mites, venereal spirochetosis (rabbit syphilis), sebaceous adenitis, cutaneous lymphoma, and thymoma.

Cheyletiella spp (nonburrowing mites): Cheyletiellosis in rabbits is a very common cause of mild-to-severe scaly dermatosis. The disease may be caused by any of the 5 currently recognized species of the mite; however, *Cheyletiella parasitivorax* is the species most commonly associated with rabbits.[25] Cheyletiellosis is zoonotic and contagious to other animal species such as dogs and cats. Diagnosis is by finding mites on skin scrapings or acetate tape preparations. In a report from South Korea, *C parasitovorax* and *Leporacarus gibbus* (another, less common, fur mite of rabbits) were found in 80 and 6, respectively, of 140 rabbits.[26] Clinical signs of pruritus and scaling were observed in 17 of 80 and 76 of 80 infested rabbits, respectively.[26]

Both these mites can cause dermatitis in humans[27] and other pets. Treatment includes *selamectin* as per treatment of ear mites (*P cuniculi*). *Lime sulfur* dips (1:32 dilution with water) 3 to 4 weekly dips is also effective but messy and cumbersome in rabbits.

Treponema paraluiscuniculi (formerly, *Treponema cuniculi*) is the organism causing venereal spirochetosis (rabbit syphilis). Clinical signs include crusts, erythema, edema, papules, vesicles, ulcers, and proliferative lesions localized to the face and perineum. In one study, lesions were found most frequently around the nose followed by the genitalia, lips, eyelids, and anus.[28] Sneezing was observed in 33% of cases with nasal lesions.[28] In cases of maternally acquired infection, lesions could be initially found mainly on the face. Lesions are painful but not pruritic. The disease may be associated with metritis, abortion, and neonatal death. Rabbit syphilis is not zoonotic. A related bacterium, *Treponema paraluisleporidarum* can cause clinical disease in both hares and rabbits, whereas *T paraluiscuniculi* only causes seroconversion in hares without causing clinical disease.[29,30]

Diagnosis is by microscopic visualization of *T paraluiscuniculi* from skin scrapes on dark field microscopy, or special silver stains to demonstrate the organisms on biopsy. Additionally, the serologic tests used to diagnose syphilis in humans can be used.

Treatment

Penicillin G at 40,000 to 80,000 IU/kg SC, weekly for 3 treatments. It is *very important* to monitor for signs of associated antibiotic enterotoxemia. Treat all in-contact rabbits.[3,4,31] Chloramphenicol has been used successfully at a dosage of 55 mg/kg q 12 h for 4 weeks.[31] Another treatment is azithromycin 30 mg/kg/d given orally every 24 hours or 12 hours for 15 days; effectiveness in a large number of rabbits has not yet been reported but this dose seems to be effective in experimental situations.[32]

Sebaceous adenitis has been reported in domestic rabbits as a cause of alopecia and nonpruritic scaly dermatosis (**Fig. 3**).[33–38] Of the 9 rabbits reported, all were adults, and 7 were males. Six rabbits showed histologic changes of sebaceous adenitis in association with mediastinal neoplasia (cyst, thymoma, thymic lymphoma) or hepatitis.[33–36] The pathogenesis is unknown but seemingly in some rabbits, there is an association with internal disease. Clinical presentation includes multifocal alopecia, erythema, follicular casts, and scaling. Diagnosis is by biopsy. Histology of the skin may show orthokeratosis, lymphocytic exocytosis, lymphocytic mural and interface folliculitis, and apoptotic cells in basal layer of epidermis and absent sebaceous glands.[33–36] The author is unaware of a favorable response reported to retinoids or glucocorticoids in the small number of rabbits treated. A case report documents a rabbit with sebaceous adenitis that was successfully treated with a combination of cyclosporine and a supplement of medium-chain triglycerides.[37] Another case report showed better success by adding topical application of a shampoo, spray, and spot-on containing the ceramide precursor phyosphingosine.[38]

Cutaneous lymphoma has been reported in rabbits.[39,40] It presents with severe alopecia, erythema, and scaling (**Fig. 4**). Prognosis is poor. An early report in rabbits noted a T-cell origin of the lymphocytes invading the epidermis,[39] whereas a more recent review of 25 cutaneous lymphomas in European pet rabbits classified the tumors as diffuse large B cell lymphomas, with 11 tumors exhibiting a T cell-rich B cell subtype.[40]

NODULAR DERMATOSES

Causes include infectious/ulcerative pododermatitis, myxomatosis, and neoplasia (trichoblastoma, fibromas, squamous cell carcinomas, and melanomas).[41–45]

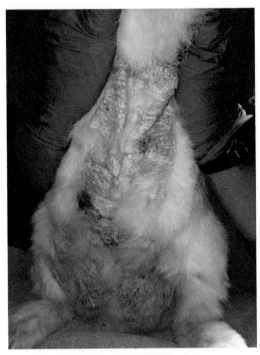

Fig. 3. A 2-year-old ovariectomized female rabbit with sebaceous adenitis.

Pododermatitis (Sore Hocks) has been reported in rabbits. It was the most common skin disease noted in a retrospective case series.[1]

Ulcerative pododermatitis is a chronic ulcerative granulomatous dermatitis of the metatarsal area seen in mainly overweight inactive rabbits kept on wet bedding, grid floors, rough cages, and/or unsanitary conditions. Hereditary factors are also thought to be involved and Rex rabbits are particularly affected because they lack protective guard hairs. It is important to remember that rabbits do not have footpads. The secondary infectious agent most commonly present is *Staphylococcus aureus*. Lesions are bilateral, in the plantar aspect of metatarsal area with a progression of lesions typified by erythema, hyperkeratosis, crusts, purulent discharge, necrosis, and associated

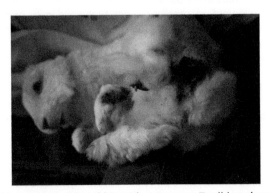

Fig. 4. A 7-year-old castrated male rabbit with cutaneous T-cell lymphoma.

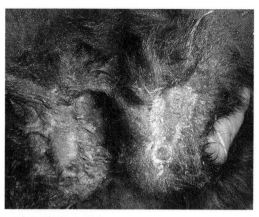

Fig. 5. Adult rabbit with pododermatitis.

with osteomyelitis and septicemia (**Fig. 5**). Treatment is difficult and based on correction of predisposing conditions, surgical drainage, topical antimicrobials, surgical dressings, and systemic antibiotics (based on culture and sensitivity). Enrofloxacin (5–15 mg/kg subcutaneously once daily) may prove helpful in early cases. Antibiotic-impregnated methylmethacrylate beads also have been reported as helpful. The earlier this disease is addressed, the better the chances of successful treatment.[3,4] Pain management may be important; meloxicam (0.1–0.5 mg/kg PO q12–24 h) or tramadol (10 mg/kg PO q24 h) may be used.[46] In an article investigating pododermatitis in pet rabbits, there was no statistical correlation between body condition score and the presence of pododermatitis but there was a statistically significant predilection in rabbits greater than 12 months of age, females, and neutered rabbits of either sex.[47]

Note that not all bacterial nodules/abscesses involve the feet—botryomycosis, a rare chronic pyogranulomatous infection reported to be caused by several bacteria, has been reported in 2 pet rabbits.[48]

Myxomatosis is caused by a myxoma virus of the poxvirus group, which is transmitted by various arthropod vectors, or through physical transport of the virus. New-World rabbits are very resistant to this disease but Old-World rabbits are extremely susceptible (and pet rabbits are Old World rabbits).[3,4] There are various

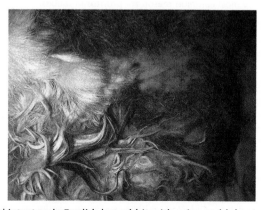

Fig. 6. A 5-year-old intact male English lop rabbit with urine scald due to degenerative narrowing of multiple intervertebral disc spaces from T11 through L1.

Box 1
Causes of urinary incontinence/scalding

Lumbosacral fractures and dislocations

Arthritis (unable to achieve proper urination posture)

Central nervous system infections
  Encephalitozoon cuniculi
  Toxoplasmosis
  Larva migrans

Urinary calculi or hypercalciuria

Ovariohysterectomy

Ectopic ureter, urinary tract infection

---

strains of this virus.[49] The incubation period can range from 8 to 21 days. Clinical signs in peracute and acute cases include edema of the head, ears, eyelids, and genitalia and milky oculonasal discharge. Firm nonpruritic and erythematous nodules (myxomas) are usually associated with less virulent strains and develop at the site of infection. Lethargy, fever, and anorexia can be present. The diagnosis is based on the clinical signs, typical microscopic lesions, and virus isolation. Supportive treatment, vector control, and a vaccine (not commercially available in the United States) may be offered/discussed with the owner; however, the prognosis is grave with morbidity and mortality approaching 100%.[3,4]

MISCELLANEOUS

Urine scald dermatitis is an erythematous, often exudative and ulcerative insult to the skin of the ventral abdomen and perineal area (**Fig. 6**) caused by extended contact with urine.[50] Although there are a number of potential causes (**Box 1**), the most common in the author's experience is a rabbit that is unable to achieve the correct posture for urinating, due to arthritis or a lumbosacral vertebral fracture caused by inappropriate handling. Treatment and prognosis are dependent on underlying disease.

CLINICS CARE POINTS

- Ectoparasites are the most common reason for pruritus in rabbits.

- Do not attempt the removal of otic crusts in *P cuniculi* infestation, instead use systemic parasiticides.

- Do not use fipronil in rabbits due to the possibility of toxicity.

- Dermatophytosis is the most common reason for nonpruritic alopecia in rabbits and is a potential zoonosis.

- Diagnostic tests for excessive scaling in a rabbit is an indication for skin scraping for ectoparasites and may include skin biopsy, thoracic radiographs, and abdominal ultrasound looking for neoplasia and/or hepatic disease.

- The serologic tests used to diagnose syphilis in humans can be used to diagnose rabbit treponematosis.

- When treating with penicillin (as well as other antibiotics) for rabbit treponematosis (rabbit syphilis), monitor the rabbit for signs of enterotoxemia.

- Domestic rabbits, which are Old World rabbits, are very susceptible to myxomatosis.

DISCLOSURE

This research did not receive any specific grant from funding agencies in the public, commercial, or not-for-profit sectors, and the author declares no conflict of interest.

REFERENCES

1. Snook TS, White SD, Hawkins MG, et al. Skin diseases in pet rabbits: a retrospective study of 334 cases seen at the University of California at Davis (1984-2004). Vet Dermatol 2013;24:613–8.
2. Hill PB, Lo A, Eden CA, et al. Survey of the prevalence, diagnosis and treatment of dermatological conditions in small animals in general practice. Vet Rec 2006; 158:533–9.
3. Jenkins JR. Skin disorders of the rabbit. Veterinary Clin North Am Exot Anim Pract 2001;4:543–63.
4. White SD, Bourdeau P, Meredith A. Dermatological problems of rabbits. Comp Cont Educ Pract Vet 2003;25:90–101.
5. d'Ovidio D, Noviello E, Santoro D. Prevalence and zoonotic risk of tropical rat mite (Ornithonyssus bacoti) in exotic companion mammals in southern Italy. Vet Dermatol 2018;29:522–5.
6. Radi ZA. Outbreak of sarcoptic mange and malasseziasis in rabbits (Oryctolagus cuniculus). Comp Med 2004;54:434–7.
7. Voyvoda H, Ulutas B, Eren H, et al. Use of doramectin for treatment of sarcoptic mange in five Angora rabbits. Vet Dermatol 2005;16:285–8.
8. Denerolle P. Sarcoptic mange in rabbits [French]. Informations Dermatologiques Vétérinaires 2008;6(21):16–20.
9. Farmaki R, Koutinas AF, Papazahariadou MG, et al. Effectiveness of a selamectin spot-on formulation in rabbits with sarcoptic mange. Vet Rec 2009;164:431–2.
10. Sobey WR, Menzies W, Conolly D. Myxomatosis: some observations on breeding the European rabbit flea Spilopsyllus cuniculi (Dale) in an animal house. J Hyg (Camb) 1974;72:453–65.
11. Mellgren M, Bergvall K. Treatment of rabbit cheyletiellosis with selamectin or ivermectin: a retrospective case study. Acta Vet Scand 2008;50:1.
12. McTier TL, Hair JA, Walstrom DJ, et al. Efficacy and safety of topical administration of selamectin for treatment of ear mite infestation in rabbits. J Am Vet Med Assoc 2003;223:322–4.
13. Kim SH, Lee JY, Jun HK, et al. Efficacy of selamectin in the treatment of cheyletiellosis in pet rabbits. Vet Dermatol 2008;19:26–7.
14. Carpenter JW, Dryden MW, Kukanich B. Pharmacokinetics, efficacy, and adverse effects of selamectin following topical administration in flea-infested rabbits. Am J Vet Res 2012;73:562–6.
15. Hansen O, Gall Y, Pfister K, et al. Efficacy of a formulation containing imidacloprid and moxidectin against naturally acquired ear mite infestations (Psoroptes cuniculi) in rabbits. Intern J Appl Res Vet Med 2005;3:281–6.
16. Pan B, Wang M, Xu F, et al. Efficacy of an injectable formulation of eprinomectin against Psoroptes cuniculi, the ear mange mite in rabbits. Vet Parasitol 2006;137: 386–90.
17. Ulutas B, Voyvoda H, Bayramli G, et al. Efficacy of topical administration of eprinomectin for treatment of ear mite infestation in six rabbits. Vet Dermatol 2005;16: 334–7.

18. Sheinberg G, Romero C, Heredia R, et al. Use of oral fluralaner for the treatment of Psoroptes cuniculi in 15 naturally infested rabbits. Vet Dermatol 2017;28: 393–395.1.

19. d'Ovidio D, Santoro D. Efficacy of Fluralaner in the Treatment of Sarcoptic Mange (Sarcoptes scabiei) in 12 Pet Rabbits. Top Companion An Med 2021;43:100528.

20. Singh SK, Jaiswal AK, Kumari S, et al. Therapeutic effects of oral fluralaner in pet rabbits with severe sarcoptic mange (Sarcoptes scabiei). Vet Parasitol 2022;304: 109693.

21. Stern LA. Fipronil toxicosis in rabbits. Vet Med 2015;110:270–4.

22. Chang CC, Wechtaisong W, Chen SY, et al. Prevalence and Risk Factors of Zoonotic Dermatophyte Infection in Pet Rabbits in Northern Taiwan. J Fungi (Basel) 2022;8:627.

23. Moriello KA, Coyner K, Paterson S, et al. Diagnosis and treatment of dermatophytosis in dogs and cats. Clinical Consensus Guidelines of the World Association for Veterinary Dermatology. Vet Dermatol 2017;28. 266–e68.

24. White SD, Vandenabeele SIJ. Rabbit and Rodent Dermatology Workshop Report. In: Hillier A, Foster AP, Kwochka KW, editors. Advances in veterinary Dermatology, vol. 5. Oxford: Blackwell; 2005. p. p373–7.

25. Barros-Battesti DM, Bassini-Silva R, Jacinavicius FC, et al. New record of Cheyletiella parasitivorax (Mégnin, 1878) (Trombidiformes: Cheyletidae) from Brazil with an illustrated key to species for the genus. Rev Bras Parasitol Vet 2020;29: e018819.

26. Kim SH, Jun HK, Song KH, et al. Prevalence of fur mites in pet rabbits in South Korea. Vet Dermatol 2008;19:189–90.

27. d'Ovidio D, Santoro D. Leporacarus gibbus infestation in client-owned rabbits and their owner. Vet Dermatol 2014;25:46–7.

28. Saito K, Hasegawa A. Clinical features of skin lesions in rabbit syphilis: a retrospective study of 63 cases (1999-2003). J Vet Med Sci 2004;66:1247–9.

29. Lumeij JT, Mikalová L, Smajs D. Is there a difference between hare syphilis and rabbit syphilis? Cross infection experiments between rabbits and hares. Vet Microbiol 2013;164:190–4.

30. Hisgen L, Abel L, Hallmaier-Wacker LK, et al. High syphilis seropositivity in European brown hares (Lepus europaeus), Lower Saxony, Germany. Transbound Emerg Dis 2020;67:2240–4.

31. Saito K, Hasegawa A. Chloramphenicol treatment for rabbit syphilis. J Vet Med Sci 2004;66:1301–4.

32. Lukehart SA, Fohn MJ, Baker-Zander SA. Efficacy of azithromycin for therapy of active syphilis in the rabbit model. J Antimicrob Chemother 1990;25(Suppl A):91–9.

33. White SD, Linder K, Shultheiss P, et al. Sebaceous adenitis in four domestic rabbits (Oryctolagus cuniculus). Vet Dermatol 2000;11:53–61.

34. Florizoone K. Thymoma-associated exfoliative dermatitis in a rabbit. Vet Dermatol 2005;16:281–4.

35. Rostaher Prélaud A, Jassies-van der Lee A, Mueller RS, et al. Presumptive paraneoplastic exfoliative dermatitis in four domestic rabbits. Vet Rec 2013;172: 155–7.

36. Florizoone K, van der Luer R, van den Ingh T. Symmetrical alopecia, scaling and hepatitis in a rabbit. Vet Dermatol 2007;18:161–4.

37. Jassies-van der Lee A, van Zeeland Y, Kik M, et al. Successful treatment of sebaceous adenitis in a rabbit with ciclosporin and triglycerides. Vet Dermatol 2009; 20:67–71.

38. Kovalik M, Thoday KL, Eatwell K, et al. Successful treatment of idiopathic sebaceous adenitis in a lionhead rabbit. J Exot Pet Med 2012;21:336–42.

39. White SD, Campbell T, Logan A, et al. Lymphoma with cutaneous involvement in three domestic rabbits (Oryctolagus cuniculus). Vet Dermatol 2000;11:61–9.

40. Ritter JM, von Bomhard W, Wise AG, et al. Cutaneous lymphomas in European pet rabbits (Oryctolagus cuniculus). Vet Pathol 2012;49:846–51.

41. Karim MR, Izawa T, Pervin M, et al. Cutaneous Histiocytic Sarcoma with Regional Lymph Node Metastasis in a Netherland Dwarf Rabbit (Oryctolagus cuniculus). J Comp Pathol 2017;156:169–72.

42. Ueda K, Ueda A, Ozaki K. Cutaneous malignant melanoma in two rabbits (Oryctolagus cuniculus). J Vet Med Sci 2018;80:973–6.

43. Budgeon C, Mans C, Chamberlin T, et al. Diagnosis and surgical treatment of a malignant trichoepithelioma of the ear canal in a pet rabbit (Oryctolagus cuniculus). J Am Vet Med Assoc 2014;245:227–31.

44. Otrocka-Domagała I, Paździor-Czapula K, Fiedorowicz J, et al. Cutaneous and Subcutaneous Tumours of Small Pet Mammals-Retrospective Study of 256 Cases (2014-2021). Animals (Basel) 2022;12:965.

45. von Bomhard W, Goldschmidt MH, Shofer FS, et al. Cutaneous neoplasms in pet rabbits: a retrospective study. Vet Pathol 2007;44:579–88.

46. Vella D. Pododermatitis. Veterinarian 2006;55–60.

47. Mancinelli E, Keeble E, Richardson J, et al. Husbandry risk factors associated with hock pododermatitis in UK pet rabbits (Oryctolagus cuniculus). Vet Rec 2014;174:429.

48. Hedley J, Stapleton N, Muir C, et al. Cutaneous botryomycosis in two pet rabbits. J Exot Pet Med 2019;28:143–7.

49. Silvers L, Inglis B, Labudovic A, et al. Virulence and pathogenesis of the MSW and MSD strains of Californian myxoma virus in European rabbits with genetic resistance to myxomatosis compared to rabbits with no genetic resistance. Virology 2006;348:72–83.

50. Klaphake E, Paul-Murphy J. Disorders of the Reproductive and Urinary Systems. In: Quesenberry KE, Orcutt CJ, Mans C, et al, editors. Ferrets, rabbits and rodents clinical medicine and surgery. St Louis: Elsevier Saunders; 2020. p. p223–5.

Ferret Dermatology

Mette Louise Halck, DVM[a],*,
Nico J. Schoemaker, DVM, PhD, Dip ECZM (Small Mammal, Avian)[b],
Yvonne R.A. van Zeeland, DVM, MVR, PhD, Dip ECZM (Avian, Small Mammal)[b]

KEYWORDS

- Parasites • Neoplasia • Endocrine disease • Skin • Integument • Pruritus
- Alopecia • *Mustela putorius furo*

KEY POINTS

- Alopecia in ferrets is common and frequently results from adrenal gland disease, hyperestrogenism, seasonal alopecia, fleas, and neoplastic conditions.
- Pruritus in ferrets does not only occur with infectious diseases but also can be associated with endocrine and neoplastic conditions, including hyperadrenocorticism, lymphoma, and mast cell tumors.
- Blue ferret syndrome is a condition in which the skin obtains a bluish tinge after clipping of the fur; it resolves within a few weeks without treatment.
- Zoonotic skin diseases in ferrets include sarcoptic mange (*Sarcoptes scabiei*), leishmaniasis, and dermatophytosis, whereas inhalation of blastomycotic spores is also possible during culturing.

INTRODUCTION

Ferrets can present with a multitude of dermatologic conditions, which can either be the result of a primary skin disease or involve a secondary manifestation of a systemic disease. This review provides an overview of dermatologic conditions that can be seen in ferrets, including their diagnosis and management.

Among the dermatologic diseases most commonly seen in ferrets are ectoparasites, cutaneous tumors, and endocrine diseases. Owing to the possibility for underlying systemic diseases, the clinical workup of a ferret with dermatologic signs should consider the ferret's signalment (eg, age, gender, and reproductive status) and consist of a detailed history (regarding the skin condition, general health, lifestyle, preventive treatments, and health of other pets and members of the household) and a thorough physical and dermatologic examination. Specific tests can subsequently be used to diagnose or rule out primary skin disease. These tests may include bacterial and/or

[a] AniCura Københavns Dyrehospital, Denmark; [b] Department of Clinical Sciences, Faculty of Veterinary Medicine, Utrecht University, Yalelaan 108, 3584 CM Utrecht, the Netherlands
* Corresponding author.
E-mail address: mettehalck@gmail.com

Vet Clin Exot Anim 26 (2023) 359–382
https://doi.org/10.1016/j.cvex.2022.12.003
1094-9194/23/© 2022 Elsevier Inc. All rights reserved.

fungal cultures, skin scrapings, cytologic evaluation of fine-needle aspirates, and histopathology of skin biopsies. In addition, a complete blood cell count, serum biochemistry, hormonal panels, and imaging should be considered if an underlying systemic disease is suspected.

FERRET SKIN AND COAT: ANATOMIC AND PHYSIOLOGIC CONSIDERATIONS

The body of the domestic ferret (*Mustela putorius furo*) is covered with thick dermis, especially on the neck and upper back because this is the area where bites are administered during play-fighting or mating.[1,2] Numerous sebaceous glands, which are under androgenic control and therefore most active during the breeding season (March to August in the northern hemisphere), give the ferret its characteristic musky odor, oily fur, and yellowish to reddish undercoat that is most noticeable in light-coated ferrets.[1,3] Furthermore, ferrets have 2 prominent scent glands located lateral to the anus, which produce a secretion when the ferret is frightened, excited, or in estrus. Because the odor will be unaffected by removal of these glands, routine anal sacculectomy (albeit performed by some breeding farms) is not recommended. Because ferrets only have eccrine sweat glands on the footpads, they are at increased risk for developing hyperthermia when exposed to high environmental temperatures.

Ferrets have long and coarse guard hairs in a variety of colors and patterns, from albino to black, depending on type.[4] A heavy shed in the spring reveals the shorter and darker summer coat.[5]

A bilaterally symmetrical, patchy, seasonal alopecia involving the tail and perineal area may be seen during the breeding season, particularly in intact females (jills).[6] Neutered individuals of both sexes display less dramatic molts.[7] Proper husbandry, including a high-quality diet of 30% to 35% animal protein and 15% to 20% fat, and avoiding excessive bathing, is important to prevent a dull, dry haircoat.[8–10]

Intact females are known to pull hair to use as bedding material, which may inadvertently be misdiagnosed as pruritic skin disease. Similarly, the typical bluish discoloration of the skin that can be seen during initial hair regrowth (eg, following hair clipping for surgery or treatment of hyperadrenocorticism) should not be mistaken for bruising or cyanosis (see section Blue Ferret Syndrome).

PARASITIC DISEASES
Fleas

Flea infestation with *Ctenocephalides felis* or *Ctenocephalides canis* is a common problem in ferrets that are housed together with cats or dogs.[11–13] Infestations with other species, including *Pulex irritans*, *Paracaras meli*, *Ceratophyllus sciurorum*, and *Ceratophyllus vison*, in contrast, are rare.[10,11] Although asymptomatic infections occur, most ferrets show mild to moderate pruritus, resulting in self-induced alopecia and trauma with a papulocrustous dermatitis on the tail base, ventral abdomen, and inner thighs.[1,11,13] Flea-bite hypersensitivity has been reported in ferrets.[14] The diagnosis is based on history and clinical signs. In case no fleas or flea excrements are found on dermatologic examination, the diagnosis is usually made based on response to treatment.[10] Effective treatments include monthly treatments with selamectin spot-on treatment (6–18 mg/kg, or 15 mg/ferret), fipronil spray (0.2–0.4 mL of a 9.7% solution), or imidacloprid (10 mg/kg or 0.4 mL/ferret), alone or in combination with 1% moxidectin.[11,15–17] Environmental eradication of fleas and treatment of other susceptible animals in the household is important to prevent reinfection.[18]

Ear mites: Otodectes cynotis

Ear mite (*Otodectes cynotis*) infections are common in ferrets. Transmission occurs via contaminated ear debris or direct contact with infected ferrets, dogs, or cats.[19,20] Otocariasis often leads to excess production of brown cerumen (**Fig. 1**A), which can be differentiated from normal ear wax by direct visualization of mites or eggs on otoscopy or microscopy (**Fig. 1**B,C).[10,14,21] Animals are mostly asymptomatic,[21,22] but may show head shaking, pruritus, self-induced alopecia, periaural crusting, excoriations, and aural hematomas as a result of scratching.[23,24] With heavy infestations, secondary bacterial or yeast infections may occur, and neurological deficits can develop in sequela to otitis media or interna.[25,26] Rarely, mites are found in alternative locations, for example, the perineum, in which case the diagnosis is made by microscopic examination via a skin scrape.[14] Treatment comprises flushing and cleaning of the ear canal followed by topical treatment using selamectin (15–45 mg/ferret every 28 days) or imidacloprid 10%/moxidectin 1.0% 2 to 3 times every 14 days.[21,24,27,28] Subcutaneous ivermectin (0.4 mg/kg every 14 days) can also be used, but it is less effective than intra-auricular ivermectin (0.4 mg/kg, diluted 1:10 in propylene glycol every 14 days), which can be used provided that the tympanic membrane is intact. Ivermectin should be avoided in pregnant jills due to its teratogenicity.[23,24] As an alternative, 1 drop of fipronil can be administered in each ear canal.[24,29] Secondary infections may warrant additional use of antifungals and/or antibiotics. Treatment of in-contact ferrets, dogs, and cats, and the environment, is important to avoid reinfection.[14,23]

Sarcoptic mange

Sarcoptes scabiei is a burrowing mite that infects dogs, cats, and ferrets by direct or indirect contact.[26,30–32] Outdoor ferrets are at higher risk for infection with *S. scabiei* because wild members of the canine family are potential sources of infection.[33] Two clinical forms exist in ferrets, that is, the pedal and generalized forms (**Fig. 2**).[31] The pedal form is characterized by alopecic and swollen feet, formation of dark brown scabs, and eventually sloughing of the claws,[33,34] and may progress into the generalized form characterized by intense pruritus and alopecia of the face, pinnae, and ventrum.[33] Severely affected ferrets can become lethargic and eventually die.[34] Because the number of mites present is relatively small, the diagnosis can be difficult, with a high risk of false-negative results.[26,31] Multiple superficial skin scrapes are indicated to increase the chance of detecting the mites, larvae, ova, and nymphs, although mites will occasionally be found upon examination of scabs that are broken into smaller pieces and treated with 10% potassium hydroxide.[14,33] Ivermectin (0.2 to 0.4 mg/kg subcutaneously every 7 to 14 days) use combined with treatment of in-contact animals, and environmental cleaning every 3 to 4 days, until eradication of the mites, is

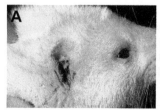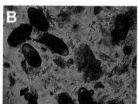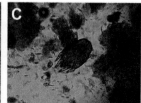

Fig. 1. (*A*) In ferrets with an *O cynotis* infection excessive brown/black debris may be seen in the ear canal. (*B, C*) *O cynotis* eggs (*B*) and an adult mite (*C*) from a ferret. (*Reprinted from*: Powers, L. V. (2009). Bacterial and parasitic diseases of ferrets. Veterinary Clinics: Exotic Animal Practice, 12(3), 531-561. With permission.)

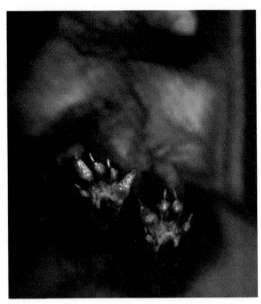

Fig. 2. *S scabiei* infection in a ferret, pedal form. (*Reprinted from*: Chapter 10 - Parasitic diseases of ferrets, Editor(s): John H. Lewington, Ferret Husbandry, Medicine and Surgery (Second Edition), W.B. Saunders, 2007, Pages 224-257, ISBN 9780702028274, https://doi.org/10.1016/B978-0-7020-2827-4.50016-4.)

recommended.[14,26,31] Ferrets with the pedal form may benefit from warm-water soaks and trimming of affected claws, alongside treatment of secondary bacterial infections.[26,31] To prevent reinfection, materials that cannot be thoroughly disinfected (eg, wooden toys, sleeping huts) should be removed and discarded.[34] Because *S scabiei* has zoonotic potential, in-contact humans should wear gloves and be carefully monitored.[14,31,35]

Demodicosis

Clinical demodicosis is uncommon in ferrets, and mostly limited to immunocompromised individuals.[14,23,36–40] Infections with both the larger, slender-bodied *Demodex canis* and shorter *Demodex criceti* have been reported.[38,41,42] Symptomatic ferrets may display no to mild pruritus, alopecia, erythematous and thickened skin, small follicular papules, and yellow-brown seborrhea with seborrheic scales (**Fig. 3**).[23,38,39] Some animals may have brown debris in the external ear canal, similar to the exudate seen in ear mite infestations.[39] Diagnosis is made by identification of the mites on skin scrape from affected areas or analysis of aural exudate.[23,39,40] Treatment options include ivermectin (0.05–0.3 mg/kg every 24 hours orally), imidacloprid 10%/moxidectin 1% spot-on treatment once monthly, and amitraz 0.0125% once weekly.[26,38,40] Because demodicosis can be hard to treat, with relapses frequently occurring, treatment is continued for weeks after negative skin scrapes are found.

Fur mites

Ulcerative facial lesions caused by the fur mite *Lynxacarus mustelae* have been reported in kits[40] (**Fig. 4**A,B). Topical treatment with permethrin powder and cleaning of the environment successfully resolved the facial lesions that were noted in these animals.[14]

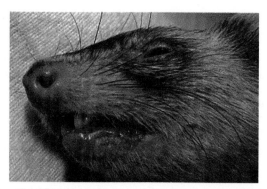

Fig. 3. Peribuccal and periocular alopecia, erythema, and skin thickening in a ferret. *Demodex* sp were found in skin scrapings from these areas. (*Reprint from*: Beaufrere, H., Neta, M., Smith, D. A., & Taylor, W. M. (2009). Demodectic mange associated with lymphoma in a ferret. Journal of exotic pet medicine, 18(1), 57-61. With permission.)

Ticks

Tick infestation is primarily a concern in ferrets exposed to outdoor environments. Generally, it results in erythema and inflammation of the site of the bite, but heavy infestations can lead to anemia.[26,31,43] Most infestations involve *Ixodes ricinus* (the castor bean tick); however, other tick species have been described in ferrets depending on geographic location.[14,31] Transmission of pathogens has not yet been documented in ferrets, but ticks can serve as vectors for *Babesia* spp, *Leishmania* spp, and other pathogens, hence posing a risk to both the ferret and in-contact humans.[14,31,34,44] Upon identifying a tick during the clinical examination, the tick should be manually removed, including head and mouth parts.[31] In addition, treatment with a tick preventative such as selamectin, fipronil, and ivermectin should be initiated.[18,26,31] Anemia, if present, will resolve with the removal of ticks.[43]

Cutaneous myiasis

Cutaneous myiasis is uncommon in ferrets and occurs mostly in ferrets exposed to flies and bot flies under warm and humid conditions.[10,26] Cutaneous myiasis can present as migratory, furuncular, or wound myiasis, depending on the infesting fly species.[14,43] *Hypoderma bovis* causes migratory myiasis, which may be associated with intense pruritus.

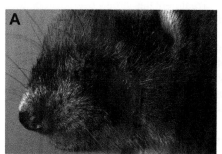
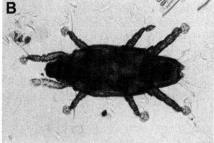

Fig. 4. (*A*) In this ferret kit and its 4 siblings ulcerative lesions were seen on the left cheeks. The jill had licked these cheeks excessively. Skin scrapings revealed that the primary cause of these lesions was the fur mite *Lynxacarus mustelae*. (*B*) *L mustelae*.

Typically, the infestation leads to granulomatous masses and sinuses in the cervical region, which results from the larvae burrowing through the skin into the lower layers of the dermis.[26]

Furuncular myiasis is the most commonly reported type of myiasis, caused by the bot fly (*Cuterebra* spp) larvae. After the egg is laid on the skin, the developing larva buries into the skin, while leaving a hole for respiration.[43] Typically, the larvae pupate in the ventral cervical, axillary, and inguinal regions or over the back.[10,26] On clinical examination, one or multiple 1- to 3-mm-diameter localized swellings can be found.[10,26,43] Upon inspecting the respiration hole, the larva can be visualized.

Wound-related myiasis, or fly strike, is caused by flesh fly larvae of *Wohlfahrtia vigil,* and primarily is a risk in young kits housed outdoor in warm and humid weather.[26] Following deposition of the eggs in an open wound, the larvae feed on the surrounding tissue, which—depending on the duration and severity—can lead to massive tissue destruction, secondary infections, and death.[43]

Following diagnosis, larvae need to be manually or surgically removed in toto. Extraction should be done gently, because remaining pieces of larvae might result in anaphylaxis.[10,34] Analgesia and sedation can be provided as needed. In addition, debridement of necrotic tissue should take place, followed by flushing of the wound or cavity with diluted chlorhexidine. In case of furuncular or migratory myiasis, the cavity can either be closed with tissue glue or left open to heal by secondary intention, while continuing daily wound care.[43] Antibiotics can be used, if indicated.[10]

Regardless of the type of myiasis, owners should be counseled on fly control and preventative measures to decrease the risk of reoccurrence.[43]

Leishmaniasis

Leishmaniasis is a potentially zoonotic, vector-borne disease caused by the protozoan organism *Leishmania infantum,* which is transferred through infected female phlebotomine sandflies (*Phlebotomus perniciosus* and *Phlebotomus ariasi*).[45,46] This disease is primarily found in Southern Europe, and mostly infects domestic dogs, although it has been described in cats, rabbits, and ferrets as well, particularly in individuals that are immunosuppressed or housed outdoors.[46–48] Cutaneous leishmaniasis in ferrets manifests as inflammatory, erythematous, papular, nonpruritic lesions, with potential local lymph node enlargement and splenomegaly.[46,47] Leishmaniasis can be diagnosed through identification of amastigotes in infected macrophages and multinucleate giant cells on cytologic, histopathologic, or immunohistochemical examination of samples collected from the dermal lesions.[46,49] Polymerase chain reaction (PCR), western blot, or enzyme-linked immunosorbent assay for specific serum IgG antibodies can also be used for confirmation of the diagnosis.[46,47] Treatment has largely been extrapolated from dogs and cats and includes the use of miltefosine and meglumine antimoniate in combination with allopurinol, which has led to good long-term results, as indicated by resolution of clinical signs and decreased antibody titers.[47,49] Monitoring for xanthinuria is recommended upon initiating treatment with allopurinol.[49] Preventive measures consist of the (off-label) use of repellents with activity against sand flies (because the use of sand fly repellents in ferrets is off-label, close monitoring for side effects is warranted), and keeping the ferret inside at times when sand flies are active.[48]

VIRAL DISEASES (CANINE DISTEMPER VIRUS)

Canine distemper virus (CDV) typically infects members of the canine family and causes fatal disease within 5 to 35 days following development of clinical signs, regardless of strain.[48] Ferrets can be infected through aerosols, fomites, or direct contact with infected animals.[31,50,51] After viral exposure, the infection is spread hematogenously, with clinical signs developing after 7 to 10 days, although incubation periods of up to 56 days have been reported.[52,53] Initial signs include lethargy, photophobia, and hyporexia. In addition, brown facial crusts due to accumulation of nasal and ocular secretions (**Fig. 5**A,B) and secondary bacterial pneumonia leading to dyspnea can be seen upon infection of the upper and lower respiratory tract.[54] Dermatologic changes characteristic for CDV infections include pruritic rashes on the chin and inguinal region, and swelling and hyperkeratosis of the footpads.[31,50,54] In rare cases, superficial pyoderma can progress into generalized desquamation.[54] Neurologic signs commonly develop in the terminal stages of the disease. Antemortem diagnosis of CDV in ferrets involves antigen detection in samples from conjunctival, tonsillar, or respiratory secretions using fluorescent antibody labeling or PCR. In addition, CDV antigens or inclusion bodies can be identified on postmortem immunohistochemistry or histopathology of affected tissues, including the tonsils, lymph nodes, urinary bladder, lung tissue, stomach, and spleen.[52,54,55] Humane euthanasia is usually recommended, although successful treatment has been reported in rare cases that were infected with a low-virulent strain and that were treated promptly using intense supportive care, vitamin A, and hyperimmune serum.[52,54,56] In case of an outbreak of CDV, healthy ferrets should be isolated and vaccinated, and the environment thoroughly disinfected.[52] Availability of CDV vaccines licensed for ferrets vary from country to country, and for some countries, a canine vaccine might be the only available option.[53] If using vaccines intended for dogs, advice from the manufacturer should be sought on the use in ferrets, because myofasciitis is a reported risk following vaccination.[57]

FUNGAL DISEASE
Dermatophytosis (Ringworm)

Dermatophytosis in ferrets is caused by *Trichophyton mentagrophytes* or *Microsporum canis,* and—in rare cases—*Microsporum nanum*.[1,10,23] Although often mentioned in books and reviews, dermatophytosis is relatively uncommon in healthy ferrets, and occurs most often in young or immunosuppressed individuals exposed to infected cats.[10,35,58,59] Upon infection of the hair shafts and stratum corneum, an annular nonpruritic alopecia develops that spreads peripherally[23,31,35] (**Fig. 6**). With severe infections, a generalized alopecia with diffuse scaling, erythema, and crusting

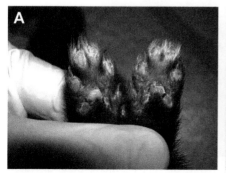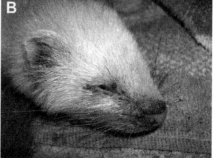

Fig. 5. Canine distemper virus infection in a ferret with hyperkeratosis and crusting of foot pads (*A*) and severe crusting dermatitis on the face (*B*). (Photograph courtesy Dr. David Perpiñán.)

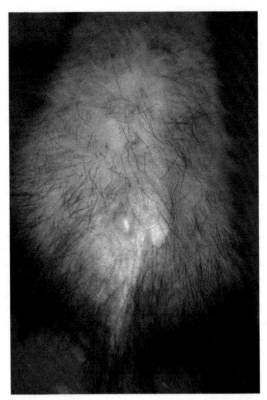

Fig. 6. This 9-month-old male ferret displays annular alopecic lesions that proved to be due to a *M canis* infection upon culture.

can develop.[23] Rarely, dermatophytosis spreads into the dermis and subcutaneous adipose tissue creating nodules with potential ulceration and granular discharge, referred to as dermatophytic pseudomycetomas (**Fig. 7**).[60] Dermatophytosis should be considered in the differential diagnosis for any animal housed with other animals

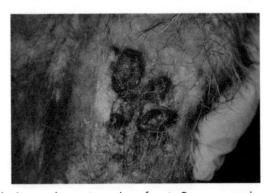

Fig. 7. Dermatophytic pseudomycetoma in a ferret. On rare occasions, these ulcerated, granular discharge-producing nodules can develop following spread of the fungal infection into the dermis and subcutaneous adipose tissue. (Photo courtesy of Seth Oster and Amelia White.)

or humans in the household that have similar annular skin lesions. Although being potentially zoonotic, spread from ferrets to humans has thus far not been documented.[10,59,61] Diagnosis is usually made by culture. On dermatophyte test media, fungal growth will appear approximately 2 to 4 weeks after culture of hair or skin scrapes from the periphery of the lesions.[62] If positive, identifying the fungus involved is recommended. Other options to diagnose dermatophytosis include identification of fungal hyphae or arthrospores on microscopy of hair or scales prepared in 10% potassium hydroxide,[26] and PCR of skin or hair samples. Similar to other animals, use of a Wood's lamp carries a high risk of false-positive and false-negative results depending on the dermatophyte species.[23] However, up to 100% of *M canis* demonstrates fluorescence.[63] Treatment includes clipping of the affected hair, using broad margins around all lesions, and the use of keratolytic shampoo.[18] Topical antifungals usually suffice and include enilconazole, clotrimazole, or miconazole cream every 12 hours, or weekly lime sulfur dips.[10,23] As systemic treatment, griseofulvin (25 mg/kg by mouth every 24 hours), itraconazole (5–10 mg/kg every 24 hours by mouth), or fluconazole (10 mg/kg every 12 hours by mouth) can be used.[31,61,63] Treatment should be continued for 2 to 4 weeks after resolution of dermal signs, or, preferably, until 2 consecutive fungal cultures with a negative outcome. Treatment of infected in-contact animals and environmental disinfection should also be initiated to minimize the risk of reoccurrence.[10,23,26,63] In addition, monitoring for signs of liver damage and bone marrow suppression is advised for animals treated with griseofulvin or itraconazole. Although most dermatophytosis cases respond favorably to treatment, dermatophytic pseudomycetomas can be difficult to treat, and carry a high risk of progressive disease leading to euthanasia or death.[61]

Fungal ear infections

Fungal otitis externa caused by malasseziosis (*Malassezia* spp) or mucormycosis (*Absidia corymbifera*) has been documented secondary to *O cynotis* in ferrets, most often transmitted from in-contact cats.[26,63] Although ear mite infections in ferrets are usually nonpruritic, concurrent fungal infections can result in intense pruritus. Malasseziosis commonly leads to generalized multifocal pustular dermatitis with hyperkeratosis and alopecia, although mucormycosis potentially spreads from the external ear canal, through the middle ear, to the inner ear, where it causes granulomatous meningoencephalitis and associated central nervous signs.[64,65] Fungal hyphae are identifiable on cytology of ear samples or skin histopathology.[65] Treatment consists of antifungal therapy combined with eradication of ear mites.[23,26,64]

Cryptococcosis

Systemic mycosis caused by *Cryptococcus* organisms (*Cryptococcus bacillisporus*, previously *Cryptococcus neoformans* varians *gattii*, or *Cryptococcus neoformans* varians *grubii*) are rare in mammals, including ferrets.[66–70] Ferrets are infected through inhalation of spores from contaminated environments. Plants like *Eucalyptus* spp are associated with an increased risk of spore formation.[66,71–73] Spore inhalation causes rhinitis and pneumonia, followed by lymphatic and hematogenous spread leading to meningoencephalitis, abscessation of the draining lymph nodes, and fungal nodules on internal organs.[66,67] Dermal presentation of cryptococcosis might be more common in ferrets than in other species, and presents as an erythematous, scaly, pruritic rash of the nasal bridge and cutaneous masses.[66,74] Identification of fungal hyphae on impression smears of cutaneous lesions, or fungal growth of aspirates from masses and abscessed lymph nodes, can be used to confirm the diagnosis.[66,73] Other diagnostic options include histopathology with immunohistochemistry or serology.[66–69,75] Surgical excision of localized masses combined with systemic anti-fungal therapy (itraconazole or fluconazole) carries a good prognosis.[66] However, in late stages of systemic fungal disease or meningitis, prognosis is generally poor.[63]

Blastomycosis

Blastomycosis can occur in immunosuppressed ferrets and is caused by inhalation of *Blastomyces dermatitidis* spores from sandy, acidic soil near water, especially in Eastern North America.[63] Interindividual transmission has not been reported, and there are no published reports documenting direct transmission from ferrets to humans.[73] Blastomycosis can present as systemic neurologic and pulmonary disease, or as ulcerative, nonhealing lesions on the skin and footpads.[76,77] Agar gel immunodiffusion assay, cytology, or histopathology can be used for diagnostic purposes.[76,77] Cultures should only take place in a professional laboratory to eliminate the zoonotic risk of infective blastomycosis spores.[63] Prognosis depends on the extent of infection at the time of diagnosis.[77] Amphotericin B (0.7–25 mg/kg intravenously, administered in smaller doses) can be used in cases nonresponsive to itraconazole,[63,73] whereas fluconazole or voriconazole can be effective in case of neurologic spread.[76] Although glucocorticosteroids can be used for anti-inflammatory purposes, mixed results and potential for further immunosuppression render their use controversial.[76]

Histoplasmosis

Histoplasmosis (*Histoplasma capsulatum*) is a rare cause of systemic mycosis in ferrets, with one case reporting formation of subcutaneous nodules.[73,78]

Systemic candidiasis

Systemic candidiasis caused by *Candida parapsilosis* has been diagnosed postmortem in a ferret with necrotizing encephalitis, lymphadenitis, and ulcerative and perivascular dermatitis.[79]

BACTERIAL INFECTIONS

Pyoderma and deeper skin infections in ferrets can be caused by a wide range of bacteria, most frequently *Staphylococcus aureus* or *Streptococcus* spp.[31,43,80] Dermal wounds created during mating or pruritus-related, self-inflicted trauma can cause bacteria to penetrate into the skin, creating abscesses.[43,81] Cervical abscesses, known as lumpy jaw, are commonly associated with *Actinomyces* spp. Diagnosis and treatment of abscesses are similar to other species, with penicillin or tetracycline being the treatment of choice for *Actinomyces* organisms.[23,81] Nontuberculous mycobacteria, notably *Mycobacterium avium* subspecies *avium*, have been cultured from a ferret with alopecia, bruises, scabs, and numerous skin nodules[82] (**Fig. 8**).

TUMORS AFFECTING THE INTEGUMENT

Neoplasia are commonly diagnosed in older ferrets, and approximately 20% of these affect the skin and/or subcutaneous tissue.[83–85] Most cutaneous tumors in ferrets are benign, with mast cell tumors and sebaceous tumors being the most frequent tumor types, each accounting for a third of the integumentary neoplasms encountered in ferrets.[86–93] Multiple tumor types can be found simultaneously in the same individual.[84,94,95] Diagnosis is made by cytology of fine-needle aspirates, or histopathology and immunohistochemistry of skin biopsies or surgically excised tumors. Staging should be performed as in other species, and treatment fine-tuned based on tumor

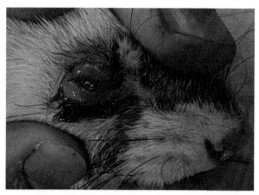

Fig. 8. Edema of the eyelids and nictitating membrane in a ferret with mycobacteriosis. (*Reprinted from*: Mentré, V., & Bulliot, C. (2015). A retrospective study of 17 cases of mycobacteriosis in domestic ferrets (Mustela putorius furo) between 2005 and 2013. Journal of exotic pet medicine, 24(3), 340-349. With permission.)

type (epithelial, mesenchymal, or round cell) and stage.[26,31] **Table 1** provides an overview of the type of integumentary tumors reported in ferrets.

ENDOCRINE DISEASES
Adrenal Gland Disease (Hyperadrenocorticism)

Steroid-producing tumors of the adrenal cortex occur in up to 70% of neutered middle-aged ferrets, most often at 3.5 years after neutering.[106,107] Prolonged exposure to daylight, as well as chronic stimulation of the adrenal gland cortex by the pituitary gland after neutering are suggested as predisposing factors.[108] Nodular hyperplasia, adenomas, and adenocarcinomas account for 56%, 16%, and 26% of adrenocortical tumors in ferrets, respectively.[106,108] Tumors are unilateral in 84% of cases, with the left adrenal gland most commonly affected.[109] In half of the patients with bilateral hyperadrenocorticism 2 tumor types are present.[109] Clinical signs result from hyperandrogenism, and include bilateral, symmetric alopecia (**Fig. 15**), thinning of the skin, vulvar enlargement, return of hormonal behavior, and urethral obstruction due to prostatic cysts or prostatitis in male ferrets.[108–110] Tumors are best visualized using abdominal ultrasonography, in which one or both adrenals can appear enlarged, rounded, heterogeneous, or hyperechoic.[110,111] Alternatively, contrast-enhanced computed tomography can be used. Blood panels may reveal elevated levels of sex steroids, for example, estradiol and androstenedione.[112,113] However, panels are not reliable for differentiating between hyperandrogenism, intact animals, and those with remnant ovarian tissue or granulosa cell tumors, and are mostly recommended for monitoring of response to treatment and signs of relapse.[111] Medical treatment is preferred to surgical treatment because it results in a longer disease-free period (16.5 months vs 13.6 months) and lower complication rate and is less invasive.[111,114] Long-acting, deslorelin acetate-containing implants usually result in resolution of dermatologic and behavioral changes within 2 weeks, and hair regrowth appears within 6 weeks postimplantation. Alternatively, leuprolide acetate depot injections (100 μg/kg subcutaneously) can be given every 3 to 4 weeks, and have been proved to be effective for 3 to 4 months.[115,116] Adrenalectomy, although leading to complete remission of clinical signs and identification of the tumor type involved through histopathology, is markedly more invasive, especially in case of right-sided

Table 1
Overview of integumentary tumors reported in ferrets

Tumor Type	Origin	Prevalence	Location	Morphologic Appearance	Malignancy Grade	Treatment	Prognosis
Sebaceous or basal cell tumor Fig. 9	Epithelial	Common, one-third of integumentary neoplasia. Average age 5.2 years; no known sex predilection	Head and neck region, although tumors may also occur on flanks, limbs, or tail	Large, warty, exophytic to pedunculated masses; ulceration can occur due to self-inflicted trauma[92,96]	Benign and slow-growing, despite grossly and histologically aggressive appearance[92,96,97]	Surgical excision	Good, although can develop into squamous cell carcinoma (rare)[96]
Apocrine scent gland (cyst) (adeno) carcinoma Fig. 10	Epithelial	Common; approximately 75% of apocrine scent gland tumors are malignant; adenomas can also occur but less frequently	Head, neck, genital areas (vulva, prepuce)	Large, firm mass, sometimes fluid-filled; should be differentiated from benign apocrine cysts[23]	Malignant with aggressive infiltration of adjacent tissues and high metastatic potential to regional lymph nodes and lungs[96,98]	Surgical excision with wide margins of at least 1 cm, which often necessitates partial to complete preputial and/or penile amputation, and use of flaps or Y-plasty to close or reconstruct the prepuce; additional radiation therapy and chemotherapy should be considered to reduce risk of metastases and eliminate local residual malignant cells	Often poor due to local infiltration; prognosis may improve upon use of radiation therapy and chemotherapy[96,97]
Mammary tumor (adenoma/ adenocarcinoma)	Epithelial	Uncommon; seen in older males (6–7 years) and younger females (2–6 years)	Mammary gland	Smaller or larger nodule in the mammary tissue, which can become ulcerated	Usually benign (30% of mammary tumors are malignant)	Surgical excision	Generally good prognosis, with surgery being curative; adenocarcinomas have potential for recurrence, especially if surgical margins are insufficient
Squamous cell carcinoma	Epithelial	Rare	Often arise from the lining of the anal sac, but can also be seen on lip, gingiva, or feet	Firm, ulcerated mass,[18] or multiple pigmented, proliferative skin lesions (papillomavirus associated)[96,99]	Malignant	Surgical excision; chemotherapy usually not effective	Guarded; local recurrence is common[18]

Tumor	Origin	Signalment/occurrence	Clinical appearance	Behavior	Treatment	Prognosis
Mast cell tumor Fig. 11	Round cell tumor	Common in older (4.5–5 years) male ferrets; account for one-third of integumentary neoplasia[92,97]	Face, ear, tail, limb, flank; in 30% of animals, multiple tumors are present	Discrete, flat, round, plaquelike, crusted, and often pruritic[94]	Benign; easily recognized on cytology (non-Wright stain) by their characteristic granules[94]	Surgical excision	Good due to low metastatic potential[92,94]
Lymphoma Fig. 12	Round cell tumor	Cutaneous form is less common than other (multicentric, gastrointestinal, mediastinal, extranodal) types[100]; appears more common in middle-aged ferrets with possible female predilection	Often involving the feet, but also reported to involve inguinal, anal, and/or periocular tissues	Focal dermal or subcutaneous masses, or more generalized, chronic dermatitis with rashlike or ulcerated appearance, alopecia, and pruritus with self-trauma (epitheliotropic lymphoma)	Highly malignant, usually T-cell type on immunohistochemistry	Chemotherapy as for other lymphomas. Palliative treatment with steroids may slow the course of disease. Epitheliotropic lymphoma (1% of lymphoma) responds poorly to corticosteroids, but may benefit from isoretinoin	Often poor prognosis due to late diagnosis, even with chemotherapy[90,100]; may develop into multicentric lymphoma, leading to clinical deterioration and euthanasia[102]
Hemangioma/ hemangiosarcoma Fig. 13	Mesenchymal	Relatively uncommon	Often on head, neck, limb, and feet[97]	Small, round, red or black masses that are well vascularized and bleed easily, if traumatized[97]	Usually benign	Surgical excision	Good for hemangioma, but hemangiosarcomas are highly aggressive and have a high recurrence rate[97]
Leiomyoma/ leiomyosarcoma	Mesenchymal, arising from smooth muscles (arrector pili muscle)	Uncommon; malignant form most common in male, middle-aged ferrets[97]	Head and back (dorsal midline)[101,102]	Raised, pink, ulcerated nodules or painful, multiple, raised, parallel, cordlike structures in the skin[97,102]	Both benign and malignant forms can occur	Surgical excision	Malignant form carries high risk for recurrence after surgical removal[101,103]
Fibroma/ fibrosarcoma	Mesenchymal	Uncommon; associated with vaccinations[104]	Dorsum and flanks (injection sites)	Subcutaneous, round mass	Generally benign, low-grade malignancies with a slow growth rate and low metastatic potential (unlike cats)	Surgical excision with wide margins[96,104]	Usually favorable
Chordoma Fig. 14	Mesenchymal, skeletal tissue	Uncommon	Usually on the tail (tip), but may develop in a vertebrae in any region of the spinal column	Irregular round, whitish gray, firm, clublike swelling	Usually low metastatic potential, although locally aggressive; metastasis to subcutaneous tissue overlying tumor as well as distant metastasis being reported[105]	Tail tip chordomas are often easily cured by tail amputation	Generally good for tumors on the tail tip, but poor when other parts of spinal column are involved due to the infiltrative nature of the tumor

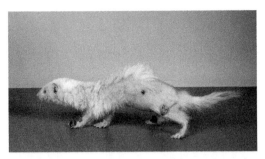

Fig. 9. In this 5-year-old female ferret with alopecia due to an adrenal tumor, multiple wartlike lesions were seen. Histology revealed these tumors to be sebaceous epithelioma. Although they appear aggressive, and thereby malignant, these tumors are considered to be benign.

hyperadrenocorticism.[106,110,111] For bilateral tumors, adrenalectomy of the largest gland combined with subtotal adrenalectomy of the contralateral gland is recommended to avoid induction of Addisonian disease (and associated treatment) postoperatively.[109]

Hyperestrogenism

Hyperestrogenism can be seen in up to 50% of ovulating unmated jills as a result of persistent estrus, but is occasionally seen in ferrets with ovarian remnants, cystic ovarian disease, ovarian neoplasia (granulosa cell tumors or thecomas), or hyperadrenocorticism.[111,117,118] In the long term, hyperestrogenism causes bone marrow suppression, pancytopenia, and nonregenerative anemia.[115] Jills with hyperestrogenism present with alopecia over the tail base, vulvar swelling, and symptoms related to pancytopenia, including pale mucous membranes, petechia and/or ecchymoses, infections, weakness, systolic murmurs, and posterior paresis.[115,119] Diagnosis is based on history, clinical signs, identification of adrenal or ovarian changes on ultrasonography, and response to treatment. Elevated serum estradiol and progesterone are not helpful in differentiating between the various diseases.[120] Acute stabilization and possible blood transfusion are often needed in critical patients, alongside hormonal treatment with human chorionic gonadotropin, or gonadotropin-releasing hormones

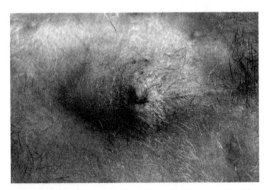

Fig. 10. A soft swelling at the entrance of the prepuce in a 6-year-old neutered male ferret was diagnosed as a basal cell carcinoma. Radical resection is an important step in the treatment of these highly malignant tumors.

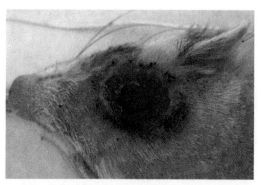

Fig. 11. An irregular mass on the head of a 4-year-old neutered female ferret was diagnosed as a mast cell tumor. Although this type of tumor is considered malignant in most companion species, in ferrets these tumors are benign.

(eg, deslorelin) to end estrous. Upon stabilization, surgical or chemical neutering should be performed.[115,121] Hyperestrogenism is best prevented by gonadectomy or subcutaneous implantation of long-acting deslorelin-containing implants, which needs to be repeated every one to two years,[122] with implants being the preferred option to avoid induction of adrenal gland disease.[106,123]

Testicular Tumors

Testicular leiomyosarcoma has been reported to cause nonpruritic alopecia of the back, neck, tail, and abdomen, which resolved after surgical castration.[124]

Hypothyroidism

Hypothyroidism is rare in ferrets and usually not associated with dermatologic changes noted in other mammals.[106]

ALLERGIC SKIN DISEASE

Allergic skin diseases are uncommon in ferrets, and most often involves contact dermatitis associated with frequent exposure to shampoos or insecticide spray, or

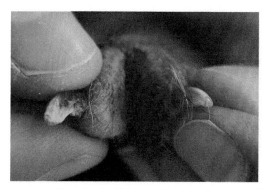

Fig. 12. Lymphomas are considered one of the most common tumors diagnosed in ferrets. This swollen tissue in the interdigital space of a 5-year-old neutered male ferret was diagnosed as cutaneous lymphoma.

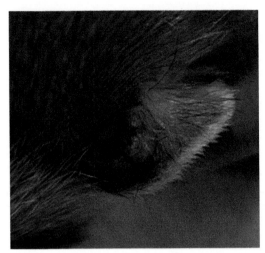

Fig. 13. Hemangiosarcoma on ferret pinna. (*Courtesy of* Peter G. Fisher, DVM, Virginia Beach, VA.)

reactions to environmental allergens.[43,125] Atopy manifests as generalized symmetric dermatitis and pruritus of the trunk, rump, and skin folds, leading to self-induced alopecia.[35,43] Despite a single case report on food hypersensitivity in a ferret, this should be ruled out as a differential.[31,35] Atopy can generally be diagnosed using histopathology of skin biopsies, intradermal allergy testing, and resolution of clinical signs following elimination of environmental allergens.[31,43] Hyposensitization with triggering allergens can be attempted, in addition to the use of antihistamines, corticosteroids, and omega-3 and -6 fatty acid supplementation to alleviate the clinical signs.[43]

MISCELLANEOUS SKIN DISEASES
Erythema Multiforme

Erythema multiforme is a rare autoimmune disease, which has currently only been reported in ferrets with concurrent adrenal disease.[43,126] Exposure to drugs, infections, or neoplasia can alter epidermal keratinocytes, making them a target for the host's

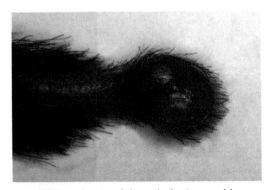

Fig. 14. A nonpruritic swelling at the tip of the tail of a 6-year-old neutered male ferret represents the typical presentation of a chordoma. When located at this region, this commonly benign tumor can easily be resected by partial amputation of the tail.

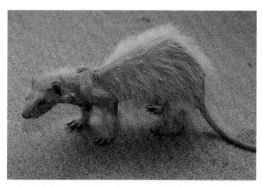

Fig. 15. Severe alopecia, as seen in the 7.5-year-old neutered female ferret, is commonly seen in ferrets with hyperandrogenism, also commonly known as hyperadrenocorticism. Severe pruritis may be seen among ferrets with this disease.

T cells, which induces keratinocyte apoptosis. Clinical signs include nonpruritic erythema, papules, and crusts, which appear 7 to 18 days postantigen exposure (**Fig. 16**A, B). The erythema starts in the inguinal region, and then spreads cranially to the axillary regions, face, ears, and foot pads. On tape cytology cornified epithelial cells

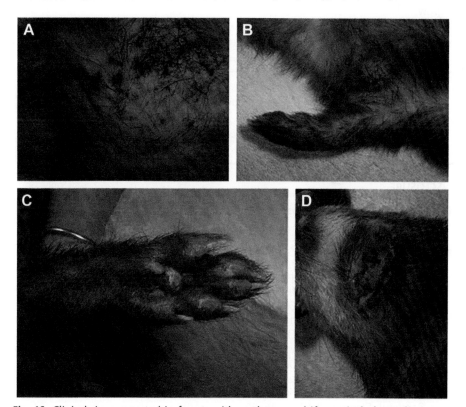

Fig. 16. Clinical signs reported in ferrets with erythema multiforme include erythematous macules and papules in the inguinal and the axillary area (A, B) and hyperkeratosis and erythema of the foot pads (C), and ear pinna (D). (*Reprinted from*: Fisher, P. G. (2013). Erythema multiforme in a ferret (Mustela putorius furo). Veterinary Clinics: Exotic Animal Practice, 16(3), 599-609. With permission.)

are found, whereas histopathological analysis shows mild to moderate hyperkeratosis, epidermal keratinocyte necrosis, and bulla formation. The symptoms can be periodically relieved with immunosuppressive doses of prednisolone, azathioprine, and cyclosporine until ineffective, after which euthanasia is warranted.[126]

Pemphigus Foliaceus-Like

Pemphigus foliaceus is an autoimmune disease attacking the desmosomes of the epidermal keratinocytes, resulting in fluid accumulation between the keratinocytes. The fluid accumulates into pustules, and gives rise to bilaterally symmetrical, yellow-brownish skin crusts on the mucogingival areas of the head (mouth, nose, chin, eyes) and prepuce; and the foot pads.[127] Mild pruritus, weight loss, and decreased activity levels were also noted.[127] The diagnosis is made on histopathology of skin biopsies showing epidermal hyperplasia, acantholysis and intra-/subcorneal pustulae, as well as a clinical response to immunosuppressive doses of prednisolone.[127]

Blue Ferret Syndrome

Blue ferret syndrome is caused when the fur on the ventral abdomen is clipped during the catagen phase of the hair growth cycle; this can cause the hair follicles to produce melanin, which gives the skin a bluish discoloration. The ferret is asymptomatic, and the discoloration resolves within a few weeks when the hair starts to regrow.[1,43]

CLINICS CARE POINTS

- Mast cell tumors in ferrets are, in contrast to those in dogs and cats, nonmalignant
- Hyperestrogenism should be suspected in the intact female ferret with nonregenerative anemia.
- Ferrets infected with ear mites (*O cynotis*) are often asymptomatic, but should be suspected with the clinical finding of brown cerumen.

DISCLOSURE

The authors have no known competing financial or personal interests affecting the work reported in this article.

REFERENCES

1. Meredith A. Ferrets: dermatoses. In: Keeble E, Meredith A, editors. BSAVA manual of rodents and ferrets. 1st edition. Quedgeley: British Small Animal Veterinary Association; 2009. p. 269–74.
2. Paterson S. Structure and function of mammal skin. In: Paterson S, editor. Skin diseases of exotic pets. Oxford, UK: Blackwell Science Ltd; 2006. p. 175–84.
3. Ivey E, Morrisey J. Ferrets: examination and preventative medicine. Vet Clin North Am Exot Anim Pract 1999;2:471–94.
4. Lewington JH. External features and anatomy profile. In: Lewington JH, editor. Ferret husbandry, medicine and surgery. 2nd edition. Saunders, Edinburgh Scotland: Elsevier; 2007. p. 15–33.
5. Fox JG, Bell JA, Broome R. Growth and reproduction. In: Fox JG, Marini RP, editors. Biology and diseases of the ferret. 3rd edition. Iowa: John Wiley & Sons; 2014. p. 187–209.

6. Fox JG, Broome R. Housing and management. In: Fox JG, Marini RP, editors. Biology and diseases of the ferret. 3rd edition. Iowa: John Wiley & Sons; 2014. p. 145–55.

7. Powers LV, Perpiñan D. Basic anatomy, physiology, and husbandry of ferrets. In: Quesenberry KE, Orcutt CJ, Mans C, et al, editors. Ferrets, rabbits, and rodents: clinical medicine and surgery. 4th edition. Missouri: Elsevier; 2020. p. 1–12.

8. Lewington JH. Nutrition Ferret husbandry, medicine and surgery, 2nd edition, 2007, Elsevier Saunders; Edinburgh Scotland, 57–85.

9. Willis LS, Barrow MV. The ferret (Mustela putorius furo L.) as a laboratory animal. Lab Anim Sci 1971;21:712–6.

10. Hoppmann E, Barron HW. Ferret and rabbit dermatology. J Exot Pet Med 2007; 16:225–37.

11. Timm KI. Pruritus in rabbits, rodents and ferrets. Vet Clin North Am Sm Anim Pract 1988;18:1077–91.

12. Wenzel U, Heine J, Mengel H, et al. Efficacy of imidacloprid 10%/moxidectin 1% (Advocate/Advantage multi) against fleas (ctenocephalides felis felis) on ferrets (Mustela putorius furo). Parasitol Res 2008;103:231–4.

13. Fehr M, Koestlinger S. Ectoparasites in small exotic mammals. Vet Clin Exot Anim 2013;16:611–57.

14. Patterson MM, Fox JG, Eberhard ML. Parasitic diseases. In: Fox JG, Marini RP, editors. Biology and diseases of the ferret. 3rd edition. Iowa: John Wiley & Sons; 2014. p. 553–73.

15. Fisher M, Beck W, Hutchinson MJ. Efficacy and safety of selamectin (Stronghold®/Revolution™) used off-label in exotic pets. Intern J Appl Res Vet Med 2007;5:87–96.

16. Powers LV. Bacterial and parasitic diseases of ferrets. Vet Clin Exot Anim 2009; 12:531–61.

17. Hutchinsin MJ, Jacobs DE, Mencke N. Establishment of the cat flea (Ctenocephalides felis) on the ferret (Mustela putorius furo) and its control with imidacloprid. Med Vet Entomol 2001;15:212–4.

18. Kelleher SA. Skin diseases of ferrets. Semin Avian Exot Pet Med 2002;11: 136–40.

19. Sweatman GK. Biology of Otodectes cynotis, the ear canker mite of carnivores. Can J Zool 1958;36:849–62.

20. Lohse J, Rinder H, Gothe R, et al. Validity of species status of the parasitic mite Otodectes cynotis. Med Vet Entomol 2002;16:133–8.

21. LeSuer C, Bour S, Schaper R. Efficacy and safety of the combination of imodacloprid 10%/moxidectin 1.0% spot-on (Advocate® spot-on for small cats and ferrets) in the treatment of ear mite infection (otodectes cynotis) in ferrets. Parasitol Res 2011;109:S149–56.

22. Orcutt C, Tater K. Dermatologic diseases. In: Quesenberry KE, Carpenter JW, editors. Ferrets, rabbits and rodents: clinical medicine and surgery. 3rd editon. Missouri: Elsevier Saunders; 2012. p. 122–31.

23. Patterson MM, Kirchain SM. Comparison of three treatments for control of ear mites in ferrets. Lab Anim Sci 1999;49:655–7.

24. Beck W. Common endo- and ectoparasitic diseases in small mammals – clinical feature, diagnosis and treatment. A review of the literature and own experiences. Tierärztl Prax 2004;32:311–21.

25. D'Ovidio D, Santoro D. Dermatologic diseases of ferrets. In: Quesenberry KE, Orcutt CJ, Mans C, et al, editors. Ferrets, rabbits, and rodents: clinical medicine and surgery. 4th edition. Missouri: Elsevier; 2020. p. 109–16.

26. Nie IA, Pick CR. Infestation of a colony of ferrets with ear mite (Otodectes cynotis) and its control. J Inst Anim Tech 1978;29:63–8.

27. Beck W. Common ectoparasitic diseases and dermatophytosis in small mammals, birds and reptiles. Prakt Tierarzt 2003;84:752–62.

28. Kramer M, Jones R, Kelleher S, et al. Selected drugs for ectoparasite control in exotic species. Exot DVM 2002;4:19–21.

29. Beck W. Otocariasis in ferret caused by *Otodectes cynotis* (Acari: Psoroptidae) – biology of *Otodectes cynotis*, pathogenesis, clinical features, diagnoses and treatment. Kleintierpraxxis 2001;46:31–4.

30. Paterson S. Skin diseases and treatment of ferrets. In: Paterson S, editor. Skin diseases of exotic pets. Oxford, UK: Blackwell Science Ltd; 2006. p. 204–20.

31. Marini RP, Otto G, Erdman S, et al. Biology and diseases of ferrets. In: Fox JG, Anderson LC, Loew FM, et al, editors. Laboratory animal medicine. 2nd edition. Amsterdam: Academic Press; 2002. p. 483–517.

32. Phillips PH, O'Callaghan, Moore E. Pedal *Sarcoptes scabiei* infestation in ferrets (*Mustela putorius furo*). Aust Vet J 1987;64:289–90.

33. Lewington JH. Parasitic diseases of ferrets. In: Lewington JH, editor. Ferret husbandry, medicine and surgery. 2nd edition. Edinburgh, Scotland: Elsevier Saunders; 2007. p. 224–57.

34. Scott DW, Miller WH, Griffin CE. Dermatoses of pet rodents, rabbits and ferrets. In: Scott DW, Miller WH, Griffin CE, editors. Muller and Kirk's small animal dermatology. 6th edition. Philadelphia: Saunders; 2001. p. 1415–58.

35. Bandi KM, Saikumar C. Sarcoptic Mange: A zoonotic ectoparasitic skin disease. J Clin Diagn Res 2013;7:156–7.

36. Martin AL, Irizarry-Rovira AR, Bevier DE, et al. Histology of ferret skin: preweaning to adulthood. Vet Dermatol 2007;18:401–11.

37. Johnson-Delaney CA. Disorders of the respiratory system. In: Johnson-Delaney CA, editor. Ferret medicine and surgery. 1st edition. Washington: CRC press; 2017. p. 311–24.

38. Sastre N, Francino O, Curti JN, et al. Detection, prevalence and phylogenetic relationships of *Demodex* spp and further skin prostigmata mites (Acari, Arachnida) in wild and domestic mammals. PLoS ONE 2016;11:1–20.

39. Beaufrere H, Neta M, Smith DA, et al. Demodectic mange associated with lymphoma in a ferret. J Exot Pet Med 2009;18:57–61.

40. Schoemaker NJ. Selected dermatologic conditions in exotic pets. Exot DVM 1999;1:5–11.

41. Zewe CM, Graham J, Lam ATH, et al. Demodecosis in a ferret caused by *Demodex canis*. Vet Dermatol 2017;28:528–9.

42. Noli C, van der Horst HHA, Willemse T. Demodecosis in ferrets (*Mustela putorius furo*). Vet Quart 1996;18:28–31.

43. Cushing EC, Patton WS. Studies on higher diptera of medical and veterinary importance: *Cochliomyia amaericana* sp. Nov., the screw-worm fly of the new world. Ann Trop Med Parasitol 1933;27:539–51.

44. Johnson-Delaney CA. Disorders of the skin. In: Johnson-Delaney CA, editor. Ferret medicine and surgery. 1st edition. Washington: CRC press; 2017. p. 325–46.

45. Giner J, Basurco A, Alcover MM, et al. First report on natural infection with *Leishmanina infantum* in a domestic ferret (*Mustela putorius furo*) in Spain. Vet Parasitol Reg Stud Rep 2020;19:1–5.

46. Giner J, Villanueva-Saz S, Alcover MM, et al. Clinical leishmaniosis in a domestic ferret (*Mustela putorius furo*) treated with miltefosine plus allopurinol: Serological and clinical follow-up. Vet Parasitol Reg Stud Rep 2021;25:1–4.

47. Giner J, Villanueva-Saz S, Alcover M, et al. Treatment and follow-up of a domestic ferret (*Mustela putorius furo*) with clinical leishmaniosis caused by *Leishmania infantum*. Vet Parasitol Reg Stud Rep 2020;21:100423.

48. Von Messling V, Springfeld C, Devaux P, et al. A ferret model of canine distemper virus virulence and immunosuppression. J Virol 2003;77:12579–91.

49. Villanueva-Saz S, Giner J, Marteles D, et al. Leishmaniosis caused by *Leishmania infantum* in ferrets: Update review. Vet Anim Sci 2022;15:100229.

50. Wyllie SE, Kelman M, Ward MP. Epidemiology and clinical presentation of canine distemper disease in dogs and ferrets in Australia, 2006-2014. Aust Vet J 2016;96:215–22.

51. Kiupel M, Perpinán D. Viral diseases of ferrets. In: Fox JG, Marini RP, editors. Biology and diseases of the ferret. 3rd edition. Iowa: John Wiley & Sons; 2014. p. 439–517.

52. Perpinán D, Ramis A, Tomás E, et al. Outbreak of canine distemper in domestic ferrets (*Mustela putorius furo*). Vet Rec 2008;163:246–50.

53. Wimsatt J, Jay MT, Innes KE, et al. Serological evaluation, efficacy and safety of a commercial modified-live canine distemper vaccine in domestic ferrets. Am J Vet Res 2001;62:736–40.

54. Perpiñan D. Respiratory diseases of ferrets. In: Quesenberry KE, Orcutt CJ, Mans C, et al, editors. Ferrets, rabbits, and rodents: clinical medicine and surgery. 4th edition. Missouri: Elsevier; 2020. p. 71–6.

55. Kubo T, Kagawa Y, Taniyama H, et al. Distribution of inclusion bodies in tissues from 100 dogs infected with canine distemper virus. J Vet Med Sci 2007;69: 527–9.

56. Rodeheffer C, von Messling V, Milot S, et al. Disease manifestations of canine distemper virus infection in ferrets are modulated by vitamin A status. J Nutr 2007;137:1916–22.

57. Garner MM, Ramsell K, Schoemaker NJ, et al. Myofasciitis in the domestic ferret. Vet Pathol 2007;44:5–38.

58. Marini RP, Adkins JA, Fox JG. Proven or potential zoonotic diseases of ferrets. J Am Vet Med Assoc 1989;195:990–4.

59. Donnelly TM, Rush EM, Lackner PA. Ringworm in small exotic pets. Semin Avian Exot Pet Med 2000;9:82–93.

60. Giner J, Bailey J, Juan-Sallés C, et al. Dermatophytic pseudomycetomas in two ferrets (*Mustela putorius furo*). Vet Dermatol 2018;29:452–4.

61. D'Ovidio D, Santoro D. Survey of zoonotic dermatoses in client-owned exotic pet mammals in southern Italy. Zoonoses Public Health 2015;62:100–4.

62. Greenacre CB. Fungal diseases of ferrets. Vet Clin Exot Anim 2003;6:435–48.

63. Moriello KA, Coyner K, Paterson S, et al. Diagnosis and treatment of dermatophytosis in dogs and cats.: Clinical consensus guidelines of the world association for veterinary dermatology. Vet Dermatol 2017;28:266-e68.

64. Hiruma M, Kume T. Mucormycotic meningoencephalitis in a ferret (case report). Kitasato Arch Exp Med 1984;57:67–73.

65. Bongiovanni L, Della Salda L, Selleri P, et al. Multifocal pustular dermatitis associated with *Malassezia* overgrowth in a ferret. J Comp Path 2017;156:107.

66. Malik R, Alderton B, Finlaison D, et al. Cryptococcosis in ferrets: a diverse spectrum of clinical disease. Aust Vet J 2002;80:749–55.

67. Skulski G, Symmers WStC. Actinomycosis and torulosis in the ferret (Mustela Furo L). J Comp Path 1954;64:306–11.
68. Greenlee PG, Stephens E. Meningeal cryptosossosis and congestive cardiomyopathy in a ferret. J Am Vet Med Assoc 1984;184:840–1.
69. Lewington JH. Isolation of *Cryptococcus neoformans* from a ferret. Aust Vet J 1982;58:124.
70. Malik R, Martin P, McGill J, et al. Successful treatment of invasive nasal cryptococcosis in a ferret. Aust Vet J 2000;78:158–9.
71. Ellis DH, Pfeiffer TJ. Ecology, life cycle and infectious propagule of *Cryptococcus neoformans*. Lancet 1990;336:923–5.
72. Ellis DH, Pfeiffer TJ. Natural habitat of *Cryptococcus neoformans* var *gattii*. J Clin Microbiol 1990;28:1642–4.
73. Fox JG. Mycotic diseases. In: Fox JG, Marini RP, editors. Biology and diseases of the ferret. 3rd edition. Iowa: John Wiley & Sons; 2014. p. 573–85.
74. Fisher D, Burrow J, Lo D, et al. *Cryptococcus neoformans* in tropical northern Australia: Predominantly variant *gattii* with good putcomes. Aust N Z J Med 1993;23:678–82.
75. Krockenberger MB, Canfield OJ, Kozel TR, et al. An immunohistochemichal method that differentiates *Cryptococcus neophormans* varieties and serotypes in formalin-fixed paraffin-embedded tissues. Med Mycol 2001;39:523–33.
76. Le K, Beaufrère H, Laniesse D, et al. Diagnosis and long-term management of blastomycosis in two ferrets (*Mustela putorius furo*). J Exot Pet Med 2019;31: 39–44.
77. Lenhard A. Blastomycosis in a ferret. J Am Vet Med Assoc 1985;185:70–2.
78. Greenacre CB, Dowling M, Nobrega-Lee M. Histoplasmosis in a group of four domestic ferrets (*Mustela putorius furo*) and a review of histoplasmosis. J Exot Pet Med 2019;29:194–201.
79. Mancinelli E, Meredith AL, Stidworthy MF. Systemic infection due to *Candida parapsilosis* in a domestic ferret (*Mustela putorius furo*). J Exot Pet Med 2014; 23:85–90.
80. King WW, Lemarié SL, Veazey RS, et al. Superficial spreading pyoderma and ulcerative dermatitis in a ferret. Vet Derm 1996;7:43–7.
81. Swennes AG, Fox JG. Bacterial and mycoplasmal diseases. In: Fox JG, Marini RP, editors. Biology and diseases of the ferret. 3rd edition. Iowa: John Wiley & Sons; 2014. p. 519–52.
82. Lipiec M, Radulski L, Iwaniak W. Case of mycobacteriosis in a pet ferret in Poland. Vet Rec Case Rep 2018;6:e000542.
83. Langenecker M, Clauss M, Hässig M, et al. Comparative investigation on the distribution of diseases in rabbits, Guinea pigs, rats, and ferrets. Tierarztl Prax Ausg K Kleintiere Heimtiere 2009;37:326–33.
84. Li X, Fox JG, Padrid PA. Neoplastic diseases in ferrets: 574 cases (1968-1997). J Am Vet Med Assoc 1998;212:1402–6.
85. Parker GA, Picut CA. Histopathologic features and post-surgical sequelae of 57 cutaneous neoplasms in ferrets (*Mustela putorius furo L.*). Vet Pathol 1993;30: 499–504.
86. Tunev SS, Wells MG. Cutaneous melanoma in a ferret (*Mustela putorius furo*). Vet Pathol 2002;39:141–3.
87. Wolfe HA, Eshar D, Higbie CT, et al. Dermal angiokeratoma in a pet ferret (*Mustela putorius furo*). Isr J Vet Med 2016;71:52–4.
88. Chambers JK, Nakamori T, Kishimoto TE, et al. Lachrymal gland basal cell adenocarcinoma in a ferret. J Comp Pathol 2016;155:259–62.

89. D'Ovidio D, Rossi G, Melidone R, et al. Subcutaneous liposarcoma in a ferret (*Mustela putorius furo*). J Exot Pet Med 2012;21:238–42.
90. Fox-Alvarez WA, Moreno AR, Bush J. Diagnosis and successful surgical removal of an aural ceruminous gland adenocarcinoma in a domestic ferret (*Mustela putorius furo*). J Exot Pet Med 2015;24:350–5.
91. Gardhouse S, Eshar D, Fromstein J, et al. Diagnosis and surgical treatment of an unusual inguinal liposarcoma in a pet ferret (*Mustela putorius furo*). Can Vet J 2013;54:739–42.
92. Kafner S, Reavill DR. Cutaneous neoplasia in ferrets, rabbits and guinea pigs. Vet Clin North Am Exot Anim Pract 2013;16:579–98.
93. Shiga T, Nakata M, Miwa Y, et al. A retrospective study (2006-2020) of cytology and biopsy findings in pet rabbits (*Oryctolagus cuniculus*), ferrets (*Mustela putorius furo*) and four-toed hedgehogs (*Atelerix albiventris*) seen at an exotic animal clinic in Tokyo, Japan. J Exot Pet Med 2021;38:11–7.
94. Vilalta L, Melendez-Lazo A, Doria G, et al. Clinical, cytological, histological, and immunohistochemical features of cutaneous mast cell tumors in ferrets (*Mustela putorius furo*). J Comp Path 2016;155:346–55.
95. Avallone G, Forlani A, Tecilla M, et al. Neoplastic diseases in the domestic ferret (*Mustela putorius furo*) in Italy: classification and tissue distribution of 856 cases (2000-2010). BMC Vet Res 2016;12:275–83.
96. Williams BH, Wyre NR. Neoplasia in ferrets. In: Quesenberry KE, Orcutt CJ, Mans C, et al, editors. Ferrets, rabbits, and rodents: clinical medicine and surgery. 4th edition. Missouri: Elsevier; 2020. p. 92–108.
97. Schoemaker NJ. Ferret oncology. Diseases, diagnostics and therapeutics. Vet Clin Exot Anim 2017;20:183–208.
98. Fox JG, Muthupalani S, Kiupel M, et al. Neoplastic diseases. In: Fox JG, Marini RP, editors. Biology and diseases of the ferret. 3rd edition. Iowa: John Wiley & Sons; 2014. p. 587–627.
99. Rodrigues A, Gates L, Payne HR, et al. Multicentric squamous cell carcinoma in situ associated with papillomavirus in a ferret. Vet Pathol 2010;45:964–8.
100. Onuma M, Kondo H, Ono S, et al. Cytomorphological and immunohistochemical features of lymphomas in ferrets. J Vet Med Sci 2008;70:893–8.
101. Rickman BH, Craig LE, Goldschmidt MH. Piloleiomyosarcoma in seven ferrets. Vet Pathol 2001;38:710–1.
102. Mialot M, Prata D, Girard-Luc A, et al. Multiple progressice piloleiomyomas in a ferret (*Mustela putorius furo*): a case report. Vet Dermatol 2011;11:100–3.
103. Mikaelian I, Garner MM. Solitary dermal leiomyosarcomas in 12 ferrets. J Vet Diagn Invest 2002;14:262–5.
104. Munday JA, Stedman NL, Richey LJ. Histology and immunohistochemistry of seven ferret vaccination-site fibrosarcomas. Vet Pathol 2003;40:288–93.
105. Munday JS, Brown CA, Richey LJ. Suspected metastatic coccygeal chordoma in a ferret (*Mustela putorius furo*). J Vet Diagn Invest 2004;16:454–8.
106. Schoemaker NJ, Schuurmans M, Moorman H, et al. Correlation between age at neutering and age at onset of hyperadrenocorticism in ferrets. JAVMA 2000;216:195–7.
107. Bakthavatchalu V, Muthupalani S, Marini RP, et al. Endocrinopathy and aging in ferrets. Vet Pathol 2016;53:349–65.
108. Wagner RA, Piché CA, Jöchle W, et al. Clinical and endocrine responses to treatment with deslorin acetate implants in ferrets with adrenocortical disease. AJVR 2005;66:910–4.

109. Weiss CA, Scott MV. Clinical aspects and surgical treatment of hyperadrenocorticism in the domestic ferret: 94 cases (1994-1996). J Am Anim Hosp Assoc 1997;33:487–93.

110. Scott DW, Harvey HJ, Yeager AE. Bilaterally symmetric alopecia associated with an adrenocortical adenoma in a pet ferret. Vet Dermatol 1991;2:165–70.

111. Schoemaker NJ, van Zeeland YR. Endocrine diseases of ferrets. In: Quesenberry KE, Orcutt CJ, Mans C, et al, editors. Ferrets, rabbits, and rodents: clinical medicine and surgery. 4th edition. Missouri: Elsevier; 2020. p. 77–91.

112. Grinblate S, Ilgaza A. Clinical symptoms and sex steroid measurements in domestic ferrets (Mustela putorius furo) with hyperadrenocorticism. Res Rural Dev 2017;1:276–80.

113. Wagner RA, Dorn DP. Evaluation of serum estradiol concentrations in alopecia ferrets with adrenal gland tumors. JAVMA 1994;205:703–7.

114. Wagner RA, Finkler MR, Fecteau KA, et al. The treatment of adrenal cortical disease in ferrets with 4.7mg deslorin acetate implants. J Exot Pet Med 2009;18: 146–52.

115. Keeble E. Endocrine diseases in small mammals. Pract 2001;nov/dec:570–85.

116. Wagner RA, Baile EM, Schneider JF, et al. Leuprolide acetate treatment of adrenocortical disease in ferrets. JAVMA 2001;218:1272–4.

117. Di Girolamo N, Huynh M. Disorders of the urinary and reproductive systems in ferrets. In: Quesenberry KE, Orcutt CJ, Mans C, et al, editors. Ferrets, rabbits, and rodents: clinical medicine and surgery. 4th edition. Missouri: Elsevier; 2020. p. 39–54.

118. Martínez A, Martínez J, Bulballa A, et al. Spontaneous thecoma in a spayed pet ferret (Mustela putorius furo) with alopecia and swollen vulva. J Exot Pet Med 2011;20:308–12.

119. Bernard SL, Leathers CW, Brobst DF, et al. Estrogen-induced bone marrow depression in ferrets. Am J Vet Res 1983;44:657–61.

120. Hauptman K, Jekl V, Dorrestein GM, et al. Comparison of estradiol and progesterone serum levels in ferrets suffering from hyperestrogenism and ovarian neoplasia. Vet Med (Praha) 2009;54:532–6.

121. Prohaczik A, Kulcsar M, Huszeniza GY. Deslorin treatment of hyperestrogenism in neutered ferrets (Mustela putorius furo): a case report. Vet Med (Praha) 2009; 54:89–95.

122. van Zeeland YR, Pabon M, Roest J, et al. Use of a GNRH agonis timplant as alternative for surgical neutering in pet ferrets. Vet Rec 2014;175:66.

123. Schoemaker NJ, Drijver E, Bandsma J, et al. Longitudinal evaluation of adrenal gland volume in chemically versus surgically neutered ferrets, Proceedings of 2018. Proc Assoc Exot Mammal Vet Ann Conf 2018;91.

124. Kammeyer P, Ziege S, Wellhöner S, et al. Testicular leiomyosarcoma and marked alopecia in a cryptorchid ferret (Mustela putorius furo). Tierärzliche Praxis Kleintiere 2014;42:406–10.

125. Cooper JE. Skin diseases of ferrets. Vet Ann 1990;30:325.

126. Fisher PG. Erythema multiforme in a ferret (Mustela putorius furo). Vet Clin North Am Exot Anim Pract 2013;16:599–609.

127. Eckerman-Ross C. Pemphigus foliaceus-like skin disease in a ferret. Exot DVM 2007;9:5.

Rodent Dermatology

Jasmine Sarvi, DVM*, David Eshar, DVM, DABVP (ECM), DECZM (SM, ZHM)

KEYWORDS

- Dermatology • Guinea pig • Chinchilla • Hamster • Mouse • Gerbil • Degu
- Black-tailed prairie dog

KEY POINTS

- Dermatologic conditions in pet rodents are one of the most common presenting complaints to the exotic veterinary practitioner.
- Acariasis, dermatophytosis, bacterial infections, endocrinopathies, neoplasia, environmental, husbandry-related, and behavioral dermatopathies are frequently encountered and are often multifactorial in nature.
- As such, a thorough history, husbandry and diagnostic evaluation is key to the successful management of dermatologic disease in pet rodents.

INTRODUCTION

Pet rodents admitted to the veterinary clinic for skin disease can present challenges for the veterinary practitioner. Dermatologic conditions in rodents are often multifactorial, typically with an underlying environmental component that must be identified. A thorough evaluation of the history and husbandry is important for achieving an accurate diagnosis and developing an effective treatment plan but specific questions pertaining to the disease (eg, whether it is pruritic) can be difficult for owners to interpret, especially in species that are fastidious groomers, are nocturnal, or spend a significant amount of time burrowing. There are also several anatomic and physiologic differences among rodent species, and an understanding of these unique characteristics is important for managing dermatologic cases. Additionally, a complete physical examination with quality diagnostic sampling may not be possible without sedation or anesthesia in small rodents. Caution is advised with the use of topical and systemic medications in rodents because few drugs are approved for their use, ingestion of medication may occur during grooming, and inappropriate antibiotic choices can result in direct toxicity or have deleterious effects on normal bacterial gut flora.

This article provides a review of common dermatologic conditions seen in pet rodents and offers practical diagnostic and therapeutic recommendations in the

Department of Clinical Sciences, College of Veterinary Medicine, Kansas State University, 1800 Denison Avenue, Manhattan, KS 66506, USA
* Corresponding author.
E-mail address: jsarvi@vet.k-state.edu

Vet Clin Exot Anim 26 (2023) 383–408
https://doi.org/10.1016/j.cvex.2022.12.004
1094-9194/23/© 2022 Elsevier Inc. All rights reserved.

management of these cases. In this article, the word "rodents" refers to guinea pigs (*Cavia porcellus*), chinchillas (*Chinchilla lanigera*), rats (*Rattus norvegicus*), mice (*Mus musculus*), Syrian and Djungarian hamsters (*Mesocricetus auratus, Phodopus sungorus*), degus (*Ocgodon degus*), Mongolian gerbils (*Meriones unguiculatus*), and black-tailed prairie dogs (*Cynomys ludovicianus*) owned as companion pets and not research or farm-raised animals, unless explicitly stated otherwise.

Unique Anatomy and Physiology

The basic structure and function of rodent skin is similar to that of other mammals but a few key differences will be discussed. Aside from guinea pigs and chinchillas, rodents have a well-developed subcutis consisting of brown adipose behind the neck, which may be gently scruffed for brief restraint.[1] All rodents lack apocrine sweat glands while eccrine sweat glands are only found in the footpads of mice, rats, and hamsters, making rodents susceptible to heat stress.[1]

Apart from gerbils, most rodents have hairless pinna, and the guinea pig also has a natural area of alopecia just behind the ears.[1,2] Rats and mice have sparsely haired tails with a thick, scaly appearance, whereas the skin overlying the tail of gerbils and degus is extremely thin and prone to degloving.[1,3,4] Chinchillas have a dense, soft coat with as many as 60 hairs per follicle.[1] This, along with a lack of sweat glands, makes the chinchilla particularly sensitive to heat and humidity.[5] Chinchillas require access to particulate dust to maintain their coat quality.[5] The dust should be purchased commercially, offered to the chinchilla in a pan once daily for bathing, and removed after use to prevent soiling and conjunctivitis.[5,6] Chinchillas also possess a unique predator avoidance adaptation referred to as "fur slip" where a large patch of fur is shed to enable escape when captured.[5]

Androgen-dependent sebaceous glands are used for scent marking, communication, and territorial behavior in many rodents but their distribution varies between species.[1] Sebaceous glands are located all along the dorsum and around the anus in guinea pigs and can result in matted, greasy hair, especially along the rump of males.[7] Syrian hamsters have darkly pigmented glands on either flank, whereas dwarf hamsters and gerbils possess a midventral sebaceous gland.[8]

Guinea pigs lack L-gulono-gamma-lactone oxidase and are unable to endogenously synthesize vitamin C (ascorbic acid),[9] which plays an important role in collagen synthesis. As such, guinea pigs require daily dietary vitamin C intake (10–25 mg/kg/d) to prevent scurvy.[10] Mild deficiencies may manifest only as dermatologic signs.[2,10]

Dermatologic Conditions

Guinea pigs

Skin disease is one of the most diagnosed conditions in guinea pigs next to dental disease, with a prevalence ranging from 33% to 50%.[11,12] In one retrospective study, pododermatitis was the most common skin condition identified in guinea pigs (47%) evaluated at a veterinary teaching hospital,[12] although a separate study found a relatively lower number of pododermatitis cases (9.4%).[11] Pododermatitis (**Fig. 1**) is considered a multifactorial condition with husbandry-related issues, including inappropriate flooring, poor sanitary conditions, hypovitaminosis C and obesity, commonly suggested as contributing factors.[2,13,14] However, White and colleagues did not find a statistical difference between the prevalence of obesity when comparing guinea pigs with and without pododermatitis. In both previously mentioned studies, ectoparasitism with *Trixacarus caviae* (**Fig. 2**) was within the top 2 most prevalent skin conditions in guinea pigs. In a separate study, *Chirodiscoides caviae* infestation was identified as a common parasitic condition reported in

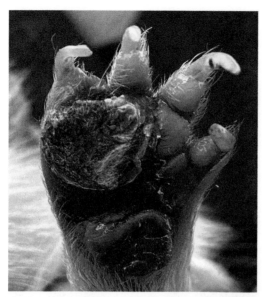

Fig. 1. Pododermatitis in a guinea pig (*C porcellus*) characterized by swelling, erythema, ulceration, and scabbing on the palmar surface of the forepaw.

guinea pigs, with up to 32% prevalence based on a survey in Italy.[15] Most guinea pigs were asymptomatic, however, with only 26.1% of affected guinea pigs showing signs of pruritus, alopecia, erythema, and scaling. Despite the frequent mention of dermatophytosis (*Trichophyton mentagrophytes/Arthroderma benhamiae*) (**Fig. 3**) in the literature,[2,6,7,13,14,16] White and colleagues interestingly only identified dermatophytes in 2 of the 293 (<1%) guinea pigs with skin disease in their study. This is in contrast to a previous study that detected *Trichophyton* spp in 7.7% of guinea pigs with skin lesions, in addition to 8.5% of clinically normal guinea pigs.[17] It is important to note that positive guinea pigs with or without clinical signs of dermatophytosis can be a source of infection for their owners, especially for children.[18] Both ectoparasites and dermatophytes tend to occur more frequently in juvenile guinea pigs, likely due to exposure from pet shops and naive immune systems.[11,17]

Subcutaneous masses are another frequent finding in guinea pigs.[11,12] Abscesses in guinea pigs may be a consequence of environmental trauma, fight wounds, or outward progression of dental disease.[7,13,19] Several organisms have been isolated from subcutaneous abscesses in guinea pigs, including *Streptococcus* spp, *Staphylococcus* spp, *Actinomyces* spp, *Fusobacterium* spp, *Pasteurella multocida*, and *Bacteroides fragilis*.[12,19] Subcutaneous abscesses should be differentiated from cervical lymphadenitis, a condition in which oral bacterial flora, typically the zoonotic pathogen *Streptococcus equi* subsp *zooepidemicus*, invade deeper tissues of the jaw through mucosal abrasions and lead to abscessation of the cervical lymph nodes.[20,21] Guinea pigs present with severe swelling of the lymph nodes in the cervical region, which can spontaneously rupture, posing a public health concern.[2] Skin tumors comprise approximately 15% of all neoplasms found in guinea pigs and trichofolliculomas are the most common (33%–89.7%).[11,22] A thorough description of dermatologic neoplasms in guinea pigs has been reviewed elsewhere.[23]

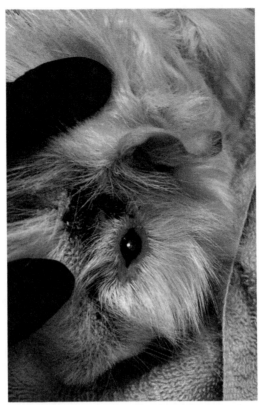

Fig. 2. Facial alopecia, excoriations, crusts, and scales in an intensely pruritic guinea pig (*C porcellus*) infected with *T caviae*.

The causes, clinical presentations, diagnostics, and therapeutic recommendations for these and other common dermatologic diseases in guinea pigs are summarized in **Table 1**.

Chinchillas

Many dermatologic conditions in chinchillas are associated with the fur rather than the skin. Fur slip, unkempt, matted fur due to improper husbandry or hypersalivation from dental disease, and fur chewing (**Fig. 4**) are common.[5,6,16,44] Characterized by excessive and repetitive grooming and biting, fur chewing is widely acknowledged as a behavioral disorder of chinchillas but the true prevalence in the pet population is unknown because most of the data pertaining to this condition is associated with farm-raised animals.[45–49] The underlying cause also remains unclear but based on recent studies, fur chewing is thought to be triggered by stress with a potential heritable component.[48,49] Fur chewing has been associated with 21% to 30% cases of dental disease in chinchillas, further suggesting that chronic stress or pain may contribute to this behavior.[50,51]

The dense fur of chinchillas predisposes them to dermatitis and pyodermas because excessive moisture, secondary to a variety of pathologic conditions or environmental factors, can get trapped beneath the fur.[13,16,51] However, the dense fur seems to provide a barrier to ectoparasitic infections, which are relatively uncommon in chinchillas compared with guinea pigs.[6,44] Similar to guinea pigs, *T mentagrophytes*

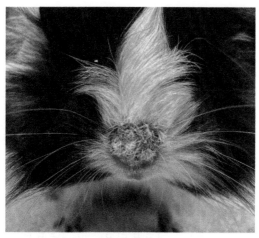

Fig. 3. Dermatophyte lesions on the nasal planum of a guinea pig (*Cavia porcellus*) caused by *A benhamiae* of the *T mentagrophytes* complex.

is the dermatophyte most frequently isolated from chinchillas, although *Microsporum* spp have also been documented to cause infection.[52,53]

Although not specifically a dermatologic condition, it is important to note that fur can accumulate around the glans penis in male chinchillas and lead to constriction injuries, acute urinary obstruction, or paraphimosis.[54] Thus, it is imperative to examine the extruded penis of male chinchillas during routine physical examinations and remove any accumulated fur or debris.

Neoplastic skin diseases in chinchillas are rare with only 3 cases of cutaneous squamous cell carcinoma and one case of mammary adenocarcinoma reported in the literature.[55,56]

In addition to those described above, other commonly reported dermatologic diseases in chinchillas, including their associated clinical signs, diagnostic and therapeutic recommendations are summarized in **Table 2**.

Small rodents—mice, rats, hamsters, gerbils, degus

A high prevalence of spontaneous skin disease is reported in pet rats (39%–47%),[62] hamsters (41%–54%),[63] and degus (36.7%).[64] Dermatologic conditions in mice and gerbils are also described commonly in the literature,[3,6,8,13,14,24,25] although much of the information regarding disease processes in these species may be based on laboratory animal research.

Ectoparasites, subcutaneous masses, environmental, and behavioral dermatopathies seem to be the most common conditions diagnosed in small rodents.[62–64] In rats and mice, mites (*Notoedres muris, Radfordia ensifera, Mycoptes musculinis, Myobia musculi, Radfordia affinis*) and less often lice (*Polyplax serrata, Polyplax spinulosa*) are the most frequently reported ectoparasites,[62,65] whereas hamsters have a predisposition for demodicosis (*Demodex aurati* or *Demodex criceti*), which is uncommon in other rodents.[8,63,64,66–68]

Skin neoplasms were one of the most common diagnoses in rats with skin disease in one study.[62] Of these tumors, the majority was histologically malignant; however, a separate study identified benign mammary gland fibroadenomas (53%) (**Fig. 5**) followed by malignant mammary gland carcinomas (12%) as the most common subcutaneous tumors of rats,[69] which were excluded in the aforementioned study.

Table 1
Dermatologic diseases of Guinea pigs

Condition	Cause	Clinical Signs	Diagnosis	Treatment
Infectious				
Ectoparasite				
Mites	*T caviae*	Intense pruritus with seizure-like spasms, alopecia, erythema, excoriations, scales, crusts, hyperkeratosis	Deep skin scraping may be negative	Selamectin 15 mg/kg topically Ivermectin 0.4 mg/kg SC q 10d × 4 doses Doramectin 0.4 mg/kg IM q 7d × 1–2 doses
	C caviae	Typically asymptomatic; pruritus, alopecia, erythema, and scaling may be observed	Skin scraping, acetate tape impression, or trichogram	Selamectin 15–30 mg topically
Lice	*Gliricola porcelli, Gyropus ovalis*	Typically asymptomatic; pruritus, alopecia, unthrifty coat may be observed	Direct visualization, skin scraping, acetate tape impression, trichogram	Imidacloprid 16–25 mg/kg + moxidectin 1.6–2.5 mg/kg topically
Fleas (uncommon)	*Ctenocephalides felis* from close contact with cats and dogs	Dull or rough hair coat, patchy alopecia, pruritus	Direct visualization of fleas or flea dirt	Selamectin 15–30 mg topically
Fungal				
Dermatophytes	*T mentagrophytes/A benhamiae; Microsporum canis* less common; zoonotic	Asymptomatic carriers common; patchy, circular alopecia, erythema, scaling, crusts, +/− pruritus	Trichogram, fungal culture Woods lamp test not useful for *Trichophyton* spp	Terbinafine (30–40 mg/kg PO q 24h) has shown better efficacy than itraconazole and fluconazole and may be preferred over topical therapy Topical dips or baths q 7d (2% miconazole shampoo, 0.2% enilconazole rinse, 2% lime sulfur, 1%–2% chlorhexidine, 1%

	Cause	Clinical Signs	Diagnosis	Treatment
				terbinafine); spot treatment not recommended Treat until 2 consecutive negative cultures
Bacterial	Various organisms; secondary to fight wounds, environmental trauma, dental disease, pododermatitis	Firm subcutaneous swelling; drainage is not common due to caseous nature of exudate	Cytology, bacterial culture of abscess capsule Skull CT to evaluate for dental disease	Thick abscess capsule and caseous nature of the exudate often necessitates surgical excision or marsupialization in conjunction with systemic antibiotics, based on culture and sensitivity Manage dental disease as indicated
Pyoderma	*Staphylococcus* spp or other bacterial invasion due to breaks in the skin barrier (ectoparasitism, urine scald, ptyalism due dental disease, unsanitary living conditions)	Alopecia, erythema, crusts, erosion, ulceration, exudate	Cytology of acetate tape prep or slide impression, bacterial culture	Topical and/or systemic antibiotics based on culture and sensitivity; identify and manage underlying disease
Pododermatitis	See noninfectious diseases			
	Secondary infections, abscessation, osteomyelitis, septic arthritis may occur in severe cases and are typically associated with *Staphylococcus* spp			

(continued on next page)

Table 1
(continued)

Condition	Cause	Clinical Signs	Diagnosis	Treatment
Cheilitis	Unknown, but abrasive feed, sharp cage materials, acidic foods, dental disease, vitamin C deficiency, and possible pox virus infections may play role	Perioral erythema, ulcers, discharge, crusts	Cytology, bacterial culture	Identify and eliminate inciting factors; antimicrobial therapy based on culture and sensitivity
Noninfectious				
Pododermatitis	Environmental, husbandry, and/or medical factors (wire flooring, abrasive substrate, poor sanitary conditions, obesity, osteoarthritis, urolithiasis, vitamin C deficiency)	Erythema, swelling, ulceration, calluses on palmar/plantar surfaces of feet, lameness; secondary infections, osteomyelitis, septic arthritis may occur in severe cases	History, cytology, bacterial culture, diagnostic imaging to evaluate for predisposing factors and extent of disease	Multimodal approach is often necessary; identify and manage predisposing factors, treat secondary bacterial infections based on culture and sensitivity, provide analgesia and anti-inflammatories, administer topical therapy (dilute chlorhexidine or iodine soaks), apply bandages as necessary
Contact dermatitis	Unsanitary or moist environment, hypersensitivity to bedding or chemical irritants, fecal matting (diarrhea, decreased grooming), urine scalding (urolithiasis, UTI, renal, neurologic, musculoskeletal, disease, obesity)	Erythema, erosion, ulceration, secondary bacterial infection on ventrum, perineal region, inner thighs, feet	History, clinical signs; blood work, urinalysis, and diagnostic imaging to rule out underlying medical conditions	Adjust husbandry, identify and treat underlying causes, analgesia, topical/systemic antimicrobials as indicated

Hormonal alopecia	Increased estrogen during pregnancy; follicular cystic ovaries	Bilateral, symmetric, noninflammatory and nonpruritic flank/dorsal alopecia, nipple hyperkeratosis, abdominal distension, lethargy, anorexia	Abdominal ultrasound	Hair generally regrows after pregnancy Ovariohysterectomy; hormone therapy has limited anecdotal success Human chorionic gonadotropin 1000 IU/ Guinea pig IM × 2 treatments, 7–10d apart Gonadotropin releasing hormone 25µg/ Guinea pig IM × 2 treatments, 14d apart Leuprolide acetate depot 100–300 µg/kg SC/IM q 3–4wk Deslorelin acetate 4.7 mg implant SC; Use of Suprelorin F (Virbac Animal Health, Fort Worth, TX) in the United States is limited to ferrets and extra-label use is prohibited
	Hyperthyroidism	Weight loss/thin body condition despite normal or increased food intake, hyperactivity, hair loss, unkempt coat, tachycardia, heart murmur, palpable cervical mass	Increased total and/or free thyroxine	Radioactive iodine, oral or transdermal thyreostatic agents (methimdazole/thimazole, carbimazole) at doses extrapolated from feline medicine; surgical thyroidectomy
	Hyperadrenocorticism	PU/PD, muscle atrophy, abdominal distension, alopecia, weight loss, obesity, lethargy	Abdominal ultrasound, ACTH stimulation test	Trilostane 2–6 mg/kg PO q 12-24h

(continued on next page)

Table 1
(continued)

Condition	Cause	Clinical Signs	Diagnosis	Treatment
Hypovitaminosis C	Inappropriate diet, inadequate dietary supplementation	Rough haircoat, seborrhea, fragile skin, poor wound healing, joint swelling, lameness, petechiae, difficult prehension, anorexia, vocalization due to pain	History, clinical signs, radiographs, serum ascorbic acid levels	Dietary vitamin C 10–25 mg/kg/d is sufficient in mild cases; provide commercial Timothy-based pellets fortified with vitamin C, vitamin C tablets (Oxbow Animal Health, Omaha, NE), and fresh produce rich in vitamin C, such as dark leafy greens and red or yellow bell peppers Severe cases may initially require parenteral ascorbic acid at 50–100 mg/kg SC/IM q 24h Vitamin C added to drinking water is unstable in light and not recommended
Barbering	Boredom, stress, dominant cage mate	Patchy alopecia with hairs broken at the shaft without skin inflammation, chewed whiskers	History, clinical signs, trichogram demonstrating broken hair shafts	Environmental enrichment (toys, exercise, treats, human bonding), separation of cage mates
Neoplasia	Trichofolliculoma, lipoma, and trichoepithelioma most common	Subcutaneous mass; trichofolliculomas often found along caudal dorsum with a central pore that may exude keratinaceous debris	Cytology, histopathology	Surgical excision is often curative for benign tumors

Adapted from Refs. [2,6,7,10–16,18,21–43]

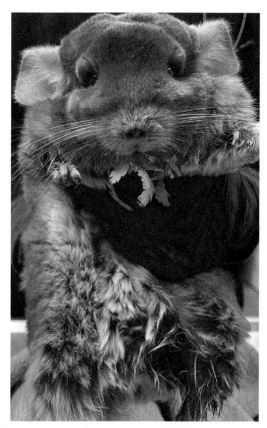

Fig. 4. Matted, unkempt coat on all 4 extremities of a chinchilla (*C lanigera*) with a history of fur chewing and dental disease.

Mammary tumors are also identified frequently in mice, but are nearly always malignant with evidence of metastasis at the time of diagnosis.[3,16] Tumors have a predilection for the skin in hamsters and gerbils as well, with various histotypes such as papillomas (**Fig. 6**),[70,71] atypical fibromas/fibrosarcomas,[71–73] mammary gland adenomas/adenocarcinomas,[70,71,73–75] squamous cell carcinoma,[73,76] and cutaneous lymphoma[71,73,77,78] been most commonly reported. Tumors may also affect the marking scent glands of hamsters and gerbils.[73,76,79] Skin neoplasms in degus have a low reported incidence compared with other small rodents, with only single cases of myxosarcoma, malignant histiocytosis, and lipoma in the literature.[64,80] Numerous other cutaneous neoplasms have been reported in small rodents and are reviewed in a separate article.[23]

Behavioral and environmental-related trauma to the skin can be attributed to the dominance hierarchies and natural behaviors observed in small rodents, in conjunction with husbandry factors.[3] Rodents housed in large groups are more likely to fight with one another and inflict wounds while dominant rodents may also barber the whiskers or muzzle of cage mates.[3] In one study, self-barbering attributed to stress and dental disease was the most common cause of skin lesions found in pet degus.[64] Stressed or bored rodents may display other stereotypic behaviors such as bar chewing and polydipsia, which can manifest as skin lesions around the mouth.[3] Mechanical skin abrasions from metal feeders, poorly devised water bottles, and abrasive bedding also occur.[3,6,64]

Table 2
Dermatologic diseases of chinchillas

Condition	Cause	Clinical Signs	Diagnosis	Treatment
Infectious				
Fungal				
Dermatophytes	*T mentagrophytes*; *Microsporum canis*, *M gypseum* (uncommon); zoonotic	Circular or patchy alopecia, scales, scabs, and pruritus, especially on face, ears, or feet	Trichogram, fungal culture	Topical and/or systemic antifungal therapy, similar to guinea pigs (see **Table 1**).
Bacterial				
Moist dermatitis, secondary pyodermas	Typically *Staphylococcus* or *Streptococcus* spp due to excessive moisture from drooling (dental disease), urine staining (unsanitary conditions, urinary disease, arthritis, obesity), high humidity	Matted fur, erythema, erosion, moist exudate, or crusting of skin	Cytology, bacterial culture	Topical and/or systemic antimicrobial therapy based on culture and sensitivity; manage underlying or predisposing conditions such as dental or urinary disease; improve husbandry
Abscesses	Typically *Staphylococcus* or *S* spp due to environmental trauma, bite wounds, or dental disease	Soft to firm subcutaneous swelling; can be missed during exam due to dense fur	Cytology, bacterial culture, skull CT to rule out dental disease	Surgical excision or marsupialization of abscess in conjunction with systemic antimicrobials based on culture and sensitivity; manage underlying dental disease
Noninfectious				
Fur chewing	Unknown, but stress (overcrowding, fighting, boredom), pain (dental disease), endocrinopathies, and genetics have been proposed	Broken hair shafts, darkened fur, hyperpigmentation; often head and extremities are spared	Observation of behavior, trichogram, blood work and diagnostic imaging to rule out underlying medical conditions	Identify and manage underlying disease, minimize stress increase environmental enrichment Fluoxetine 10 mg/kg PO q 24h × 90d has not shown to be effective

Fur slip	Predation, rough handling, trauma	Well circumscribed alopecia, unaffected skin	Observation of trauma, clinical signs	Treatment typically not necessary; hair regrowth may occur within 4–6 mo
Unkempt coat	Lack of access to particulate dust, high ambient temperature (<80 F/26.7 C), humidity (>50%) or unsanitary living conditions	Thickened, matted fur	History, clinical signs	Correct husbandry; offer commercial chinchilla dust for 30 min daily
Pododermatitis	Environmental, husbandry, medical factors (abrasive flooring, unsanitary conditions, obesity, osteoarthritis, urinary disease)	Erythema, ulcers, hyperkeratotic lesions on the bottoms of the feet; may progress to abscessation and osteomyelitis in severe cases	History, cytology, bacterial culture, diagnostic imaging	Identify and manage predisposing factors; multimodal approach often necessary as with guinea pigs (see **Table 1**).
Fur ring	Accumulation of fur around glans penis	Excessive grooming, stranguria, pollakiuria, urinary obstruction, paraphimosis, lethargy, anorexia	Clinical signs, physical examination	Lubrication and manual removal of fur; sedation or anesthesia may be necessary

Adapted from Refs. [5,6,13,14,16,25,44–54,57–61]

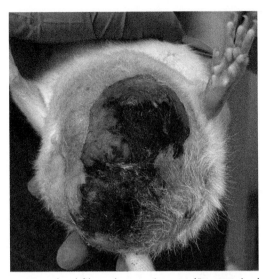

Fig. 5. Ulcerated mammary gland fibroadenoma in a rat (*R norvegicus*).

Table 3 summarizes the causes, clinical presentations, diagnostic and therapeutic recommendations for the dermatologic conditions mentioned above as well as other common skin diseases of rats, mice, hamsters, gerbils, and degus.

Black-Tailed Prairie Dogs

Although dermatologic disease seems to be one of the most frequent health concerns in captive prairie dogs,[111] information regarding the prevalence and outcomes of these conditions is sparse and limited to case reports and anecdotal observations.

Demodicosis, successfully treated with amitraz, has been described in pet prairie dogs presenting for hair loss over the dorsum.[112] Anecdotally, dermatophytosis (*T mentagrophytes*) has also been reported.[81]

Bacterial infections (*Staphylococcus aureus*) may occur secondary to environmental trauma or fight wounds.[14] Development of abrasions and alopecia on the nose (bald

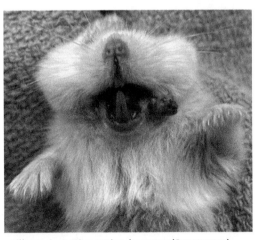

Fig. 6. Cutaneous papilloma in a Djungarian hamster (*P sungorus*).

Table 3
Dermatologic diseases of rats, mice, hamsters, gerbils, degus

Condition	Cause	Clinical Signs	Diagnosis	Treatment
Infectious				
Ectoparasites				
Mites	*N muris, R ensifera* (rats); *M musculinis, M musculi, R affinis* (mice)	Alopecia, pruritus, excoriations, ulcers, crusts, rough coat, papular lesions (*N muris*)	Acetate tape impression, skin scraping	Ivermectin 0.2–0.4 mg/kg SC q 7–14d Selamectin 10–24 mg/kg topically Moxidectin 0.5 mg/kg topically once or 2 mg/kg PO q 15d
	D aurati, D. criceti (hamsters), *D merioni* (gerbils), *D* spp (degus) typically associated with immunosuppressive conditions	Alopecia, scaling, crusting, ulceration, ± pruritus	Skin scraping	Ivermectin 0.3 mg/kg PO q 24h Selamectin 30 mg/kg + sarolaner 5 mg/kg topically q 7d × 4–6wk Fluralaner 25 mg/kg PO q 60d Topical amitraz 0.013%–0.025% q 7–14d
	Ornithonyssus bacoti; may infect humans and rarely transmit zoonotic agents (*Bartonella henselae*)	Alopecia, erythema, pruritus, rough haircoat	Macroscopic detection of red-orange mites, skin scraping	Moxidectin + imidacloprid 0.5 mg/kg topically q 15d × 2 treatments
Lice	*P serrata, P spinulosa* (mice, rats)	Pruritus, dermatitis, restlessness	Macroscopic visualization of lice and nits, acetate tape impression, trichogram	Similar as for mites
Fungal				
Dermatophytes (rare)	*T mentagrophytes, Microsporum* spp less common; zoonotic	Clinical disease is rare; Patchy, circular alopecia, erythema, scaling, crusts may be seen	Trichogram, fungal culture	As with other rodents (see **Table 1**).

(continued on next page)

Table 3
(continued)

Condition	Cause	Clinical Signs	Diagnosis	Treatment
Bacterial				
Pyoderma, abscesses	Breaks in skin barrier as with other species	Alopecia, erythema, crusts, moist dermatitis, subcutaneous swelling	Cytology, bacterial culture	As with other rodents
Cutaneous botryomycosis/ pseudomycetoma (Hamsters)	Atypical pyogranulomatous reaction to bacteria, typically *Staphylococcus* spp	Subcutaneous nodules, ± drainage of purulent material with white granules	Cytology, bacterial culture, histopathology	Systemic antibiotic therapy based on culture and sensitivity; may not be effective without surgical excision of masses
Non-infectious				
Environmental trauma	Meetal feeders, cage wires, sharp water bottle nozzles, abrasive bedding, chemical irritants, stereotypic behavior, fighting	Alopecia, abrasions, erythema, swelling, puncture/laceration wounds	History, clinical signs	Topical and systemic antimicrobials as indicated, identify and manage husbandry related factors, increase environmental enrichment, remove aggressive animals
Tail slip (gerbils, degus)	Improper handling	Degloved, raw, exposed tail	History, clinical signs	Surgical amputation is recommended to prevent necrosis
Barbering	Dominant cage mate; self-barbering due to stress, boredom, anxiety or pain	Typically all but one animal with broken whiskers and alopecia around muzzle; self-barbering spares head and neck	History, clinical signs	Another animal usually resumes dominance after removal of dominant animal; environmental enrichment (larger cage, burrowing substrate, exercise, addition of amicable conspecific,

			Diagnosis	Treatment
				appropriate light/dark cycle); identify and manage underlying painful conditions
Facial eczema/sore nose/ nasal dermatitis (gerbils)	Irritation due to increased porphyrin secretion from stress (high humidity, overcrowding, illness)	Erythema, alopecia, moist dermatitis, scabs around the nares, ± secondary bacterial infection	History, clinical signs, cytology, bacterial culture	Topical and/or systemic antimicrobials as indicated, facial cleansing with topical disinfectants (dilute chlorhexidine); maintain dry (<50% humidity) environment; provide sand bath once signs resolve for prevention
Ulcerative dermatitis (mice)	Immune mediated vasculitis of unknown cause; common in black mouse strain (C57BL/6)	Intense pruritus, alopecia, crusts, ulcers, necrosis, fibrosis, skin contracture especially over dorsal neck and face; secondary bacterial infections	Rule out infectious and environmental etiologies based on husbandry, skin scraping, bacterial/fungal culture, and histopathology	Multimodal approach consisting of toenail trimming, topical therapy (0.005% sodium hypochlorite solution once daily), and dietary vitamin E supplementation (3000 IU/ kg) may reduce pruritus and skin lesions; maropitant citrate (1 mg/kg IP × 5d) may also be effective Topical and systemic antibiotics, corticosteroids, antihistamines, and lidocaine show limited success

(continued on next page)

Table 3
(continued)

Condition	Cause	Clinical Signs	Diagnosis	Treatment
Hyperadreno-corticism (hamster)	Primary adrenal gland tumor or pituitary adenoma	Symmetric alopecia, thin skin, hyperpigmentation, comedones, polyuria, polydipsia, polyphagia, pot-bellied appearance	Clinical signs, increased plasma cortisol, serum alkaline phosphatase, and ultrasound findings may raise suspicion; confirmatory function tests (Adrenocorticotropic hormone stimulating test, low dose dexamethasone suppression test) are not described in hamsters and require large volume of blood	Metyrapone (8 mg PO/d) or mitotane (5 mg PO/d) may not be fully successful; outcomes of surgical adrenalectomy have not been described
Neoplasia	Mammary fibroadenoma, carcinoma (rats), adenocarcinoma, fibrosarcoma (mice)	Subcutaneous masses found anywhere from neck to inguinal region along ventrum (rats, mice) or dorsum (mice)	Cytology (may not exfoliate well), histopathology	Surgical excision, though mammary tumors frequently recur in rats; early ovariectomy (4–7 mo age) may prevent occurrence in rats; effects of sterilization at time of surgical resection have not been studied; prognosis is poor in mice due to high likelihood of malignancy and metastasis
	Zymbal's gland tumors (rats)	Firm subcutaneous mass below ear		
	Various others (papilloma, squamous cell carcinoma, lymphoma, fibroma, fibrosarcoma)	Cutaneous masses; papillomas have predilection for head; tumors may also affect flank glands (hamsters, gerbils)	Cytology, histopathology	Surgical excision may be curative with some neoplasms

Adapted from Refs.[3,4,6,8,14,16,23–25,62–79,81–110]

Table 4
Dermatologic diseases of black-tailed prairie dogs

Condition	Cause	Clinical Signs	Diagnosis	Treatment
Infectious				
Ectoparasites	*Demodex* spp	Bilateral, symmetric dorsal alopecia	Skin scraping	Amitraz sponge bath (250 ppm) for 3–5 min q 4d × 60d
Noninfectious				
Behavioral dermatopathy	Incessant rubbing against cage, excessive grooming due to stress, boredom, lack of companionship	Alopecia, abrasions on nose (bald nose)	History, clinical signs	Group housing in a large, smooth-walled cage with appropriate bedding and tunnels for natural digging and burrowing behaviors
Idiopathic necrosis	Unknown, but associated with cystocentesis; proposed causes include sensitivity to 70% alcohol, escaped urine, or prolonged exposure on heat source	Necrotic dermatitis along ventrum	History, clinical signs, histopathology	Wound cleaning (dilute cholorhexidine solution), topical 1% silver sulfadiazine, systemic antimicrobial therapy
Neoplasia (Uncommon)	Cases of lipoma, SCC, lymphoma, basal cell tumor, leiomyoma, adenocarcinoma reported	Skin mass ± ulceration	Cytology, histopathology	The effects and outcomes of surgical excision, chemotherapy and/or radiation have not been studied

Adapted from Refs.[14,81–83,111–114]

nose) is described in prairie dogs that incessantly rub against cage wiring.[14] Pet prairie dogs lacking companionship may also self-mutilate or groom excessively.[111] Group housing in a large, smooth-walled cage with soft bedding and tunnels to allow natural digging and burrowing behaviors can provide adequate enrichment to prevent environmental or self-inflicted trauma.[14]

An incidence of necrotic dermatitis along the ventrum was reported in several prairie dogs after routine cystocentesis.[82] Although the underlying cause was not identified, proposed causes included hypersensitivity to one or more of the products used (eg, 70% alcohol), escaped urine, or prolonged heat exposure on water blankets and heat packs.

Tumors of the skin and subcutis are rarely reported in prairie dogs[83] but cases of lipoma,[111] adenocarcinoma,[111] malignant lymphoma,[111,113] basal cell tumor,[83] squamous cell carcinoma,[83] and cutaneous leiomyoma[114] have been documented.

Reported dermatologic diseases of prairie dogs are summarized in **Table 4**.

SUMMARY

Rodents are frequently inflicted with dermatologic diseases caused by ectoparasites, infectious agents (dermatophytes and bacteria), hormonal imbalances, tumors, inappropriate husbandry, and behavioral disorders. The clinical presentation for skin disease varies greatly depending on the underlying cause but alopecia, pruritus, unkempt coat, self-mutilation, erythema, crusts, ulcers, masses, or asymptomatic animals may be seen. Because many skin conditions in rodents are multifactorial in nature, it is important to obtain a thorough history to identify any underlying husbandry deficiencies or predisposing environmental factors. A diagnostic workup may involve microscopic evaluation of skin scrapings, acetate tape impressions, or hair plucks, bacterial culture and sensitivity, dermatophyte culture, and fine needle aspiration for cytology or surgical excision for histopathology of subcutaneous masses. Furthermore, bloodwork, diagnostic imaging, or urine testing should be considered in some circumstances to evaluate the extent of disease and rule out other medical conditions that may be contributing to dermatologic disease. Therapy is aimed at managing the underlying cause (if identified), treating secondary bacterial infections, providing analgesia when appropriate, and optimizing husbandry.

CLINICS CARE POINTS

- An understanding of the unique anatomic and physiologic differences related to the skin is important for treating skin disease in rodents.
- Practitioners working with rodents should be familiar with their basic husbandry and environmental needs because many skin diseases are associated with an underlying husbandry deficiency.
- A thorough physical examination and diagnostic evaluation often requires anesthesia.
- Currently, a lack of licensed antiparasitics, antimicrobials, and other drugs for use in rodents in most countries necessitates extra-label use of many of the pharmaceuticals recommended for skin disease.
- Topical and systemic drugs should be used with caution in rodents because ingestion of medication may occur during normal grooming, accurate dosing may not be possible in extremely small patients, and inappropriate antibiotic choices can result in direct toxicity or have deleterious effects on normal bacterial gut flora.

DISCLOSURE

The authors have no conflicts of interest to disclose. This research did not receive any specific grant from funding agencies in the public, commercial, or not-for-profit sectors, and the authors declare no conflict of interest.

REFERENCES

1. Meredith A. Chapter 14: Structure and function of mammal skin. In: Paterson S, editor. Skin diseases of exotic pets. Oxford: Blackwell Science; 2006. p. 251–63.
2. Pignon C, Mayer J. Chapter 21: Guinea pigs. In: Quesenberry KE, Orcutt CJ, Mans C, et al, editors. Ferrets, rabbits, and rodents. 4th edition. St. Louis: Elsevier; 2021. p. 270–97.
3. Frohlich J. Chapter 25: Rats and mice. In: Quesenberry KE, Orcutt CJ, Mans C, et al, editors. Ferrets, rabbits, and rodents. 4th edition. St. Louis: Elsevier; 2021. p. 345–67.
4. Jekl V. Chapter 23: Degus. In: Quesenberry KE, Orcutt CJ, Mans C, et al, editors. Ferrets, rabbits, and rodents. 4th edition. St. Louis: Elsevier; 2021. p. 323–33.
5. Mans C, Donnelly TM. Chapter 22: Chinchillas. In: Quesenberry KE, Orcutt CJ, Mans C, et al, editors. Ferrets, rabbits, and rodents. 4th edition. St. Louis: Elsevier; 2021. p. 298–322.
6. Hoppman E, Mori M. Rodent dermatology. J Exot Pet Med 2007;16:238–55.
7. Meredith A. Chapter 19: Skin diseases and treatment of guinea pigs. In: Paterson S, editor. Skin diseases of exotic pets. Oxford: Blackwell Science; 2006. p. 232–50.
8. Miwa Y, Mayer J. Chapter 26: Hamsters and gerbils. In: Quesenberry KE, Orcutt CJ, Mans C, et al, editors. Ferrets, rabbits, and rodents. 4th edition. St. Louis: Elsevier; 2021. p. 368–84.
9. Nishikimi M, Kawai T, Yagi K. Guinea pigs possess a highly mutated gene for L-gulono-gamma-lactone oxidase, the key enzyme for L-ascorbic acid biosynthesis missing in this species. J Biol Chem 1992;267(30):21967–72.
10. Harkness JE, Turner PV, Woude SV, et al. Specific diseases and conditions. In: Harkness JE, Turner PV, Woude SV, et al, editors. Biology and medicine of rabbits and rodents. 5th edition. Ames: Wiley-Blackwell; 2010. p. 249–394.
11. Minarikova A, Hauptman K, Jeklova E, et al. Diseases in pet guinea pigs: a retrospective study in 1000 animals. Vet Rec 2015;177(8):200.
12. White SD, Guzman DS, Paul-Murphy J, et al. Skin diseases in companion guinea pigs (Cavia porcellus): a retrospective study of 293 cases seen at the Veterinary Medical Teaching Hospital, University of California at Davis (1990-2015). Vet Dermatol 2016;27:395 –e100.
13. de Matos R, Kalivoda K. Chapter 21: Dermatoses of exotic small mammals. In: Scott DW, Miller WH, Griffin CE, editors. Muller & Kirk's small animal dermatology. 7th edition. St Louis: Elsevier; 2013. p. 844–83.
14. Ellis C, Mori M. Skin diseases of rodents and small exotic mammals. Vet Clin North Am Exot Anim Pract 2001;4(2):493–542.
15. d'Ovidio D, Santoro D. Prevalence of fur mites (Chirodiscoides caviae) in pet guinea pigs (Cavia porcellus) in southern Italy. Vet Dermatol 2014;25(2):135–7, e37-e38.
16. Haskins S, Mitchell MA. Chapter 2: Integumentary system. In: Mitchell MA, Tully TN, editors. Current therapy in exotic pet practice. St. Louis: Elsevier; 2016. p. 17–75.

17. Kraemer A, Mueller RS, Werckenthin C, et al. Dermatophytes in pet guinea pigs and rabbits. Vet Microb 2012;157:208–13.
18. Kraemer A, Hein J, Heusinger A, et al. Clinical signs, therapy and zoonotic risk of pet guinea pigs with dermatophytosis. Mycoses 2013;56(2):168–72.
19. Minarikova A, Hauptman K, Knotek Z, et al. Microbial flora of odontogenic abscesses in pet guinea pigs. Vet Rec 2016;179(13):331.
20. Barrios-Arpi LM, Morales-Cauti SM. Cytomorphological characterization of lymphadenopathies in guinea pigs: study of 31 clinical cases. J Exot Pet Med 2020;32:1–5.
21. Meredith A, Johnson-Delaney CA. Chapter 6: Guinea pigs. In: BSAVA manual of exotic pets: a foundation manual. 5th edition. Quedgeley: British Small Animal Veterinary Association; 2010. p. 52–64.
22. Kanfer S, Reavill DR. Cutaneous neoplasia in ferrets, rabbits, and guinea pigs. Vet Clin North Am Exot Anim Pract 2013;16(3):579–98.
23. Hocker SE, Eshar D, Wouda RM. Rodent oncology: diseases, diagnostics, and therapeutics. Vet Clin North Am Exot Anim Pract 2017;20(1):111–34.
24. Fehr M, Koestlinger S. Ectoparasites in small exotic mammals. Vet Clin Exot Anim 2013;16:611–57.
25. Palmeiro BS, Roberts H. Clinical approach to dermatologic disease in exotic animals. Vet Clin North Am Exot Anim Pract 2013;16(3):523–77.
26. Eshar D, Bdolah-Abram T. Comparison of efficacy, safety, and convenience of selamectin versus ivermectin for treatment of Trixacarus caviae mange in pet guinea pigs (Cavia porcellus). J Am Vet Med Assoc 2012;241:1056–8.
27. Singh SK, Dimri U, Ahmed QS, et al. Efficacy of doramectin in Trixacarus caviae infestation in guinea pigs (Cavia porcellus). J Parasit Dis 2013;37(1):148–50.
28. Kim SH, Jun HK, Yoo MJ, et al. Use of a formulation containing imidacloprid and moxidectin in the treatment of lice infestation in guinea pigs. Vet Dermatol 2008; 19:187–8.
29. Fisher MA, Beck W, Hutchinson MJ. Efficacy and safety of selamectin (Stronghold®/RevolutionTM) used off-label in exotic pets. Int J Appl 2007;5:87–96.
30. Mieth H, Leitner I, Meingassner JG. The efficacy of orally applied terbinafine, itraconazole and fluconazole in models of experimental trichophytoses. J Med Vet Mycol 1994;32(3):181–8.
31. Bertram CA, Müller K, Klopfleisch R. Genital tract pathology in female pet guinea pigs (Cavia porcellus): a retrospective study of 655 post-mortem and 64 biopsy cases. J Comp Pathol 2018;165:13–22.
32. Pilny A. Ovarian cystic disease in guinea pigs. Vet Clin North Am Exot Anim Pract 2014;17(1):69–75.
33. Bean AD. Ovarian cysts in the guinea pig (Cavia porcellus). Vet Clin North Am Exot Anim Pract 2013;16(3):757–76.
34. Beregi A, Zorn S, Felkai F. Ultrasonic diagnosis of ovarian cysts in ten guinea pigs. Vet Radiol Ultrasound 1999;40(1):74–6.
35. Collins BR. Endocrine diseases of rodents. Vet Clin North Am Exot Anim Pract 2008;11(1):153–62.
36. Schuetzenhofer G, Goericke-Pesch S, Wehrend A. Effects of deslorelin implants on ovarian cysts in guinea pigs. Schweiz Arch Tierheilkd 2011;153(9):416–7.
37. Mayer J. The use of GnRH to treat cystic ovaries in a guinea pig. Exot DVM 2003;5(5):36.
38. Girod-Rüffer C, Müller E, Marschang RE, et al. Retrospective study on hyperthyroidism in guinea pigs in veterinary practices in Germany. J Exot Pet Med 2019; 29:87–97.

39. Künzel F, Hierlmeier B, Christian M, et al. Hyperthyroidism in four guinea pigs: clinical manifestations, diagnosis, and treatment. J Small Anim Pract 2013; 54(12):667–71.

40. DiGeronimo PM, Brandão J. Updates on thyroid disease in rabbits and guinea Pigs. Vet Clin North Am Exot Anim Pract 2020;23(2):373–81.

41. Mayer J, Wagner R, Taeymans O. Advanced diagnostic approaches and current management of thyroid pathologies in Guinea pigs. Vet Clin North Am Exot Anim Pract 2010;13:509–23.

42. Zeugswetter F, Fenske M, Hassan J, et al. Cushing's syndrome in a guinea pig. Vet Rec 2007;160(25):878–9.

43. Zaheer OA, Beaufrère H. Treatment of hyperadrenocorticism in a guinea pig (*Cavia porcellus*). J Exot Pet Med 2020;34:57–61.

44. Meredith A. Chapter 16: Skin diseases and treatment of chinchillas. In: Patterson S, editor. Skin diseases of exotic pets. Oxford: Blackwell Science; 2006. p. 195–203.

45. Tisljar M, Janić D, Grabarević Z, et al. Stress-induced cushing's syndrome in fur-chewing chinchillas. Acta Vet Hung 2002;50(2):133–42.

46. Ponzio MF, Busso JM, Ruiz RD, et al. A survey assessment of the incidence of fur-chewing in commercial chinchilla (*Chinchilla lanigera*) farms. Anim Welf 2007;16:471–9.

47. Franchi V, Aleuy O, Tadich T. Fur-chewing and other abnormal repetitive behaviors in chinchillas (*Chinchilla lanigera*), under commercial fur-farming conditions. J Vet Behavi 2015;11:60–4.

48. Ponzio MF, Monfort SL, Busso JM, et al. Adrenal activity and anxiety-like behavior in fur-chewing chinchillas (*Chinchilla lanigera*). Horm Behav 2012; 61(5):758–62.

49. González C, Yáñez JM, Tadich T. Determination of the genetic component of fur-chewing in chinchillas (*Chinchilla lanigera*) and its economic impact. Animals 2018 21;8(9):144.

50. Jekl V, Hauptman K, Knotek Z. Quantitative and qualitative assessments of intraoral lesions in 180 small herbivorous mammals. Vet Rec 2008;162(14):442–9.

51. Longley L. Chapter 10: Rodents: dermatoses. In: Keeble E, Meredith A, editors. BSAVA manual of rodents and rerrets. Gloucester. British Small Animal Veterinary Associations; 2009. p. 107–22.

52. d'Ovidio D, Santoro D. Survey of zoonotic dermatoses in client-owned exotic pet mammals in southern Italy. Zoonoses Public Health 2015;62:100–4.

53. Marietto-Goncalves GA. Ringworm by Microsporum canis in longtailed chinchilla (*Chinchilla lanigera*). Acta Vet Bras 2015;9:274–8.

54. Mans C, Donnelly TM. Update on diseases of chinchillas. Vet Clin North Am Exot Anim Pract 2013;16(2):383–406.

55. Szabo Z, Reavill DR, Kiupel M. Squamous cell carcinoma in chinchillas: a review of three cases. J Exot Pet Med 2019;28:115–20.

56. Konell AL, Gonçalves KA, Sousa RS, et al. Mammary adenocarcinoma with pulmonary, hepatic and renal metastasis in a chinchilla (*Chinchilla lanigera*). Acta Sci Vet 2018;18:310.

57. Crossley DA. Dental disease in chinchillas in the UK. J Small Anim Pract 2001; 42(1):12–9.

58. Martel A, Donnelly T, Mans C. Update on diseases in chinchillas: 2013-2019. Vet Clin North Am Exot Anim Pract 2020;23(2):321–35.

59. Tynes VV. Behavioral dermatopathies in small mammals. Vet Clin North Am Exot Anim Pract 2013;16(3):801–20.

60. Vergneau-Grosset C, Ruel H. Abnormal repetitive behaviors and self-mutilations in small mammals. Vet Clin North Am Exot Anim Pract 2021;24(1):87–102.

61. Galeano MG, Ruiz RD, de Cuneo MF, et al. Effectiveness of fluoxetine to control fur-chewing behaviour in the chinchilla (*Chinchilla lanigera*). Appl Anim Behav Sci 2013;146:112–7.

62. White SD, Bourdeau PJ, Brément T, et al. Companion rats (*Rattus norvegicus*) with cutaneous lesions: a retrospective study of 470 cases at two university veterinary teaching hospitals (1985–2018). Vet Dermatol 2019;30:237 -e72.

63. White SD, Bourdeau PJ, Brément T, et al. Companion hamsters with cutaneous lesions; a retrospective study of 102 cases at two university veterinary teaching hospitals (1985–2018). Vet Dermatol 2019;30(3):243 –e74.

64. Jekl V, Hauptmann K, Knotek Z. Diseases in pet degus: a retrospective study in 300 animals. J Small Anim Pract 2011;52:107–12.

65. Reeves WK, Cobb KD. Ectoparasites of house mice (*Mus musculus*) from pet stores in South Carolina, U.S.A. Comp Parasitol 2005;72:193–5.

66. Owen D, Young C. The occurrence of Demodex aurati and Demodex criceti in the Syrian hamster (*Mesocricetus auratus*) in the United Kingdom. Vet Rec 1973;92(11):282–4.

67. Estes PC, Richter CB, Franklin JA. Demodectis mange in the golden hamster. Lab Anim Sci 1971;21:825–8.

68. Beck W, Hora F, Pantchev N. Case series: Efficacy of a formulation containing selamectin and sarolaner against naturally acquired mite infestations (*Demodex sp., Ornithonyssus bacoti*) in degus (*Octodon degus*). Vet Parasitol 2021;293: 109430.

69. Vergneau-Grosset C, Keel MK, Goldsmith D, et al. Description of the prevalence, histologic characteristics, concomitant abnormalities, and outcomes of mammary gland tumors in companion rats (*Rattus norvegicus*): 100 cases (1990-2015). J Am Vet Med Assoc 2016;249(10):1170–9.

70. Rother N, Bertram CA, Klopfleisch R, et al. Tumours in 177 pet hamsters. Vet Rec 2021;188(6):e14.

71. Kondo H, Onuma M, Shibuya H, et al. Spontaneous tumors in domestic hamsters. Vet Pathol 2008;45:674–80.

72. Baba Y, Takahashi K, Nakamura S. Androgen-dependent atypical fibromas spontaneously arising in the skin of Djungarian hamsters (*Phodopus sungorus*). Comp Med 2003;53(5):527–31.

73. Rowe SE, Simmons JL, Ringler DH, et al. Spontaneous neoplasms in aging Gerbillinae. A summary of forty-four neoplasms. Vet Pathol 1974;11(1):38–51.

74. Kondo H, Onuma M, Shibuya H, et al. Morphological and immunohistochemical studies of spontaneous mammary tumours in Siberian hamsters (*Phodopus sungorus*). J Comp Pathol 2009;140(2–3):127–31.

75. Yoshimura H, Kimura-Tsukada N, Ono Y, et al. Characterization of spontaneous mammary tumors in domestic Djungarian hamsters (*Phodopus sungorus*). Vet Pathol 2015;52(6):1227–34.

76. Vincent A, Ash L. Further observations on spontaneous neoplasms in the Mongolian gerbil, *Meriones unguiculatus*. Lab Anim Sci 1978;28(3):297–300.

77. Harvey RG, Whitbread TJ, Ferrer L, et al. Epidermotropic cutaneous t-cell lymphoma (mycosis fungoides) in Syrian hamsters (*Mesocricetus auratus*). A report of six cases and the demonstration of T-cell specificity. Vet Dermatol 1992; 3:13–9.

78. Jackson TA, Heath LA, Hulin MS, et al. Squamous cell carcinoma of the midventral abdominal pad in three gerbils. J Am Vet Med Assoc 1996;209:789–91.

79. Van Hoosier GL Jr, Trentin JJ. Naturally occurring tumors of the Syrian hamster. Prog Exp Tumor Res 1979;23:1–12.

80. Murphy J, Crowell T, Hewes K. Spontaneous lesions in the degu (Rodentia Hystricomorpha: Octodon degus. In: Montali R, Migaki G, editors. The comparative pathology of zoo animals. Washington DC: Smithsonian Institution Press; 1980. p. 437–44.

81. Johnson-Delaney C. Special rodents: prairie dogs. In: Johnson-Delaney C, editor. Exotic companion medicine handbook. Lake Worth: Zoological Education Network; 2005. p. 17–25.

82. Heckel BM, Eshar D, Almes KM. Idiopathic dermal necrosis in black-tailed prairie dogs (Cynomys ludovicianus). Comp Med 2018;68(3):204–7.

83. Thas I, Garner MM. A retrospective study of tumours in black-tailed prairie dogs (Cynomys ludovicianus) submitted to a zoological pathology service. J Comp Pathol 2012;147:368–75.

84. Meredith A. Chapter 20: Skin diseases and treatment of hamsters. In: Paterson S, editor. Skin diseases of exotic pets. Oxford: Blackwell Science; 2006. p. 251–63.

85. Meredith A. Chapter 22: Skin diseases and treatment of mice. In: Paterson S, editor. Skin diseases of exotic pets. Oxford: Blackwell Science; 2006. p. 275–87.

86. Wing SR, Courtney CH, Young MD. Effect of ivermectin on murine mites. J Am Vet Med Assoc 1985;187(11):1191–2.

87. Beco L, Petite A, Olivry T. Comparison of subcutaneous ivermectin and oral moxidectin for the treatment of notoedric acariasis in hamsters. Vet Rec 2001; 149(11):324–7.

88. Miedel EL, Hankenson FC. Chapter 5: Biology and diseases of hamsters. In: Fox JG, Andersen LC, Otto GM, et al, editors. Laboratory animal medicine. 3rd edition. San Diego: Academic Press; 2015. p. 209–45.

89. Tani K, Iwanaga T, Sonoda K, et al. Ivermectin treatment of demodicosis in 56 hamsters. J Vet Med Sci 2001;63(11):1245–7.

90. Pollicino P, Rossi L, Rambozzi L, et al. Oral administration of moxidectin for treatment of murine acariosis due to Radfordia affinis. Vet Parasitol 2008;151:355–7.

91. Pullium JK, Brooks WJ, Langley AD, et al. A single dose of topical moxidectin as an effective treatment for murine acariasis due to Myocoptes musculinus. Contemp Top Lab Anim Sci 2005;44:26–8.

92. Gönenç B, Sarimehmetoğlu HO, Iç_a A, et al. Efficacy of selamectin against mites (Myobia musculi, Mycoptes musculinus and Radfordia ensifera) and nematodes (Aspiculuris tetraptera and Syphacia obvelata) in mice. Lab Anim 2006; 40(2):210–3.

93. Brosseau G. Oral fluralaner as a treatment for Demodex aurati and Demodex criceti in a golden (Syrian) hamster (Mesocricetus auratus). Can Vet J 2020; 61(2):135–7.

94. Hasegawa T. A case report of the management of demodicosis in the golden hamster. J Vet Med Sci 1995;57(2):337–8.

95. d'Ovidio D, Noviello E, Santoro D. Tropical rat mite (Ornithonyssus bacoti) infestation in pet Syrian hamsters (Mesocricetus auratus) and their owner. Vet Dermatol 2017;28(2):256–7.

96. d'Ovidio D, Noviello E, Santoro D. Prevalence and zoonotic risk of tropical rat mite (Ornithonyssus bacoti) in exotic companion animals in southern Italy. Vet Dermatol 2018;29(6):463–4.

97. Bradley JM, Mascarelli PE, Trull CL, et al. Bartonella henselae infections in an owner and two Papillon dogs exposed to tropical rat mites (*Ornithonyssus bacoti*). Vector Borne Zoonotic Dis 2014;14:703–9.

98. Grosset C, Bellier S, Lagrange I, et al. Cutaneous botryomycosis in a Campbell's Russian dwarf hamster (*Phodopus campbelli*). J Exot Pet Med 2014;23(4): 389–96.

99. Eshar D, Mayer J, Keating JH. Dermatitis in a Siberian hamster (*Phodopus sungorus*). Bacterial pseudomycosis. Lab Anim 2010;39:71–3.

100. Martorell J, Gallifa N, Fondevila D, et al. Bacterial pseudomycetoma in dwarf hamster, *Phodopus sungorus*. Vet Dermatol 2006;17:449–52.

101. Kastenmayer RJ, Fain MA, Perdue KA. A retrospective study of idiopathic ulcerative dermatitis in mice with a C57BL/6 background. J Am Assoc Lab Anim Sci 2006;45:8–12.

102. Lawson GW, Sato A, Fairbanks LA, et al. Vitamin E as a treatment for ulcerative dermatitis in C57BL/6 mice and strains with a C57BL/6 background. Contemp Top Lab Anim Sci 2005;44(3):18–21.

103. Perkins SN, Hursting SD, Phang JM, et al. Calorie restriction reduces ulcerative dermatitis and infection-related mortality in p53-deficient and wildtype mice. J Invest Dermatol 1998;111:292–6.

104. Mader JR, Mason MA, Bale LK, et al. The association of early dietary supplementation with vitamin E with the incidence of ulcerative dermatitis in nice on a C57BL/6 background: diet and ulcerative dermatitis in mice. Scand J Lab Anim Sci 2010;37:253–9.

105. Michaud CR, Qin J, Elkins WR, et al. Comparison of 3 topical treatments against ulcerative dermatitis in mice with a C57BL/6 background. Comp Med 2016; 66(2):100–4.

106. Adams SC, Garner JP, Felt SA, et al. A "pedi" cures all: Toenail trimming and the treatment of ulcerative dermatitis in mice. PLoS One 2016;11(1):e0144871.

107. Williams-Fritze MJ, Carlson Scholz JA, Zeiss C, et al. Maropitant citrate for treatment of ulcerative dermatitis in mice with a C57BL/6 background. J Am Assoc Lab Anim Sci 2011;50(2):221–6.

108. Bauck LB, Orr JP, Lawrence KH. Hyperadrenocorticism in three teddy bear hamsters. Can Vet J 1984;25:247–50.

109. Planas-Silva MD, Rutherford TM, Stone MC. Prevention of age-related spontaneous mammary tumors in outbred rats by late ovariectomy. Cancer Detect Prev 2008;32:65–71.

110. Hotchkiss CE. Effect of the surgical removal of subcutaneous tumors on survival of rats. J Am Vet Med Assoc 1995;206:1575–9.

111. Thas I, Wagner RA, Thas O. Clinical diseases in pet black-tailed prairie dogs (*Cynomys ludovicianus*): a retrospective study in 206 animals. J Small Anim Pract 2019;60:153–60.

112. Jekl V. Demodicosis in nine prairie dogs (*Cynomys Ludovicianus*). Vet Dermatol 2006;17(4):2803.

113. Miwa Y, Matsunaga S, Nakayama H, et al. Spontaneous lymphoma in a prairie dog (*Cynomys ludovicianus*). J Am Anim Hosp Assoc 2006;42(2):151–3.

114. Sano Y, Matsuda K, Minami S, et al. Cutaneous angioleiomyoma in a black-tailed prairie dog (*Cynomys iudovicianus*). J Comp Pathol 2014;151:126–9.

Reptile Dermatology

Graciela Aguilar, DVM,
Mark A. Mitchell, DVM, MS, PhD, DECZM (Herpetology)*

KEYWORDS

- Reptile • Dermatology • Infectious • Neoplasia • Husbandry • Nutrition • Deficiency

KEY POINTS

- Dermatologic conditions in reptiles are a primary reason they are presented to veterinarian hospitals.
- Many diagnostic tests used for dermatologic workups have low-test sensitivity; a parallel testing strategy can improve the sensitivity of the tests.
- Emerging fungal diseases are being reported in both wild and captive reptiles.
- Squamous cell carcinoma is a common skin cancer in reptiles, and may be associated with husbandry practices (eg, ultraviolet B exposure).

INTRODUCTION

Diseases of the integument are common in both captive and wild reptiles. In a recent study, the prevalence of dermatologic diseases in bearded dragons (*Pogona vitticeps*) presented to veterinary hospitals in Europe was 22.4% (168/529).[1] Calculating a 95% confidence interval (18.8–25.9) for this study confirms that diseases of the integument are common, accounting for as much as a quarter of all case presentations. This is similar to reports in dogs, where the prevalence of skin disease for dogs presented to veterinarians was found to be 17% to 21.4% (795/3707).[2] This commonality between species suggests that veterinarians should be sure to thoroughly evaluate the integument of their reptilian patients to ensure they are identifying potential dermatologic conditions.

Because reptiles routinely present to veterinarians with skin disease, it is important for us to approach these cases using a thorough approach to the patient because the integument can be associated with both primary and secondary disease processes. Using a hypothetical-deductive approach can help the veterinarian in diagnosing the case. This strategy allows the clinician to set specific hypotheses for each identified problem and work toward identifying system or systems that are involved. This is especially important for skin diseases in reptiles because many of these diseases lead

Department of Veterinary Clinical Sciences, Louisiana State University, School of Veterinary Medicine, 1909 Skin Bertman Drive, Baton Rouge, LA 70803, USA
* Corresponding author.
E-mail address: mmitchell@lsu.edu

Vet Clin Exot Anim 26 (2023) 409–424
https://doi.org/10.1016/j.cvex.2022.12.005
vetexotic.theclinics.com

to secondary issues that must be addressed. An example of this is with the emerging fungal diseases, *Nannizziopsis guarroi* and *Ophidiomyces ophiodiicola*.[3] Although these pathogens seem to originate at the surface of the skin, they soon penetrate the integument and can involve the musculoskeletal system and gain systemic access. These pathogens can lead to dehydration and secondary opportunistic bacterial infections. If the veterinarian only focuses on the "skin lesions" in these cases, they will not likely have a positive resolution.

REPTILE INTEGUMENT

Before reviewing the methods for diagnosing and managing cases with reptile skin disease, it is important to understand the differences between the integuments of reptiles and domestic species, where most of our understanding for managing these cases arise. Reptiles have a keratinized skin modified into scales, which cannot be scraped off like fish scales.[4] Evolutionarily, this unique feature allowed the reptiles to adapt to a terrestrial lifestyle.[5] Reptile skin functions as a mechanical shield to protect members of this taxa from desiccation, abrasion, ultraviolet radiation, and infectious diseases.[4–6] From this basic adaptation, interspecific differences have evolved for different functions in reptiles[5]; therefore, it is difficult to generalize one "normal reptile skin." However, similar to any other vertebrate group, the reptile's integument consists of the epidermis and dermis.[6] The epidermis consists of 3 layers: *stratum corneum*, *stratum intermedium*, and *stratum germinativum*. The *stratum corneum* is heavily keratinized and includes 6 to 8 cellular layers. These layers are compounds of 2 different types of keratin: alpha keratin (α-keratin) and beta keratin (β-keratin). The α-keratin is present in the softer and flexible areas, such as the hinges and the space between scales.[7] Mites and bacterial infections are commonly found in these areas.[4] The β-keratins include the hard and brittle areas, such as the horns of Jackson's chameleon (*Chamaeleo jacksonii*) and scutes of hard-shelled turtles. The shell of the soft-shell turtle (*Apalone* spp) is composed of α-keratin.[8,9] The variation between the epidermal thicknesses also depends on the body location; dorsal areas are thick for protection and ventral areas are thinner to allow for freedom of movement.[6] The *stratum intermedium* contains a lipid-rich film that makes the skin a water-permeable barrier. Finally, the *stratum germinativum* is the deepest layer and comprises the cuboid cells responsible for producing the scales. Additionally, this inner stratum is where melanocytes can be found.[4,7,10]

The dermis underlies the epidermis and contains a single aglandular layer. This layer contains the connective tissue, blood vessels, lymphatics, nerves, and chromatophores. The chromatophores are responsible for displaying color change characteristics of the reptiles.[6,9] Additionally, the osteoderms are located within the dermis. Osteoderms are the protective bony plates found in the dermis of chelonians, plated and girdled lizards, skinks, and crocodilians. Because of their bony density, they can be seen on radiographs and may obscure the examination of the coelomic cavity.[7] In chelonians, the osteoderms are fused with the ribs and spinal column to form the shell.

The skin of reptiles can also have a limited number of accessory components. For example, reptile skin glands are in minimal numbers and often site and species specific. Scent glands can be found in squamates and are associated with the vent/cloaca. Lizards from the family Iguanidae have prefemoral pores that function as sexual scent glands and can be used to differentiate males from females.[9] Musk or Rathke's glands are present in all turtles except tortoises (Testudinidae) and some emydid turtles.[11] Cutaneous sensation in the keratinized skin of reptiles is reduced compared with birds and mammals, which places these animals at a higher risk from thermal burns.[4]

The process of skin renewal in reptiles is called ecdysis, or the shedding of the skin. Ecdysis is a normal physiologic process that is controlled by the thyroid gland and follows 2 main phases: resting and renewal.[9] The resting phase is the period between periods of shedding. This phase is shorter in young animals compared with older reptiles; however, environmental temperatures, humidity, and skin diseases (eg, parasites, thermal/ultraviolet burns) can influence the length of this phase. In the renewal phase, there is a mitotic division of the *stratum germinativum*, creating a new epidermis to replace the outer epidermis. This renewal phase also includes the spectacles (eye caps) of squamates. The separation between the old and new epidermis is achieved through enzyme-induced lysis. Snakes shed the entire skin altogether, whereas the rest of the reptiles shed it in small sections. During this process, which takes around 2 weeks, the skin is more vulnerable to trauma, infection, parasites, and toxins. Additionally, animals can manifest aggression, hide, or refuse to eat. Multiple factors can affect the normal ecdysis process and cause dysecdysis.

ANAMNESIS AND PHYSICAL EXAMINATION

The anamnesis, or history, and physical examination are the 2 most important tools that a veterinarian has to manage a case. Shortchanging either of these procedures may lead the veterinarian down the wrong diagnostic path. The information gained from the anamnesis can help to guide the veterinarian with characterizing the signalment of the patient, husbandry and nutrition practices for the patient, biosecurity methods, and the client's experience level with that species of reptile. Unfortunately, reptiles will continue to present for dermatologic conditions associated with deficient husbandry (eg, too high/low humidity) and nutrition (eg, hypovitaminosis A) practices until we develop better evidence to assist pet reptile owners. Fortunately, there is good "best husbandry and nutrition practices" information available on the Internet and in the lay literature for different reptile species but it requires the client and veterinarian to do some investigating to determine the value of the information. The authors look for patterns in the experiential based information in determining its value when evidence-based information is not available. By not obtaining a complete anamnesis, the veterinarian increases the likelihood of missing important data to guide them through the physical examination and with selecting appropriate diagnostic tests. Thus, it is essential for veterinarians to develop systematic methods (eg, history intake forms) to gather the appropriate historical information for a case, regardless of who collects the data (eg, veterinarian, technician, front staff), to provide essential data and lay the groundwork for pursuing a diagnosis.

As noted previously, when performing a physical examination on a reptile with skin disease, it is important to conduct a thorough examination of the entire patient and not only focus on the skin issue. Because many skin diseases are systemic in nature, identifying any anomalies on the physical examination can further aid in the diagnosis and determine the extent of the disease. When assessing the skin on the physical examination, it is important to evaluate the entire animal starting from the head and continuing to the tail. The skin should be palpated for alterations in texture, any obvious swellings, ulcers, erosions, or damage to indicate a break in the skin barrier. All anomalies should be recorded as a component of the physical examination in the medical record and evaluated, in conjunction with the anamnesis, to develop a problem list and identify the systems, beyond the integument, that are affected in the reptile patient. This information can then be used to develop a list of differential disease diagnoses and create a diagnostic plan.

DIAGNOSTIC TESTS

The diagnostic approach for reptile dermatologic cases can use the same methods commonly performed for mammals. The diagnostic plan should follow a stepwise strategy and collect samples in a methodical manner to minimize the likelihood of missing a potential diagnosis. The authors prefer to start the diagnostic workup using a noninvasive strategy (eg, skin cytology, impression smears) and rely on more invasive methods (eg, biopsy) if the initial diagnostics are unrewarding. It is important to set a hypothesis on your expectations for each test result. This can help minimize misclassification bias, especially for tests with lower sensitivity. In these cases, a diagnostic test that is subject to a higher false-negative rate could lead the veterinarian down the wrong path if they do not consider this limitation in the test. It is important to recognize that the test characteristics (eg, sensitivity, specificity, positive and negative predictive values) for dermatologic tests in reptiles have not been investigated, so we must rely on the experiential learning we have gained over time and the evidence that may exist in other species to develop an understanding of the potential risks for misclassification (eg, false negative, false positive) for a test.

Skin cytology and impression smears can be collected by directly placing a glass microscope slide against a lesion; this should be done multiple times over the length of the slide to increase the sensitivity of this method. Skin scrapes using a #15 scalpel blade can also be used to collect samples for cytologic review. The skin scraping typically provides more information than the impression smears because they can obtain deeper tissue samples. Regardless, the slide should be heat fixed or air-dried based on the best practice for a preferred stain. The authors use Gram stain (Polysciences Inc., Warrington, PA, USA) to evaluate the bacterial and fungal flora associated with the lesion; these slides should be heat fixed before staining. The results should be considered a screening test, and the authors look for changes in the distributions of the organisms. If there seems to be a novel organism (eg, uniform abundance of a Gram-negative rod), then this may guide the veterinarian to pursue culture or molecular methods to identify the pathogen. Although this strategy is typically done in veterinary hospitals for different species, it is important to note that agreement between culture and Gram stain may only be fair.[12] Again, this should reinforce to the veterinarian why setting a hypothesis for each test is important. For example, if the Gram stain sample is found to have uniform Gram-negative rods and the culture does not isolate a Gram-negative rod (eg, failed growth due to overgrowth with a Gram-positive bacteria), then instead of assuming the Gram stain is wrong, a third test, molecular testing (eg, skin microbiome testing), could be pursued to identify the Gram-negative bacteria in the lesion. When attempting to evaluate cell types from a lesion, a Diff Quik stain (Polysciences Inc.,Warrington, PA, USA) can be used to evaluate the epithelial cells, white blood cells, and red blood cells, among other cells. Although both of these stains potentially have moderate (to low) sensitivity, the specificity for these tests is higher. Therefore, there is a lower likelihood for false-positive results, so if you "see something," it is likely real.

Acetate tape impressions can also be collected from reptiles for cytologic analysis but these are typically reserved for evaluating ectoparasites such as mites (eg, *Ophionyssus natricis*). The sensitivity for this test is typically high because you can see the ectoparasites and apply the tape directly over the mites. The mites can also be collected using mineral oil soaked cotton-tipped applicators. The tape or oil can be applied to a slide and reviewed under light microscopy. The shed skin from reptiles experiencing dysecdysis (difficulty shedding) can also be reviewed under light microscopy.

Diagnostic imaging is not routinely used for assessing dermatologic lesions in most vertebrates but does have value in chelonians. Radiographs or computed tomography scans can provide insight into the extent of disease in the osteoderms (eg, fractures, osteomyelitis) of a chelonian. In chelonian cases presented with traumatic injuries to the shell, these imaging modalities can also provide insight into the secondary impacts on the soft tissue structures (eg, pulmonary contusion) within the coelom.

For cases where superficial skin sampling is unrewarding (eg, impression smears, skin scrapes) or the skin lesion is a mass, a full-thickness biopsy should be collected. A punch biopsy or incisional biopsy can be used to collect these samples. If an infectious disease is suspected with the mass, then a sample should be collected for culture before the tissue is placed in formalin and fixed for review under a light microscope. To conclusively diagnose a skin infection, it is preferred to isolate the organism in culture, or confirm it using molecular techniques, and see the pathogen and inflammatory process in the tissues under light microscopy.

Historically, microbiologic culture has been a standard component of the diagnostic workup of dermatologic cases in human and veterinary medicine. However, culture is a moderately sensitive diagnostic method because of the potential for false negatives resulting from sample collection and handling to the methods used for culture. How many times have you had to tell a client the culture was negative, when there was obvious disease? Because of this, it is important to educate your clients to this risk before sample submission so they are aware of this limitation. To overcome some of these limitations, newer technologies, such as matrix-assisted laser desorption/ionization time-of-flight mass spectrometry (MALDI-TOF MS), have been pursued. This method is commonly used in many commercial diagnostic laboratories because of its efficiency and cost. However, although it has an improved sensitivity over standard culture identification methods,[13] it still has limitations. Recently, a study evaluated the challenges of identifying aerobic bacteria from the skin of reptiles using MALDI-TOF MS.[14] Overall, the authors found that the MALDI-TOF MS performed well, characterizing 93.5% of the bacteria characterized as categories 1 (85.1%) and 2 (8.4%). The struggle with identification was associated with the category 3 isolates (6.5%). Molecular techniques were used to characterize these isolates, and although some isolates were also identified correctly using MALDI TOF MS, several could not be identified. These results should remind veterinarians of the limitations of this diagnostic test and to discuss pursuing other techniques (eg, 16S rRNA sequencing) to confirm a potential pathogen.

Complete blood counts and biochemistry testing can be useful diagnostic tools when working up a reptile dermatologic case. As for the other tests, understanding the limitations of these tests is key to gaining the most value from the results. With more than 10,000 species of reptiles, one of the primary challenges we face when interpreting these results is having limited reference data. In many cases, there is a degree of subjectivity when interpreting these results, as we often need to rely on closely related species for reference values. If reference values are available, it is important to review how the data was collected and processed. Small sample sizes and highly variable reference intervals remain an issue. Understanding these limitations, the authors primarily use the results of these blood tests to assess the physiologic status of the patient and determine whether the disease is systemic in nature (eg, an elevated white blood cell count). Again, each of these tests has individual value but the true value of these tests is in their collective value. A patient with a white blood cell count indicating a systemic inflammatory response, with cytologic impressions from crusting and ulcerative skin lesions demonstrating an inflammatory response (eg, heterophils and macrophages present) with a possible pathogen (eg, uniform fungal hyphae), should direct the clinician to consider a systemic infection and the pursuit of additional directed diagnostics (eg, polymerase chain reaction [PCR], culture) and treatment (eg, antifungals).

COMMON CAUSES OF SKIN DISEASE IN REPTILES
Bacterial Disease

Bacterial dermatitis is considered the most common cause of dermatitis in reptiles.[9] Lesions are commonly identified in reptiles secondary to traumatic injuries or husbandry/nutritionally related issues. Gram-negative bacteria tend to be the most common organisms isolated from skin lesions, with many genera being opportunistic pathogens from within the reptile's enclosure or a component of their skin microflora: *Aeromonas* spp, *Citrobacter* spp, *Escherichia coli*, *Edwardsiella* spp, *Klebsiella* spp, *Proteus* spp, *Pseudomonas* spp, *Salmonella* spp, and *Serratia* spp. However, a diverse range of bacteria has been associated with bacteria dermatitis, including Gram-positive cocci (*Micrococcus* spp, *Staphylococcus* spp, and *Streptococcus* spp), Gram-negative cocci (Neisseria spp), *Mycobacterium* spp, and anaerobic bacteria (*Bacteroides* spp, *Fusobacterium* spp, *Peptostreptococcus* spp, and *Clostridium* spp).[6,9] Skin discoloration is typically one of the first clinical signs associated with bacterial dermatitis in squamates, with the skin becoming erythematous because of the inflammatory process (**Fig. 1**). In chelonians, bacterial dermatitis tends to be patchy, with changes starting in the superficial keratin. Over time, the infections continue

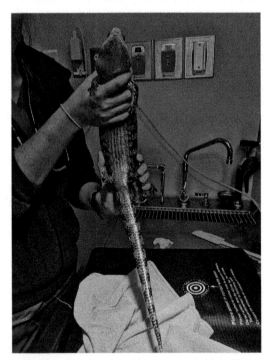

Fig. 1. Erythematous skin discoloration in a blue-tongued skink (*Tiliqua scincoides*).

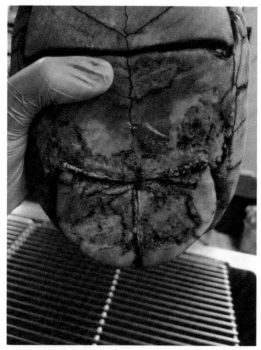

Fig. 2. Chronic-active ulcerative plastron dermatitis in a red-eared slider (*Trachemys scripta elegans*).

into erosive or ulcerative lesions (**Fig. 2**). Severe cases will involve the musculature and septicemia. Treatment should be focused on the severity of disease and the culture results but usually includes topical disinfectants (eg, betadine, chlorhexidine), topical or systemic antibiotics, and a bandage to protect the wound during the healing process. When necrosis is present, the wound should be surgically debrided.[9,15]

Although some dermatitis lesions remain open as ulcers, many develop into abscesses. These lesions are characterized by being hard, swollen, and well-circumscribed masses. Because the central core of these lessons contains bacteria, inflammatory cells, and fibrosis, some authors suggest the term fibriscesses.[6] Abscesses in reptiles have a unique caseous configuration because of having decreased myeloperoxidase activity in their heterophils.[9] When collecting a culture from a reptile abscess, the wall of the abscess is the preferred site. Because of the caseous nature of reptile abscesses, it is recommended to remove them surgically. If the abscess is local or focal, this can be done under sedation and with a local anesthetic; however, general anesthesia is recommended for multifocal abscesses or abscesses that involve muscle and/or bone. Systemic antibiotics are not considered necessary for focal abscesses. Ultimately, these lesions are best handled topically following surgical removal of the abscess using disinfectants (eg, betadine, chlorhexidine) and topical ointments/creams (eg, silver sulfadiazine). For large well-encapsulated abscesses, a primary closure may be considered after completely irrigating the surgical site and removing the abscess en toto.[15]

Two well-described bacterial dermatitides of reptiles serve as important examples of how husbandry conditions can lead to life-threatening skin disease: "Blister disease" and septic cutaneous ulcerative disease (SCUD). "Blister disease" (scale rot, necrotizing dermatitis) is a frequent condition reported in snakes housed on unhygienic or contaminated substrates and in lizards due to high environmental humidity.[14] The lesions start as sterile "blisters" (vesicles and bullae) in the ventral scales, the site of contact with the substrate. Over time the lesions progress, leading to ulceration, necrosis, abscess formation, and septicemia. Once again, Gram-negative bacteria (eg, *Aeromonas* spp and *Pseudomonas* spp) are commonly isolated from these lesions.[7] Microbiologic culture and antimicrobial sensitivity testing should be pursued to confirm the pathogen and the best option for antimicrobial treatment. The culture swab should be inserted into one of the blisters to increase the likelihood of obtaining the pathogen; swabbing the ventral surface of the skin is likely to result in a contaminated sample and an increased likelihood of missing the pathogen (false-negative result). Treatment should be focused on eliminating the predisposing factor (eg, cleaning the environment/substrate, correcting deficiencies in temperature and humidity), topical therapy, and systemic therapy with an antimicrobial identified as appropriate from antimicrobial sensitivity testing. Topical therapy should include sharp debridement of necrotic tissues under sedation/anesthesia.[9,15] The authors use wet-to-dry bandaging for 48 to 72 hours to decontaminate the affected areas. Chlorhexidine or saline are used on the wet gauze for these bandages, and we secure them to the skin using Tegaderm (3M products, St. Paul, MN, USA). Once the lesions are effectively dried, the authors use a silver hydrogel (SilvaSorb, Medline Industries, Inc., Mundelein, IL, USA) to protect the viable tissues while providing additional topical antimicrobial therapy (silver).

SCUD is common in aquatic turtles housed in unhygienic water and is characterized by ulcers and erosions on the shell surface.[9] The lesions often change in color from the normal shell and scute loss is common.[15] Over time, the infection can penetrate into the deeper levels of the dermis and cause osteomyelitis. SCUD is considered a syndrome that can involve several species of bacteria, including *Serratia* spp, *Aeromonas hydrophila*, *Beneckea chitinivora*, and *Mycobacterium kansaii*, rather than a specific disease caused by *Citrobacter freundii*.[1] Ultimately, microbiome testing using next-generation sequencing of samples collected from the shell lesions would be best to determine the bacterial populations associated with these lesions. Diagnosis is typically based on the anamnesis and physical examination but shell biopsy for histopathology and culture are needed for a definitive diagnosis. Treatment should focus on improving the water quality (eg, reducing organic load, regular water changes, improved filtration), dry docking aquatic species, debridement of lesions, wet-to-dry bandaging to control infection, and topical (eg, silver-based products) and systemic antimicrobials (based on culture and sensitivity testing).[16] Recent study using bacteriophages in combination with antimicrobials were used to manage a multidrug-resistant *C freundii* infection in a loggerhead sea turtle (*Caretta caretta*).[17] Although not commercially available, these types of treatments may be viable options for threatened/endangered species.

Mycotic Disease

Fungal dermatitis is becoming more common in both wild and captive reptiles. In captive reptiles, a variety of fungal pathogens have been isolated from skin lesions, including *Aspergillus* spp, *Candida* spp, *Fusarium* spp, *Geotrichum* spp, *Mucor* spp, *Oospora* spp, *Paecilomyces* spp, *Penicillium* spp, *Trichoderma* spp, and *Trichophyton* spp.[9] These infections were primarily considered secondary to environmental or husbandry deficiencies, overcrowding, and immunosuppression.[7,18] However, *Emydomyces testavorans*, *Chrysosporium* spp, *Nannizziopsis* spp, *Paranannizziopsis* spp, and *Ophidiomyces* spp are being isolated from both wild-caught and captive reptiles and are considered to be obligate fungal pathogens.[3,9,19,20] These latter fungal organisms are also contributing to the loss of wild reptiles and will affect future conservation plans for some species. The distribution of these fungi was originally limited to certain regions of the world but more recent findings of them in Asia (eg, Taiwan) suggest they are truly ubiquitous.[21] These findings should further reinforce the importance of taking a stepwise approach to managing our reptilian patients and the importance of a hypothetical deductive approach. When things do not make sense, we need to pursue the case further. The majority of these emerging fungal cases were likely initially treated as bacterial infections because only bacterial cultures were commonly selected as a diagnostic. These cases required the veterinarian to pursue biopsy and ultimately fungal culture and molecular testing to confirm these fungi.

Among these obligate pathogenic fungi, 2 emerging diseases are common in captive reptiles: yellow fungus disease (YFD) and snake fungal disease (SFD). YFD has been associated with necrotizing dermatitis in captive green iguanas (*Iguana iguana*) and bearded dragons (*P vitticeps*). *N guarroi* is one species found to serve as a primary agent of YFD in these captive lizards. Lesions progress from white nodules to crusty yellow discolored scales and ultimately evolve to severe necrotic lesions.[22] The causative agent for SFD, or ophidiomycosis, is *O ophiodiicola*. This fungal pathogen has been well recognized in both wild and captive snakes. Lesions start as mild dermatitis with hyperkeratosis (**Fig. 3**) but develop into crusts, premature shedding, subcutaneous nodules, and corneal opacities. These lesions can quickly penetrate the dermis and affect bones; on the face, these lesions can lead to severe disfigurement. Severe cases of ophidiomycosis have been associated with mortality.[23]

Dermatomycosis can be challenging to diagnose. First, the lesions and clinical signs can be confused with a bacterial infection. Lesions start as moist, exudative erythematous ulcers or blisters and crusts but can develop into granulomas, necrosis, and osteomyelitis.[7] Second, diagnosing fungi can be challenging because the veterinarians need to submit a specific request for a fungal culture, and some fungi are challenging to culture. Cytologic sampling of a lesion can be used to help in determining the possibility of a fungal involvement; however, it is subject to misclassification

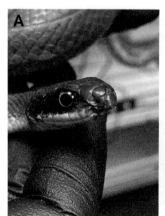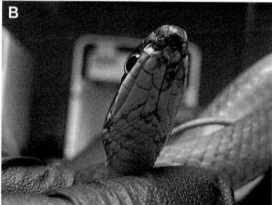

Fig. 3. Crusting and erythema on rostrum (*A*) and mandible (*B*) of a blackmask racer (*Coluber constrictor latrunculus*). This wild snake was presented with these lesions. Unfortunately, it did not respond to treatment and the lesions were confirmed to be attributed to *O ophiodiicola*.

(false-negative result). Ultimately, biopsy with histopathology and molecular testing are helpful in confirming a diagnosis of a fungal infection.[9]

Fungal dermatoses require long-term therapy and correction of any predisposing husbandry and/or environmental factors. Local infections can be surgically removed (eg, granulomas) or treated with antiseptic products (dilute iodine solution, chlorhexidine 2%) and antifungal cream (eg, miconazole, ketoconazole).[9,24] Systemic antifungal agents are recommended for cases that are generalized or deep; however, signs of toxicity should be carefully monitored. The authors have used both itraconazole 5 to 10 mg/kg SID-BID and voriconazole 5 mg/kg SID-BID successfully to manage systemic fungal infections in reptiles. However, voriconazole is preferred because it seems to be safer and associated with lower mortalities in lizards.[25] Additionally, the administration of terbinafine at 20 mg/kg PO SID to q48h may be beneficial to treat dermatomycoses caused by *N guarroi* in bearded dragons.[26]

Viral Disease

Historically, viral skin diseases were not commonly diagnosed in captive reptiles. However, economic factors and a requirement for specific testing methods (eg, PCR) to make a diagnosis may have played a role in these limited findings.[15] Today, new viruses are being reported in reptiles on a regular basis, so it is important to include these pathogens in our differential diagnoses lists. Several viruses are well known for causing dermatosis in reptiles. Herpesvirus and papillomavirus have been associated with the tumor-forming disease fibropapillomatosis in green turtles (*Chelonia mydas*).[27] Ranavirus has been isolated from lizards with purulent to ulcerative-necrotizing dermatitis and hyperkeratosis and in soft-shelled turtles (*Pelodiscus sinensis*) and box turtles (*Terrapene carolina*) with cervical edema and ulcers.[28,29] Poxvirus has been found to cause gray-white or brownish wart-like skin lesions in captive crocodilians (*Caiman crocodilus* and *Crocodylus niloticus*).[6] West Nile Virus has been shown to produce "pix" or lymphohistiocytic proliferative cutaneous lesions (**Fig. 4**) in American alligators (*Alligator mississippiensis*).[30] Diagnosis of viral dermatitis typically requires biopsy, histopathology, and molecular testing (eg, PCR testing).

Parasitic Disease

Ectoparasites are commonly associated with dermatologic problems in captive reptiles because of poor biosecurity (eg, mixing wild and captive reptiles), high stocking densities, and inappropriate husbandry (eg, wrong substrate).[9,18] Acarids (eg, ticks and mites) are the most common reptile ectoparasites encountered in the authors'

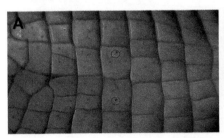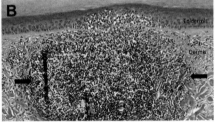

Fig. 4. West Nile virus infection in alligators (*Alligator mississippiensis*) results in a lymphoproliferative reaction that causes lesions that affect the retail quality of the leather. Note the circular lesions (*red circles*) that can be seen grossly in the leather (*A*). These lesions are attributed to the severe lymphoproliferative lesions (between *arrows*) that develop in the dermis and expand into the epidermis (*B*).

practice. Heavy ectoparasite infestations can lead to anemia, pruritus, discomfort, severe dermatitis, secondary infections, dysecdysis, and behavioral changes (prolonged soaking in water and frequently rubbing in cage furnishings). Additionally, these ectoparasites can also serve as vectors for bacterial and viral pathogens. Overall, more than 250 species of mites have been reported to be parasitize reptiles.[31]

O natricis is the primary mite parasite of snakes, although it will also infest lizards. This black parasite is primarily found under the scales, around the nares, in the infraorbital pits, and in the periorbital conjunctiva.[14] Snake mites have been associated with the transmission of inclusion body disease (arenavirus) in captive snake colonies.[32] Additionally, *O natricis* has been reported to cause a papular vesiculobullous eruption in humans.[33] The lizard mite (*Ophionyssus acertinus*) only infests lizards. This large red parasite tends to congregate in the skin folds around the lizard's neck and at the base of its tail.[15] Both of these parasites ingest blood meals from their hosts. In contrast, trombiculid mites (*Hirstiella* spp) consume cellular fluid from their host. This mite is a parasite during its larval stage in reptiles, creating necrotic debris, and is zoonotic.[9]

Ixodes spp, *Hyalomma* spp, *Haemaphysalis* spp, *Amblyomma* spp, *Aponomma* spp, *Argasidae* spp, and *Ornithodoros* spp are ticks that have been found to infest reptiles.[9,34–37] Imported reptiles can introduce exotic ticks and should be inspected closely for the presence of these ectoparasites.[34,35,38–41] Leeches may be encountered on turtles from outdoor ponds. There are several examples of nematodes (*Kalicephalus* spp and *Paratrichosoma* spp), cestodes, and filarid/filarial worms causing dermatoses in reptiles by migrating in the subcutaneous space. These parasites must be removed surgically.[42]

Medical therapy for ectoparasites includes a combination of treating the affected animals and the environment. For *O natricis*, ivermectin (0.2 mg/kg, SC or oral q 14 days; or 10 mg/L water sprayed topically, q 7 days) and Provent-a-mite (Pro products, Mahopac, NY, USA) can be used to treat the reptiles, whereas Provent-a-mite and predatory mites (*Hypoaspis* spp) can be used to eliminate the mites from the reptile's environment. It is also important to remove and replace the substrate. Because the life cycle of the mite is 40 days, it is important to treat and reinspect the animals after that time to ensure the treatment was successful. Ticks can be removed manually but you should be careful to extract the mouthparts.

Nutritional Diseases

Vitamin A is a fat-soluble vitamin that is important for maintaining epithelial health and several biological processes, including vision, growth, reproduction, and immune function.[43] For example, a recent study has shown the beneficial effect of this liposoluble vitamin for tail regeneration in lizards (*Podarcis muralis*).[44] Hypovitaminosis A is a well-recognized disease of captive reptiles; however, it is also one of the most overdiagnosed diseases of captive reptiles. Hypovitaminosis A is frequently attributed to nutritional deficiencies in captive chelonians and chameleons (panther chameleon, *Furcifer pardalis*; veiled chameleon, *Chamaeleo calyptratus*).[7] The primary pathogenesis associated with this nutritional deficiency is squamous metaplasia. Affected animals develop hyperkeratosis and parakeratosis of the skin, secondary dermatitis, conjunctivitis, blepharoedema, blepharitis, aural abscesses, blindness, and rhinitis.[43,45] Diagnosis can be guided by the anamnesis and clinical signs; however, confirmation should be done using an appropriate diagnostic method (eg, high-performance liquid chromatography). Plasma, liver, skin, and fat can all be used to measure vitamin A concentration in a reptile.[46] In addition, histopathology can be used to confirm the presence of squamous metaplasia. Treatment can be accomplished using a single parenteral injection of vitamin A (2000–5000 IU/kg vitamin A), followed by dietary adjustment.[47] Care should be taken with parenteral doses, as higher or serial doses can lead to hypervitaminosis A.

Neoplasia

The number of cases of cutaneous neoplasia in reptiles has been on the rise because reptiles are living longer. This finding is likely due to the improved husbandry methods being provided to captive reptiles. However, some forms of cutaneous neoplasia, such as squamous cell carcinoma, may actually be the direct result of some husbandry factors, such as exposure to ultraviolet radiation. In addition to squamous cell carcinoma, other cancers associated with the skin of reptiles include fibrosarcoma, myxosarcoma, liposarcoma, chromatophoroma, mast cell tumor, lymphoma, lymphosarcoma, plasma cell tumors, and leukemia.[9] Any abnormal skin mass on a reptile should be pursued using the same diagnostic methods described for domestic pets. Fine-needle aspirates and biopsies can be typically used to confirm the type of cancer. Treatment will be dependent on the type of tumor. To date, treatment options are limited for reptiles and results variable. The authors recommend consulting with a medical oncologist when devising a treatment plan for neoplasia in reptiles.

OTHER DISEASES

Ultraviolet B (UVB) radiation has been found to increase circulating plasma 25-hydroxyvitamin D_3 concentrations in several reptiles.[48–51] In captivity, this spectrum of light is typically provided using commercial light bulbs. Because there is no oversight of these bulbs, the amount of UVB produced can vary, with many bulbs producing levels (closer to the bulb surface) that are much higher than sunlight. Although the production of vitamin D is important to the overall health of the reptile, the UVB can also cause side effects, especially at high doses. In mammals, increased UVB exposure is associated with cataract formation and skin cancer.[52] Although no studies have confirmed these same lesions can develop in reptiles, a case series in captive bearded dragons (P vitticeps) found a pattern of squamous cell carcinoma developing on the dorsum and head, areas commonly exposed to potentially high sources of UVB from commercial light bulbs.[53] Ultimately, a nonexperimental study (case-control or cohort study) should be pursued to evaluate this risk. Although there seems to be important benefits from these commercial UVB sources, it is important for veterinarians to reduce the risk of side effects. Recent studies in leopard geckos (Eublepharis

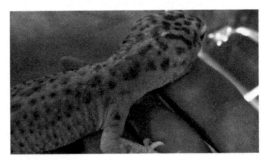

Fig. 5. Leopard gecko (E macularius) undergoing complete ecdysis following exposure to weekly ultraviolet B radiation without shelter. The geckos shed their entire skin every week during the 4-week study. Providing shelter eliminated the shedding altogether, while still allowing the geckos to increase their 25-hydroxyvitamin D concentrations.

macularius) found that the positive benefits associated with UVB exposure (eg, increased 25-hydroxyvitamin D$_3$) can be achieved exposing the animals to lower doses of UVB, including increasing the distance between the animal and bulb, as well as the amount of time the animal is exposed to the UVB.[49] Preliminary research with leopard geckos exposed to 50μwatts/cm^2 or lesser for 12 h/d found that the geckos would undergo ecdysis on a weekly basis, similar to a sunburn in humans (**Fig. 5**). However, when the exposure time was 2 hours per day, none of the geckos underwent ecdysis. To reduce the likelihood of side effects with UVB, it is important for veterinarians to educate their clients on the risks of these bulbs and reduce the overall exposure by limiting exposure time and dose. The authors currently recommend UVB exposure being limited to no more than 2 hours per day to reduce this risk. If there are concerns that this exposure time is too short, we recommend measuring the reptile's plasma 25-hydroxyvitamin D$_3$ concentration to determine if it is low; this is similarly done in humans if there is a concern a patient has low vitamin D.

SUMMARY

Reptiles have adapted a unique integument that has allowed them to be a very successful taxon; however, disruptions on their normal skin layers can lead to dermatologic problems. The appropriate anamnesis and physical examination are fundamental to diagnosing the correct disease. To ensure the likelihood for a proper diagnosis in a reptile case, the authors recommend considering the specific limitations for the available diagnostic tests in this group and carrying out the testing order from the least invasive to the most invasive tests. Bacterial, mycotic, viral, and parasitic infections, as well as nutritional and neoplastic conditions, can causes dermatopathies in reptiles; therefore, it is essential to become familiar with each group's different etiologic agents or underlying pathologic conditions, the clinical signs, and treatments to guarantee the best management of these cases.

CLINICS CARE POINTS

- Gram stains and microbiologic culture may not have a high level of agreement; thus, clinicians should consider the patient presentation when interpreting the results.
- When treating fungal disease in reptiles with azoles, monitor the patients closely for changes in mentation and appetite.
- Consider next-generation sequencing for samples collected from skin lesions of patients previously treated with antibiotics because microbiologic culture may be negative in these cases.
- When treating *O natricis* infestations, be sure to treat both the reptile and the environment.

DISCLOSURE

The authors' research is supported by Fluker Farms (Port Allen, LA, USA) but they made no contributions to the writing of this article.

REFERENCES

1. Schmidt-Ukaj S, Hochleithner M, Richter B, et al. A survey of diseases in captive bearded dragons: a retrospective study of 529 patients. Vet Med (Praha) 2017; 62(9):508–15.

2. Hill P, Lo A, Eden C, et al. Survey of the prevalence, diagnosis and treatment of dermatological conditions in small animals in general practice. Vet Rec 2006; 158(16):533–9.

3. Mitchell MA, Walden MR. *Chrysosporium* anamorph *Nannizziopsis vriesii*: an emerging fungal pathogen of captive and wild reptiles. Vet Clin North Am Exot Anim Pract 2013;16(3):659–68.

4. O'Malley B. General anatomy and physiology of reptiles. In: O'Malley B, editor. Clinical anatomy and physiology of exotic species: structure and function of mammals, birds, reptiles, and amphibians. Elsevier Saunders; 2005. p. 17–39.

5. Chang C, Ping WU, Baker RE, et al. Reptile scale paradigm: Evo-Devo, pattern formation and regeneration. Int J Dev Biol 2009;53(5–6):813–26.

6. Scheelings TF, Hellebuyck T. Dermatology-skin. In: Divers SJ, Stahl SJ, editors. Mader's reptile and amphibian medicine and surgery. 3rd edition. St. Louis, MO: Elsevier; 2019. p. 699–711.

7. Palmeiro BS, Roberts H. Clinical approach to dermatologic disease in exotic animals. Vet Clin North Am Exot Anim Pract 2013;16(3):523–77.

8. Goodman G. Structure and function of reptile skin. In: Paterson S, editor. Skin diseases of exotic pets. Oxford, UK: Blackwell Science; 2006. p. 75–9.

9. Perry SM, Sander SJ, Mitchell MM. Integumentary system. In: Mitchell MA, Tully TN, editors. Current therapy in exotic pet practice. St. Louis, MO: Elsevier; 2016. p. 17–76.

10. Kuriyama T, Murakami A, Brandley M, et al. Blue, black, and stripes: evolution and development of color production and pattern formation in lizards and snakes. Front Ecol Evol 2020;8:1–14.

11. Vitt LJ, Caldewell JP. Anatomy of amphibians and reptiles. In: Vitt LJ, Caldewell JP, editors. Herpetology: an introductory biology of amphibians and reptiles. 4th edition. Elsevier Inc; 2013. p. 1710–1.

12. Evans EE, Mitchell MA, Whittington JK, et al. Measuring the level of agreement between cloacal Gram's stains and bacterial cultures in Hispaniolan Amazon parrots (*Amazona ventralis*). J Avian Med Surg 2014;28(4):290–6.

13. Randall LP, Lemma F, Koylass M, et al. Evaluation of MALDI-ToF as a method for the identification of bacteria in the veterinary diagnostic laboratory. Res Vet Sci 2015;101:42–9.

14. Brockmann M, Aupperle-Lellbach H, Gentil M, et al. Challenges in microbiological identification of aerobic bacteria isolated from the skin of reptiles. PLoS One 2020;15(10):e0240085.

15. Hoppmann E, Barron HW. Dermatology in reptiles. J Exot Pet Med 2007;16(4): 210–24.

16. Meyer J, Selleri P. Dermatology-shell. In: Divers SJ, Stahl SJ, editors. Mader's reptile and amphibian medicine and surgery. 3rd edition. Elsevier; 2019;vol. 31. 714–720.e2.

17. Greene W, Chan B, Bromage E, et al. The use of bacteriophages and immunological monitoring for the treatment of a case of chronic septicemic cutaneous ulcerative disease in a loggerhead sea turtle *Caretta caretta*. J Aquat Anim Health 2021;33(3):139–54.

18. Harkewicz KA. Dermatology of reptiles: a clinical approach to diagnosis and treatment. Vet Clin N Am Exot Anim Pract 2001;4(2):441–61.

19. Woodburn DB, Miller AN, Allender MC, et al. *Emydomyces testavorans* , a new genus and species of onygenalean fungus isolated from shell lesions of freshwater aquatic turtles. J Clin Microbiol 2019;57(2):1–11.

20. Schmidt V. Fungal infections in reptiles —An emerging problem. J Exot Pet Med 2015;24:267–75.

21. Sun PL, Yang CK, Li WT, et al. Infection with *Nannizziopsis guarroi* and *Ophidiomyces ophiodiicola* in reptiles in Taiwan. Transbound Emerg Dis 2022;69(2): 764–75.

22. Gentry SL, Lorch JM, Lankton JS, et al. Koch's postulates: confirming *Nannizziopsis guarroi* as the cause of yellow fungal disease in *Pogona vitticeps*. Mycologia 2021;113(6):1253–63.

23. Davy CM, Shirose L, Campbell D, et al. Revisiting ophidiomycosis (snake fungal disease) after a decade of targeted research. Front Vet Sci 2021;8:1–10.

24. Wissman MA, Parsons B. Dermatophytosis of green iguanas (*Iguana iguana*). J Small Exot Anim Med 1993;2:133–6.

25. Van Waeyenberghe L, Baert K, Pasmans F, et al. Voriconazole, a safe alternative for treating infections caused by the *Chrysosporium anamorph* of *Nannizziopsis vriesii* in bearded dragons (*Pogona vitticeps*). Med Mycol 2010;48(6):880–5.

26. McEntire MS, Reinhart JM, Cox SK, et al. Single-dose pharmacokinetics of orally administered terbinafine in bearded dragons (*Pogona vitticeps*) and the antifungal susceptibility patterns of *Nannizziopsis guarroi*. Am J Vet Res 2022; 83(3):256–63.

27. Mashkour N, Jones K, Wirth W, et al. The concurrent detection of chelonid alphaherpesvirus 5 and *Chelonia mydas* papillomavirus 1 in tumoured and non-Tumoured green turtles. Animals 2021;11(697):697.

28. Ball I, Stöhr AC, Mathes K, et al. Ranavirus infections associated with skin lesions in lizards. Vet Res 2013;44(1):84.

29. Wytamma W, Schwarzkopf L, Lee F, et al. Ranaviruses and reptiles. PeerJ 2018;6: e6083.

30. Nevarez JG, Mitchell MA, Morgan T, et al. Association of West Nile virus with lymphohistiocytic proliferative cutaneous lesions in American alligators (*Alligator mississippiensis*) detected by RT-PCR. J Zoo Wildl Med 2008;(4):562–6.

31. Fitzgerald K, Vera R. Ascariasis. In: Mader D, editor. Reptile medicine and surgery. 2nd edition. Saunders: Elsevier; 2006;15(3). p. 720–38.

32. Chang L-W, Jacobson ER. Inclusion body disease, a worldwide infectious disease of boid snakes: a review. J Exot Pet Med 2010;19(3):216–25.

33. Amanatfard E, Reza MY, Barimani A. Human dermatitis caused by *Ophionyssus natricis*, a snake mite. Iran J Parasitol 2014;9(4):594–6.

34. Burridge MJ. Ticks (Acari: Ixodidae) spread by the international trade in reptiles and their potential roles in dissemination of diseases. Bull Entomol Res 2001; 91(1):3–23.

35. Mihalca AD. Ticks imported to Europe with exotic reptiles. Vet Parasitol 2015; 213(1–2):67–71.

36. Sánchez-Montes S, Isaak-Delgado AB, Guzmán-Cornejo C, et al. Rickettsia species in ticks that parasitize amphibians and reptiles: novel report from Mexico and review of the worldwide record. Ticks Tick Borne Dis 2019;10(5):987–94.

37. Mendoza-Roldan J, Ribeiro SR, Castilho-Onofrio V, et al. Mites and ticks of reptiles and amphibians in Brazil. Acta Tropica 2020;208:105515.

38. Kenny MJ, Shaw SE, Hillyard PD, et al. Ectoparasite and haemoparasite risks associated with imported exotic reptiles. Vet Rec 2004;154(14):434–5.

39. Gonzlez-Acua D, Beldomnico PM, Venzal JM, et al. Guglielmone. Reptile trade and the risk of exotic tick introductions into southern South American countries. Exp Appl Acarol 2005;35(4):335–9.

40. Barradas PF, Mesquita JR, Lima C, et al. Pathogenic rickettsia in ticks of spur-thighed tortoise (*Testudo graeca*) sold in a Qatar live animal market. Transbound Emerg Dis 2020;67(1):461–5.

41. Phipps LP, Hernandez-Triana L, Johnson N, et al. Importation of an exotic tick into the UK on a leopard tortoise. Vet Rec 2021;189(5):208–9.

42. Cooper JE. Dermatology. In: Mader D, editor. Reptile medicine and surgery. 2nd edition. Saunders: Elsevier; 2006;15(3):p. 196–216.

43. Mans C, Braun J. Update on common nutritional disorders of captive reptiles. Vet Clin North Am Exot Anim Pract 2014;17(3):369–95.

44. Alibardi L. Vitamin A administration in lizards during tail regeneration determines epithelial mucogenesis and delays muscle and cartilage differentiation. J Exp Zool B Mol Dev Evol 2020;334(1):59–71.

45. Boyer T. Hypovtaminosis A and hypervitaminosis A. In: Mader D, editor. Reptile medicine and surgery. 2nd edition. St. Louis, MO: Elsevier Saunders; 2006;15(3):p. 831–5.

46. Boykin KL, Mitchell MA. Evaluation of vitamin A gut loading in black soldier fly larvae (*Hermetia illucens*). Zoo Biol 2021;40(2):142–9.

47. Kirchgessner M, Mitchell MA. Chelonians. In: Mitchell MA, Tully TN, editors. Manual of exotic pet practice. St. Louis, MO: Saunders Elsevier; 2009;18(1): p. 207–49.

48. Acierno M, Mitchell MA, Roundtree M, et al. Evaluating the effect of ultraviolet B radiation on 1,25 hydroxyvitamin D levels in red-eared sliders (*Trachemys scripta elegans*). Am J Vet Res 2006;67(12):2046–9.

49. Acierno M, Mitchell MA, Roundtree M, et al. Effects of ultraviolet radiation on plasma 25-hydroxyvitamin D concentrations in corn snakes (*Elaphe guttata guttata*). Am J Vet Res 2006;69(2):294–7.

50. Gould A, Molitor L, Rockwell K, et al. Evaluating the physiologic effects of short duration ultraviolet B radiation exposure in leopard geckos (*Eublepharis macularius*). J Herpetol Med Surg 2018;28(1):34–9.

51. Hoskins A, Thompson D, Mitchell MA. Effects of artificial ultraviolet B radiation on plasma 25-hydroxyvitamin D3 concentrations in juvenile Blanding's turtles (*Emydoidea blandingii*). J Herpetol Med Surg 2022;32(3):225–9.

52. Watson MW, Mitchell MA. Vitamin D and ultraviolet B radiation considerations for exotic pets. J Exot Pet Med 2014;23(4):369–79.

53. Hannon DE, Garner MM, Reavill DR. Squamous cell carcinomas in inland bearded dragons (*Pogona vitticeps*). J Herpetol Med Surg 2011;21(4):101–6.

Amphibian Dermatology

Norin Chai, DVM, MSc, PhD, DECZM (Zoo Health Management)

KEYWORDS

- Amphibians • Skin disease • Dermatosepticemia • *Brucella* • *Ranavirus*
- Herpesvirus • Fungi • Ectoparasite

KEY POINTS

- Many of amphibian skin diseases are related to captive husbandry.
- Coinfections are frequent, and the most common clinical skin presentations include hyperemia, discoloration, dermal mass, ulceration, and necrosis.
- Severe symptoms and death are more due to the loss of homeostasis functions of the skin than to the infectious agents themselves.

INTRODUCTION

Amphibians are globally distributed except in the polar regions of Antarctica. There are three orders of amphibians: Anura, Caudata, and Gymnophiona. The AmphibiaWeb database currently contains 8483 amphibian species.[1] Dermatologic semiology is poorly specific in amphibians as many diseases may be expressed by an abnormal skin gross appearance. The integument is one of the most important organs in amphibians. It provides protection and mechanical and biological defense functions. It is also a sensory organ with mechanical and chemical sensitivity. It also plays critical roles in thermoregulation, fluid balance, respiration, transport of essential ions, and sex recognition. Thus, any skin lesion can impede these vital functions.[2] This review emphasizes the main conditions encountered in amphibian dermatology.

Clinical Anatomy and Physiology

The epidermis is relatively thin and limited to the *stratum corneum, central stratum spinosum*, and *stratum germinativum*.[3] Epithelial cells and chromatophores lie in the *stratum germinativum*. The dermis is largely composed of connective tissue formed by collagenous fibers in two layers: the spongious dermis (made of connective fibers, blood capillaries, and skin glands) and the compact dermis (made of large number of collagen fibers). Resident immune cells are spread over these layers. Mast cells play an important role in inflammatory and antiparasitic responses via degranulation of biologically active compounds, such as histamine. The presence of macrophages and lymphocytes in healthy skin tissue is not uncommon.[3] A unique feature to note

Yaboumba, 10 Boulevard de Picpus, Paris 75012, France
E-mail address: norin.chai@yaboumba.org

Vet Clin Exot Anim 26 (2023) 425–442
https://doi.org/10.1016/j.cvex.2023.01.001
1094-9194/23/© 2023 Elsevier Inc. All rights reserved.

vetexotic.theclinics.com

is the separation of spongious and compact dermis by the Eberth–Katschenko layer.[4] This noncellular layer is composed entirely of glycosaminoglycans and glycoconjugates, wherein hyaluronan and dermatan sulfate have been reported as the key constituents. Hyaluronan molecules are proposed to reduce water evaporation. Glands within the dermal layer include granular glands, mucosal glands, and small mixed glands. Some studies have demonstrated that electrical stimulation or chasing a frog for 5 to 10 minute stimulates the release of mucosal and granular gland contents.[5] In practice, long restrain may stimulate this release as well. Mucosal glands secrete mucus to maintain the moisture, permeability, and elasticity of the skin.[6] The mucus plays also a role in physical and chemical defense against pathogen invasion. The granular glands produce secretions containing amines, alkaloids, cardiotoxins, and peptides (especially antimicrobial peptides [AMPs]) which have antibacterial, antifungal, and cytolytic activities. These glands may secrete serous fluid, or toxic substances, and are also called serous or parotoid/venom glands. Frog skin is the most abundant natural source of AMPs found on earth.[7] A lack of AMPs on frog skin has been shown to be detrimental to adult *Xenopus laevis* defense against the fungal pathogen *Batrachochytrium dendrobatidis*.[8] Toxic alkaloid in the Dendrobatidae family is believed to originate largely from insects in the diet. They are primarily involved in predation avoidance and defense against microbes.[9] The shedding of epidermis in most amphibia is periodic, controlled by the thyroid and the pituitary gland. A single outer layer of cells of the *stratum corneum* separates nearly simultaneously over the whole body. Depending on the species and the environment, 2 hours to 10 days may be required for the shedding process. Molting is often swallowed by animals. Skin wound healing in amphibians has similar stages as with mammals, including hemostasis, inflammation, proliferation, and remodeling. However, the healed skin lacks patent mucous and granular glands and thus would not have the same physiologic capabilities as intact skin (see **Fig. 7**D). Many premetamorphic amphibian species are capable of regenerating complete limbs. This "epimorphic" regeneration ability is affected at metamorphosis.[10]

Clinical Notes Box

Clinical note 1: Restraint must always be done with wet gloves to protect both the handler from skin secretions and the animal from capture lesions.

Clinical note 2: The skin of amphibians is very permeable. This permeability also allows the administration of drugs (antibiotics, anesthetics, and so forth) through this route.

Clinical note 3: If skin vascular supply is impeded by trauma, infections, and tissue necrosis, wound healing will be impeded. Good wound care involves debridement, management of exudate, and treatment of underlying infection. Wet-to-dry bandages are not recommended.

Clinical Examination and Diagnostic Sampling

Many of the diseases observed in captive amphibians are related to husbandry issues. Proper examination of the husbandry practices and environment is completely part of the diagnosis process. The clinician should also know the specific requirements of the patient and its normal phenotype. Body posture, responses to stimuli, shedding (**Fig. 1**A), including gular and pulmonary movements, skin texture (**Fig. 1**B), and hydration status are evaluated. The close examination is performed with gloves and the animal in a damp tissue (**Fig. 1**C). Gentle impression smears and skin scrape can be made on skin lesion (**Fig. 1**D–F). Samples should be evaluated immediately before desiccation and stained after for cytology. A Gram stain and acid-fast stain are

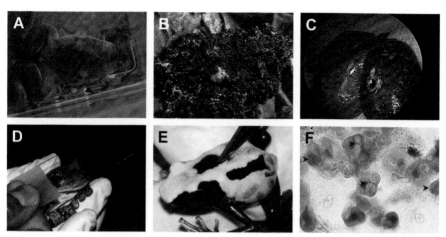

Fig. 1. (*A*) Over shedding in a *X laevis*. (*B*) Isolated ulcer in a *Theloderma corticale*. (*C*) Evaluation with the use of magnification tools and light source. We can see here different stages of ulcers on a *X laevis*. (*D*) Impression smears on the rostrum of a milk frog (*Trachycephalus resinifictrix*). (*E*) Skin scrape are performed moderately with the blunt edge of a scalpel blade, here on a *Dendrobates tinctorius*. (*F*) A skin scraping from of a tomato frog with chytridiomycosis, after immersion in lactophenol blue. Many zoosporangia are easily seen (*arrows*). (*Courtesy of* Norin Chai, France, with permission.)

indicated if fungi or bacteria and atypical mycobacteria infections are suspected. However, results must be interpreted with cautious as they may reflect secondary colonization by ubiquitous organisms. Biopsy samples are collected on anesthetized animal and submitted for cultures and histopathology. The clinician is encouraged to refer to several reviews on anesthesia and soft tissues surgery techniques in amphibians.[11,12]

Bacterial Infections

Clinical signs seem rapidly and associated with weakness, anorexia, edema, ascites, skin discoloration (**Fig. 2**A), petechiae, and hemorrhagic skin ulcers. Most causing agents are common environmental bacteria including Gram-negative bacteria such as *Aeromonas* spp, *Pseudomonas* spp, *Proteus* spp, and *Escherichia coli* that are routinely cultured from otherwise healthy captive amphibians.[13] Immunosuppression and skin disruption caused by viral or fungal infection, poor husbandry, and toxic and traumatic environment will allow the bacteria to overgrow and cause disease; thus, the original pathogen may often be difficult to detect. Ubiquitous bacteria can invade tissues from the environment or the normal gut in 1 to 3 hours after a primary infection or skin trauma has occur.[14] An infected amphibian may be an infectious source for others. Selected bacterial infections are summarized in **Table 1**.

Bacterial Dermatosepticemia

The constant erythema symptoms gave birth to the term "red-leg disease," although "bacterial dermatosepticemia" is more appropriated as many other noninfectious diseases may cause ventral erythema. *Aeromonas hydrophila* is frequently isolated in these cases, but many other bacteria have been implicated. Bacterial dermatosepticemia is acute to peracute systemic bacterial infection (**Fig. 2**B, C). The pathogenesis is close to disseminated intravascular coagulation in mammals.[13] In general, death,

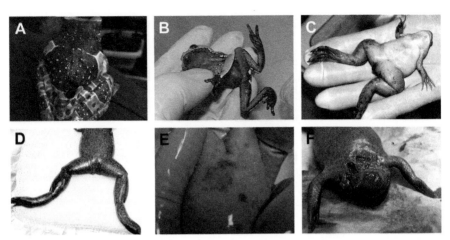

Fig. 2. (*A*) Discoloration due to non-mycobacterial bacterial dermatitis in a *T resinifictrix*. Skin discoloration is often a sign of bacterial dermatitis. The skin may take on a gray, brown, or black color. The infection becomes systemic after several weeks of evolution. (*B*) Bacterial dermatosepticemia on a *P bicolor* and on a *X laevis* (*C*). Some lesions of mycobacteriosis in *Xenopus* spp with subcutaneous hemorrhages on a hind leg very similar to a "Red legs" (*D*), disseminate erythema (*E*), and typical mycobacterial granuloma on the lower mandible (*F*). (*Courtesy of* Norin Chai, France, with permission.)

due to both sepsis and impedance of the skin vital functions (especially osmotic imbalance), follows ecchymosis and convulsions. Generalized congestion is observed at necropsy. Samples are taken as quickly for culture and identification. The histological lesions encountered are multiple areas of necrosis and coagulation with clusters of bacteria. In facilities, the main treatment involves isolation of the affected animals and improvement of the environmental conditions. Treatment will start with fluid therapy by soaking the animal in a shallow layer of well-oxygenated, chlorine-free water that is at the species-specific preferred body temperature.[13] A good fluid choice is the isotonic amphibian Ringer's solution (6.6 g NaCl, 0.15 g KCl, 0.15 g $CaCl_2$, and 0.2 g $NaHCO_3$ mixed thoroughly in 1 L distilled water). Antibiotics treatment will be started after establishing an antibiogram. Amphibian formulary and routes of delivery may be found elsewhere.[15]

Mycobacteriosis

Many species of commensal and saprophytic mycobacteria have been isolated from amphibians. These organisms determine a chronic granulomatous infection that can potentially extend to all internal organs.[16] Most mycobacterial infections are subclinic and chronic, but epizootic outbreaks in zoos and facilities are not uncommon.[16] A recent publication described die-off captive frogs in a zoo involving a new strain of *Mycobacterium marinum*, where clinical signs included nonhealing proliferative and ulcerative skin lesions, cloacal prolapse, hind limb weakness, weight loss, and sudden death.[17] The skin is almost always affected (**Fig. 2**D–F). Histologically, granulomas contain acid-fast bacilli highlighted by specific staining (Ziehl–Neelsen) are evident. Mycobacteria species identification requires molecular techniques (polymerase chain reaction [PCR]), in particular 16S RNA.[16] Any weight loss or decrease in performance must be thought of as mycobacteriosis.[16,18] An effective treatment has not been reported in amphibians, and eradication strategies have typically included depopulation and repopulation; however, the investigators have described a method for saving

Table 1
Selected bacterial diseases

Bacteria	Species Affected and Skin Symptoms	Management
Bacterial dermosepticemia *Aeromonas* sp, *Citrobacter* sp, *Salmonella* sp, *Proteus* sp, *Flavobacterium* sp, *Pseudomonas* sp, *Escherichia coli* *Staphylococcus* sp, *Streptococcus* sp, *Enterococcus* sp	Most species Erythema and/or white or pale-colored skin progress into large subcutaneous hemorrhages. Edema, ulceration, tissue lysis (generalized or localized to extremities), necrosis, and over sloughing.	Sick animals are isolated. Samples for culture and sensitivity. Targeted antibiotics concurrent with an antifungal drug. Supportive care. Improve husbandry.
Mycobacteriosis *Mycobacterium abscessus, M chelonae, M fortuitum, M marinum, M xenopi, M gordonae, M szulgai, M liflandii, M ranae, M thamnospheos, M xenopi*	Observed in various species. Petechiation, subcutaneous hemorrhages, erosions, nodules, abscesses, nodules, tubercles, or just dots of different sizes.	No widely accepted treatments.
Chlamydiosis *Chlamydophila pneumoniae*	Giant barred frog (*Mixophyes iteratus*) Petechiation, sloughing of skin, ulcers, and cutaneous depigmentation.	Diagnosis with cell culture, histology, and PCR testing. Oral administration of tetracycline-class antibiotics.
Atypical Brucella *B inopinata* BO1 and *Brucella-like* BO2	Red-eyed tree frog (*Agalychnis callidryas*) Hind leg abscess Big-eyed tree frog (*Leptopelis vermiculatus*) Subcutaneous abscesses White's tree frog (*Litoria caerulea*) Fluid-filled skin on the lower back. Waxy tree frogs (*P sauvagii*) Discoloration, subcutaneous mass.	Surgical debridement, targeted antibiotics after antibiotic susceptibility. The lesions were drained and treated with enrofloxacin but required a second drainage before resolution. Enrofloxacin 10 mg/kg im sid q 30 d, soaking in amphibian Ringer solution, oxygenation (5 L/min) for 15 min q 48 h.

valuable strains from a *Mycobacterium liflandii* infection in a population of *Silurana tropicalis*.[18]

Chlamydiosis

Beside cutaneous signs (see **Table 1**), a recent complete overview of amphibian chlamydiosis showed the presence of a granulomatous inflammatory process commonly affecting liver, spleen, and kidney.[19] However, in some cases, there are no signs of inflammation associated with infection.[19,20] In a die-off of anurans in Switzerland, *Chlamydia* spp has been isolated, proof that amphibians can carry and spread the bacteria. However, the absence of histopathologic lesions and the low number of positive samples rather indicate that this mass mortality was caused by something else.[20] Still, there are reports where *Chlamydia pneumoniae* has induced skin disease in anurans.[21]

Brucellosis

Atypical *Brucella* may induce localized infection in several frog species with skin and soft tissue abscesses, panophthalmitis, spinal arthropathy, swollen paravertebral ganglia, and involvement of several internal organs (systemic disease).[22,23] These "atypical" isolates differ from classical *Brucella* by host tropism, phenotypic traits, or phylogenetic distance.[23] *Brucella* isolates obtained from amphibians are most closely related to *Brucella inopinata* BO1 and *Brucella*-like BO2 strains based on results from multilocus sequence analyses.[22] If some isolates may cause high mortality, others have been isolated from clinically normal frogs suggesting that they are either commensal organisms or these animals were subclinical carriers. In a series of cases of atypical *Brucella* in captive Australian green tree frogs (*Litoria caerulea*), *Brucella* organisms were cultured from cloacal swabs mostly and skin swabs were consistently negative.[23] In another series of cases of atypical *Brucella* in captive Waxy tree frogs (*Phyllomedusa sauvagii*), a single swab of the skin and cloaca identified *Brucella* strain oaks.[24] Cases of atypical brucellosis with skin lesions are described in **Table 1**.[22–24]

Clinical Note for Bacterial Infections

With signs of septicemia, the animal is isolated and individually monitored. An immediate evaluation of the husbandry should be performed. Ulcers and abscesses respond well to surgery and appropriate antibiotic therapy, both topical and parenteral. Antimicrobial therapy should target Gram-negative bacteria, although *B dendrobatidis* as mixed infection is common.

Viral Infections

Ranavirus

Ranavirus is a genus of double-stranded DNA viruses of the family Iridoviridae. Three species of *Ranavirus* are known to infect amphibians: *Ambystoma tigrinum* virus, common midwife toad virus, and frog virus 3 (FV3).[25] To date, almost half of the research on ranaviruses (44%) focused on the FV3 lineage.[25] Arenavirus has been recognized as responsible of die-offs in numerous amphibian species and has been found in at least 105 species in 18 families of amphibians worldwide.[26] In captivity, high host density, elevated viral titers, and stress induced from unsanitary conditions definitively increase adult mortality.[27] However, deaths may be due to individuals succumbing to secondary invaders (bacterial and fungal) rather than to the primary virus. Systemic hemorrhage and cellular necrosis often result in organ failure within only a few days to 2 to 3 weeks of exposure. Although asymptomatic infections may occur, clinical signs include erratic swimming, lethargy, buoyancy problems, anorexia, swelling of the legs and body, and death.[26,27] Skin lesions are listed in **Table 2**.[13,26,27] *Ranavirus* infection is listed as "Notifiable Pathogen" by the World Organization for Animal Health. Antemortem samples may be screened for *Ranavirus* using conventional PCR (cPCR) and quantitative PCR (qPCR). Histopathology will show characteristic basophilic intracytoplasmic inclusion bodies.

Herpesvirus

Herpesviruses are large double-stranded DNA viruses that can infect a wide range of hosts. All known amphibian herpesviruses are in the genus *Batrachovirus*. Until recently, only two batrachoviruses were known: ranid herpesvirus 1 (RaHV-1), the etiologic agent of the Lucké adenocarcinoma of leopard frogs (*Lithobates pipiens*) and RaHV-2, isolated from the urine of a tumor-bearing frog (adenocarcinoma). In 1994, a herpesvirus-associated proliferative skin disease was identified in *Rana dalmatina* in Italy.[28] In 2015 and 2017, two new batrachoviruses inducing obvious skin lesions

Table 2
Selected viral diseases

Virus	Species Affected and Skin Symptoms	Management
Ranaviruses	Amphibians worldwide. Irregular patches of discoloration, necrotizing and ulcerative dermatitis, and erythematous skin particularly around the mouth or base of the hindlimbs. Hemorrhages and swellings are the most common gross lesions noted in the larvae, cutaneous erosions and ulcerations are more frequently seen in adult anurans in Europe and adult caudates in North America. In experimentally challenged tiger salamanders (*A tigrinum*) lesions with white polypoid that would cover in time nearly 90% of the body have been described.	PCR testing. Supportive care and control of secondary bacterial infection. Quarantine of infected animals is recommended.
Ranid herpesvirus 3 (RaHV3)	Spring frog (*R dalmatina*) and common frog (*R temporaria*) Dermal edema, proliferative dermatitis characterized by epidermal hyperplasia with prominent, multifocal, firm skin patches ranging from 1 to 3 mm diameter. Lesions extend from over the dorsal and ventral aspects of the body to both flanks.	Intranuclear inclusions. Diagnosis is through light and electron microscopy and PCR
Bufonid herpesvirus 1	Common toad (*B bufo*) Abnormal skin shedding, multifocal raised, dark brown, patchy areas scattered over the dorsum.	Virus detected by histology, electron microscopy and PCR.

have been discovered in Switzerland: RaHV-3 in free-ranging common frogs (*Rana temporaria*) and bufonid herpesvirus 1 in free-ranging common toads (*Bufo bufo*), respectively.[29,30] An RHV3-specific PCR assay was carried out afterward and suggests that the herpesvirus strains that infected *R dalmatina* in Italy in 1994 and *R temporaria* in Switzerland in 2015 are very closely related viruses.[29] They seem also to have common pathogenetic pathways and the lesions induced are very similar.[29] All the lesions described for these viruses are summarized in **Table 2**.

Clinical Note for Viral Diseases

Diagnostic of a viral disease includes PCR testing, transmission electron microscopy, and virus isolation. To date, there is no reliable treatment for these infections and a quarantine of infected animals is recommended. As most of the cases are presented with mixed infections, treatment for secondary invaders may limit the severity of the disease.

Fungal Infections

Mycosis often reveals a state of immunosuppression (intercurrent disease, poor maintenance conditions, and so forth). Except for chytridiomycosis, fungal infections are rarely encountered if an amphibian's husbandry is appropriate. Skin injuries promote the development of mycosis.

Chytridiomycosis

Amphibian chytridiomycosis is a fungal disease caused by *B dendrobatidis* (*Bd*) and *Batrachochytrium salamandrivorans* (*Bs*) (Chytridiomycota, Rhizophydiales). In the past decade, *Bd* has been the most studied amphibian pathogens; an extended review on Amphibian chytridiomycosis has been recently published.[31] For diagnosis, cPCR and qPCR are routinely done on skin swabs from mouthparts of live anuran larvae and from the ventral pelvic patch, hind legs, and feet of live postmetamorphic, freshly dead, frozen or ethanol-preserved post-metamorphic amphibians. **Table 3** summarizes the main skin lesions and proposes selected treatments. Newly acquired animals should be maintained in quarantine in separate containers for at least 2 months and skin swabs should be collected for PCR assay on arrival and 7 weeks later. A thorough necropsy including PCR (ideally qPCR) on the appropriate tissues must be performed on any animals that die.

Other Fungal Infections

There are many other pathogenic fungal skin diseases in amphibians. Selected fungal infections are summarized in **Table 3**.[13–15,31–33]

Saprolegnia is a ubiquitous saprophyte of aquatic amphibians. It develops on the skin (**Fig. 3**A, B) and gills, usually on preexisting lesions (**Fig. 3**C). Diagnosis is based on skin sampling and direct observation (characteristic hyphae on wet mounts).[13] A report described saprolegniasis in a Chinese Giant Salamander (*Andrias davidianus*) with lesions that resolved spontaneously without treatment but with improvement of the husbandry.[32]

Infestation with *Mucor amphibiorum* is highly pathogenic even in an immunocompetent individual. Contamination occurs through ingestion. This endemic Australian zygomycete has been associated with disease in wild species in Australia and captive populations in Europe, causing disseminated granulomatous disease and fatal ulcerative mycosis. Diagnosis is based on histology and culture. No treatment has been described.

Infestation with *Basidiobolus ranarum* has been reported in dwarf African clawed frogs (*Hymenochirus curtipes*), Canadian toads (*Bufo hemiophrys*) and Wyoming toads (*Bufo baxteri*). Affected toads had darkened dorsal skin, ventral hyperemia, and increased shedding, with death occurring 5 to 7 days after the onset of clinical signs.[2]

Chromomycosis are infections caused by several taxa of pigmented fungi with skin lesions or more commonly, systemic granulomatous lesions within visceral organs. The animal slowly dies in several months. Contamination occurs by ingestion or through a skin wound. It is a zoonotic agent so euthanasia is recommended.[13]

Several mesomycetozoeans, fungal-like organisms, are pathogenic for amphibians, mainly *Amphibiocystidium*, *Amphibiothecum* (Dermocystida), and *Ichthyophonus* (Ichthyophonida). Dermocystids are now recognized as two distinct genera, *Amphibiothecum* (previously *Dermosporidium*) and *Amphibiocystidium*.[13,33] Diagnosis is based on histopathology or finding characteristic spores through microscopic examination of material from the lesions.

Table 3
Selected fungi diseases

Fungi	Species Affected and Skin Symptoms	Management
Chytridiomycosis *B dendrobatidis* (Bd) *B salamandrivorans* (Bs)	*Bd* infects anurans, urodeles, and caecilians. *Bs* seems restricted to salamanders and newts. Skin lesions: roughness, erythema, hyperplasia, small skin ulcers, excessive shedding, and necrosis of digits/feet. In anuran larvae, clinical signs are generally limited to depigmentation of the mouthparts. *Bs* infection induces multifocal superficial erosions and extensive epidermal ulcerations, excessive shedding of the skin.	Supportive care and treatment with itraconazole: 0.005% (50 mg/L) bath, 5 min/d for 10 d (most situations); 0.01% bath, 30 min/d for 11 d (terrestrial African caecilians).
Saprolegniasis *Saprolegnia* sp	Aquatic frogs and tadpoles and Salamander species, Caecilians. Erythematous or ulcerated skin with fluffy or cotton-like texture. Mild inflammatory response.	Improve husbandry. Bath treatment with itraconazole, benzalkonium chloride. Isolated lesions respond to topical miconazole, dilute benzalkonium chloride, potassium permanganate.
Mucor sp	Reported in Anuran species Lethargy and multifocal hyperemic nodules with visible fungal growth particularly on the ventral integument. Systemic infection with nodules and granulomas in a variety of internal organs. Progressive weight loss. Death.	Cytology on smears, histology, culture. To date, no successful treatment.
B ranarum	Reported in Wyoming toad (*B baxteri*). Ventral epithelial, erythema and sloughing, and toe ulcerations.	Diagnosis is based on culture and histology. Treatment based on benzalkonium chloride and itraconazole. Copper, malachite green, and formalin are not effective.
Chromomycosis *Phialophora* sp, *Fonsecaea* sp, *Rhinocladiella* sp, *Cladosporium* sp	Various wild and captive anurans. Cutaneous clinical forms: swelling, dermal papules, nodules and ulcers, or granulomas of the skin, sometimes with gray to black pigmentation.	Cytology on smears, histology (pigmented hyphae), and culture. Treatment generally unsuccessful. Euthanasia is recommended. On a in a cane toad (*Bufo marinus*), a combination of electrosurgery and 5 mg/kg oral itraconazole given every 48 h for 30 d showed resolution at 2 y after treatment.
Mesomycetozoans *Amphibiothecum* sp (formerly *Dermosporidium* sp), *A* sp, and *Ichthyophonus* sp	Various anurans species. Dermal nodules filled with spores typically located in the ventral dermis in general. It may heal within 4–8 wk.	Standard supportive care.

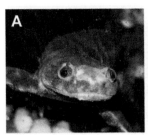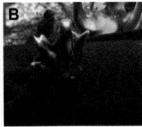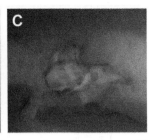

Fig. 3. Saprolegniasis on a *Paramesotriton* spp (A) and the foreleg of an *A mexicanum* (B). (C) Fungal infection on an *A mexicanum* after a trauma. (*Courtesy of* Norin Chai, France, with permission.)

Clinical Note for Fungal Infections

Fungal infections can look grossly like bacterial infections, so culture and cytology are recommended. In house cytologic examination of stained or unstained skin smears and skin fragments for the detection of zoosporangia provides rapid diagnosis while waiting for PCR testing results. Specific treatment is associated with supportive care and husbandry improvement.

Parasitic Infections

Amphibians host a wide array of protists (flagellata, amebae, sporozoans, and ciliates) and macroparasites (eg, helminths, arthropods, and leeches). Selected parasitic infections are summarized in **Table 4**.[13,14,34]

Trichodina spp are ciliated protozoa considered to be nonpathogenic ectocommensal of amphibians, fish, and invertebrates. These organisms become pathogenic if they are present in large populations on the skin or gills and usually indicate poor husbandry, overcrowding, or another disease process. Skin infections can be diagnosed by lesional skin scrapes. Gill infections can be diagnosed via wet mount of gill tissue or a gill biopsy.[34] *Epistylis* spp are freshwater protozoan parasites primarily described as ectoparasites of fish. The presence of *Epistylis* infection is a strong indicator of poor water quality with a high organic load. In these cases, *Epistylis* may cause in aquatic amphibians, skin ulcers, and discoloration.[35] These parasitic infestations predispose to secondary bacterial or fungal infections.

Ciliates, opalinids, and flagellates are commonly found on the skin of amphibians, and most of these organisms are commensal and nonproblematic. Flagellates such as the dinoflagellate genera *Piscinoodinium* or the flagellate *Ichthyoboda* may cause serious skin or gill lesions if present in high numbers.[14,35]

Microsporidial septicemia with ulcerative dermatitis has been described in a giant tree frog (*Phyllomedusa bicolor*). The animal presented a progressive ulcerative erythematous dermatitis on the dorsal skin lateral to the vertebral column and on the left hind leg. Tissue imprints revealed a mass of microsporidial spores. Chloramphenicol sodium succinate (5–10 mg/kg ICe) for 18 days in combination with topical oxytetracycline hydrochloride and polymyxin B for 21 days led to healing of the lesions.[36]

A recent paper describes an acute mortality in Tiger salamander (*Ambystoma californiense*) and long-toed salamander (*Ambystoma macrodactylum croceum*) caused by *Ribeiroia ondatrae* a digenetic trematode.[37] *R ondatrae* is mostly known causing malformations in a wide range of amphibians. In this die-off, gross lesions were restricted to the integument. The disease is characterized by a severe metacercarial infection, leading to a granulocytic inflammation with skin erosions, ulcers, and necrosis.[37]

Table 4
Selected parasitic diseases

Parasites	Species Affected and Skin Symptoms	Signs and Comments
Ciliated protozoa Trichodinads Trichodina xenopodus, T uricola, T pediculus, T fultoni	Aquatic amphibians. Ulcerative skin lesions, discoloration, excessive cutaneous mucus production, and reddened gills. Frogs with skin infestations may be observed rubbing against solid objects in an attempt to dislodge the parasites.	Immersion of the animal in a saltwater bath. For frogs, immersion in a sodium chloride bath (10–25 g/L for 5–30 min or 4–6 g/L for 24 h) has been reported to kill the parasite successfully. Immersion in distilled water for 2–3 h may be effective.
Flagellates Piscinoodinium or Ichthyobodo	Aquatic amphibians Lesions are always external, ranging from a fuzzy, dusty appearance to gray discoloration on the skin and gills that may progress to with dense white dusting of the skin.	Diagnosis with skin scraping Prognosis is guarded. Regular water changes are essential. Baths of malachite Green or diluted formalin may be prescribed. Metronidazole is effective when administered orally.
Trematodes R ondatrae	Salamanders. Skin discoloration, dermal erosions and ulcers with crust formation.	No treatment described. Death due to numerous invading cercariae, which penetrated the epidermis and then encysted as metacercariae, leading to dermal disruption and secondary septicemia or metabolic imbalances.
Nematodes Pseudocapillaroides xenopi	Epidermis of Xenopus sp sloughing of the epidermis, erythema, ulcers, and death.	Topical ivermectin, alternated monthly with oral fenbendazole
Leeches Larvae of trombiculid mites ("chiggers") Amblyomma ticks	Anurans, salamanders Skin with focal congestion and hemorrhage	Scrapings or biopsies of the lesions show the presence of parasites. Manual removal (if possible). Treatment for external leeches: hypertonic saline bath Treatment for chiggers: long-term oral or topical ivermectin
Copepods L cyprinacea	Various amphibian species Protrusion of thread-like Y-shaped projections on the gills, ventrum, front limbs, all the body (consistent with embedded, gravid female Lernaea sp)	Under anesthesia, remove the anchor worms using micro forceps by gripping the anchor worm near the epidermis or gill filaments. Follow-up treatment: immersion bath of lufenuron at 0.1 mg/L, repeated once a week for 5 wk, with complete water changes every 7 d to coincide with fresh immersion baths. Ivermectin baths (10 mg/L for 60 min) also seem to be effective.

The diverse species of nematodes are the most represented helminths in amphibians. Some genera are well known for causing integument diseases. *Pseudocapillaroides xenopi* and *Dracunculus* spp are a group of subcutaneous parasitic nematodes. Studies have shown that tadpoles are experimentally susceptible to infection with *Dracunculus insignis*, *Dracunculus ophidensis*, and *D medinensis*.[38] Filariae can infest tissues, blood, and lymph vessels, and microfilariae can kill debilitated amphibians.

Leeches are rarely a problem of the established amphibian but may sometimes be seen in freshly imported or otherwise wild-caught specimens.[13] Trombiculid mites are occasionally encountered in terrestrial anurans and salamanders.

Anchor worms (*Lernaea cyprinacea*) are parasitic copepod crustaceans that have been reported in various amphibian species (**Fig. 4**A, B). A recent paper describes an epizootic infestation in axolotls occurred in commercially bred animals contaminated by goldfish (*Carassius auratus*).[39]

Skin Neoplasia and Hyperplasia

In the author experience, skin tumors are common in captive amphibians, but reports of neoplasia are relatively rare when compared with other classes of animals. A comprehensive review on amphibian neoplasia may be found elsewhere.[40] Potential causes may include an infectious etiology, such as herpesvirus, toxic etiologies, traumatic or environmental irritant etiologies, such as water conditioners and cleaners or ultraviolet radiation, or genetic predisposition,[13,40] although usually the cause is unknown. One recent paper describes squamous cell carcinoma in a group of Solomon Island leaf frogs (*Ceratobatrachus guentheri*) in which despite all the exhaustive investigations, no specific etiology could be identified.[41] The diagnosis is confirmed with histopathology, and management attempts include surgical excision or debulking after evaluation of the mass by radiographic and ultrasonic examination. For more information, the clinician may refer to a review on soft tissue surgery in Amphibians.[12] Cryosurgery, radiosurgery, and diode laser surgery may be used in amphibians. When possible, complete surgical excision is usually curative as metastasis seems to be uncommon.[13] Examples of neoplasia surgical excision may include debulking surgery of a mandibular hyperplasia in an African clawed frog (*X laevis*), complete excision of a

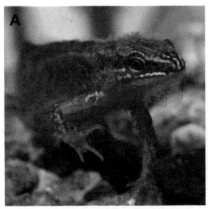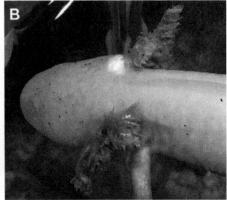

Fig. 4. (*A*) Massive anchor worms (*L cyprinacea*) infestation in wild palmate newt (*Lissotriton helveticus*) and (*B*) in an *A mexicanum*. (*Courtesy of* Yves Thonnerieux (*A*) and Norin Chai (*B*), France, with permission.)

pedicled lobular capillary hemangioma-like in an axolotl (*Ambystoma mexicanum*) by radiosurgery and excision of a dermal fibroma in a Riobamba marsupial frog (*Gastrotheca riobambae*).[12]

Traumatic Injuries

Rostral trauma against walls (**Fig. 5**A, C, and E), rough substrate and furniture (woods, sharp rocks) (**Fig. 5**B), and cage-mate aggression (especially during the breeding season) (**Fig. 5**D) are sources of injuries. Rostral abrasions are entry points for infectious agents (see **Fig. 5**C); wound treatment should be started as soon as possible. Healing is slow. Treatment includes gentle lavage and debridement with sterile 0.9% saline solution and application of topical agents, such as silver sulfadiazine or benzalkonium chloride. Anecdotal reports indicate that the use of silver nitrate rod application (**Fig. 6**A, B), electric (**Fig. 6**C, D) or chemical cauterization with formulation that contains policresulen (Lotagen) can be successful. Other formulations may be interesting to use: one with 2-octyl cyanoacrylate (Orabase), one with carboxymethyl glucose sulfate polymers (Dermapliq), and the one with becaplermin (Regranex Gel). The use of cold laser therapy has not been reported in the literature, but may hold promise for managing amphibian skin wounds (**Fig. 7**A–D). Antibiotic ointment, with an antifungal (miconazole or ketoconazole), may be applied. Ophthalmic ointments are often successfully used by the author. Antibiotics are warranted for large, nonhealing or infected wounds. However, in all cases, the husbandry will be improved and the origin of stress must be identified.

Environmental Conditions

Amphibians' physiology is heavily influenced by the environment. Anthropogenic factors, such as pesticides, impair immunity and can reduce chemical skin defenses. In some instances, the chemicals exert a direct effect on the skin epidermal cells.[4] High levels of chlorine and ammonia are commonly implicated in the deaths of amphibians.[13] Signs of chemical exposure can include disseminated or contact erythema, skin hyperplasia, petechiation, increased mucus production, cutaneous ulceration,

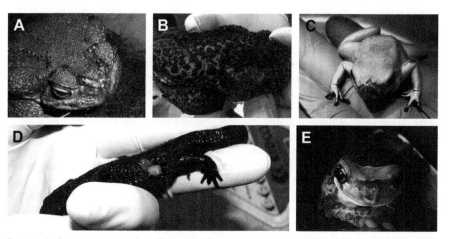

Fig. 5. Injuries against rough rocks in a *Bufo paracnemis* presented with rostral (*A*) and side (*B*) abrasion. Vesicle on a rostral abrasion in a *Phyllobates terribilis* (*C*). Cage-mate aggression on a *Paramesotrition* sp (*D*). A deep rostral abrasion in a *T resinifictrix* (*E*). (*Courtesy of* Norin Chai, France, with permission.)

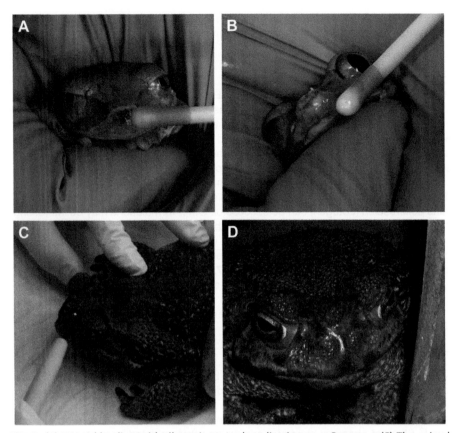

Fig. 6. (*A*) Wound healing with silver nitrate rod application on a *Rana* spp. (*B*) The animal just after application. It is a good method of cauterization on noninfectious wounds. (*C*) Electric cauterization of the animal on **Fig. 5**A. (*D*) The animal, on week after. Topical benzalkonium chloride has also been applied. (*Courtesy of* Norin Chai, France, with permission.)

excessive agitation, lethargy, convulsions, flaccid paralysis, avoidance, postural, or escape behaviors.[13,14] A level above 0.2 parts per million (ppm) is suspicious for a diagnosis of ammonia toxicosis, and a level above 1 ppm should consider ammonia as one etiology for clinical signs. A complete water change is the best therapy for ammonia intoxication.[13] The diagnosis is confirmed by physico-chemical measurements. Treatment of dermatologic irritation involves removing the animal to a clean enclosure and providing supportive therapy.

Overexposure to UV-B radiation results in damage to the epidermal layer of larval and adult frogs. Skin damage is characterized by epidermal shedding and sore formation. It is suggested that UV radiation breaches the skin barrier and induces host immunosuppression, causing the frog to be more susceptible to both pathogen invasion and exposure to chemical contaminants.[42]

Inappropriate water sources, water quality or temperature, are common causes of dehydration. Signs of severe dehydration in amphibians include a dry or wrinkled appearance to the skin, dark coloration, sunken eyes, and dry mucus in the mouth. Rehydration is accomplished by placing the animal in a shallow layer of well-oxygenated, chlorine-free water.

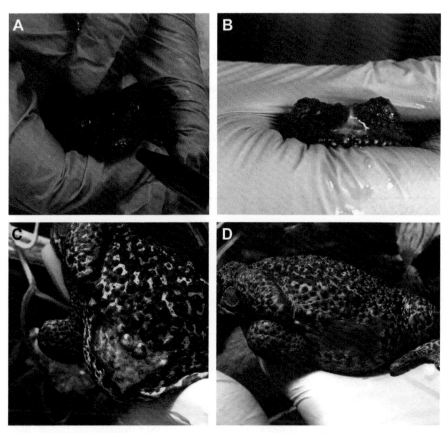

Fig. 7. (A) Cold laser therapy on rostral abrasion in a *T corticale*. (B) The same animal 1 month later. (C) The animal of **Fig. 5**B, 1 day one laser therapy session (D). The animal, 1 month later. In both cases, topical benzalkonium chloride has also been applied. The parameters of the sessions were: Wavelength: 660, 800, 970; Mode: continuous, pulsed; Power: 0.8 W; Duration: 1′36″; Energy: 77 J; Surface treated: 4 cm²; Irradiance: 0.2 W/cm²; Fluency: 19.25 J/cm². (*Courtesy of* Norin Chai, France, with permission.)

SUMMARY

The specificity of dermatologic semiology in Amphibians is relatively low as all inflammation and/or infections may be expressed by a skin lesion. For instance, excess vitamin D and calcium supplementation or kidney damage may lead to a dermatitis by mineralization of the basement membrane. The author has seen skin discoloration with hepatitis and digestive neoplasia in *Litoria* sp and *Trachycephalus* sp Amphibian dermatology should be considered more as internal medicine than an isolated discipline.

CLINICS CARE POINTS

- As the skin of amphibians is very permeable, most of drugs (antibiotics, anesthetics, and so forth) may be administrated pour on.

- Antimicrobial therapy should take into account that mixed infection with Gram-negative bacteria and *B dendrobatidis* are common.
- Ulcers and abscesses respond well to surgery and appropriate antibiotic therapy, both topical and parenteral.
- Complete surgical tumor excision is usually curative as metastasis seems to be uncommon.
- Clinicians should not hesitate to use ophthalmic ointments, cold laser therapy for managing amphibian skin wounds.
- Rehydration is best accomplished by placing the animal in a shallow layer of well-oxygenated, chlorine-free water.
- A complete water change with supportive care is the best therapy for environmental intoxication.

DISCLOSURE

The author has nothing to disclose.

ACKNOWLEDGMENTS

The authors specially thank Mr Yves Thonnerieux for his kind authorization to use his picture.

REFERENCES

1. AmphibiaWeb: Information on amphibian biology and conservation. Berkeley, California: Available at: http://amphibiaweb.org. Accessed June 24, 2022.
2. Pessier AP. An overview of amphibian skin disease. Semin Avian Exot Pet Med 2002;11:162–74.
3. Haslam IS, Roubos EW, Mangoni ML, et al. From frog integument to human skin: dermatological perspectives from frog skin biology. Biol Rev 2014;89:618–55.
4. Varga JFA, Bui-Marinos MP, Katzenback BA. Frog Skin Innate Immune Defences: Sensing and Surviving Pathogens. Front Immunol 2019;9:3128.
5. Brunetti AE, Hermida GN, Iurman MG, et al. Odorous secretions in anurans: morphological and functional assessment of serous glands as a source of volatile compounds in the skin of the treefrog *Hypsiboas pulchellus* (Amphibia: Anura: Hylidae). J Anat 2016;228:430–42.
6. Larsen EH, Ramløv H. Role of cutaneous surface fluid in frog osmoregulation. Comp Biochem Physiol 2013;165:365–70.
7. Ladram A, Nicolas P. Antimicrobial peptides from frog skin: biodiversity and therapeutic promises. Front Biosci 2016;21:1341–71.
8. Ramsey JP, Reinert LK, Harper LK, et al. Immune defences against *Batrachochytrium dendrobatidis*, a fungus linked to global amphibian declines, in the South African clawed frog, *Xenopus laevis*. Infect Immun 2010;78:3981–92.
9. Hovey KJ, Seiter EM, Johnson EE, et al. Sequestered alkaloid defences in the *Dendrobatid* poison frog oophaga pumilio provide variable protection from microbial pathogens. J Chem Ecol 2018;44:312–25.
10. Yannas IV, Colt J, Wai YC. Wound contraction and scar synthesis during development of the amphibian *Rana catesbeiana*. Wound Repair Regen 1996;4:31–41.
11. Sladakovic I, Divers SJ. Amphibian Anesthesia. In: Divers SJ, Stahl SJ, editors. Mader's reptile and Amphibian. Medicine and surgery1509, 3rd Editions. St Louis, Missouri: Elsevier Saunders; 2019. p. 480–5.

12. Chai N. Surgery in Amphibians. Vet Clin Exot Anim 2016;19(1):77–95.
13. Whitaker BR, Wright KM. Amphibian medicine. In: Divers SJ, Stahl SJ, editors. Mader's reptile and Amphibian. Medicine and surgery. 3rd Editions. St Louis, Missouri: Elsevier Saunders; 2019. p. 992–1013.
14. Poll CP. Wound Management in Amphibians: Etiology and Treatment of Cutaneous Lesions. J Exot Pet Med 2009;18(1):20–35.
15. Whitaker BR, McDermott CT. Amphibian Formulary. In: Divers SJ, Stahl SJ, editors. Mader's reptile and Amphibian. Medicine and surgery. 3rd Editions. St Louis, Missouri: Elsevier Saunders; 2019. p. 992–1013.
16. Chai N. Mycobacteriosis in amphibians. In: Miller E, Fowler ME, editors. Fowler's zoo and wild animal medicine volume 7. St Louis, Missouri: Elsevier Saunders; 2011. p. 224–30.
17. Milnes EL, Delnatte P, Lentini A, et al. Mycobacteriosis in a Zoo Population of Chinese Gliding Frogs (*Rhacophorus dennysi*) Due to *Mycobacterium marinum*. J Herpetological Med Surg 2020;30(1):14–20.
18. Chai N, Bronchain O, Panteix G, et al. Propagation method of saving valuable strains from a *Mycobacterium Liflandii* infection in Western Clawed Frogs (*Silurana tropicalis*). J Zoo Wildl Med 2012;43(1):15–9.
19. Eisenberg T, Fawzy A, Kaim U, et al. Chronic wasting associated with *Chlamydia pneumoniae* in three *ex situ* breeding facilities for tropical frogs. Antonie van Leeuwenhoek 2020;113:2139–54.
20. Blumer C, Zimmermann DR, Weilenmann R, et al. Chlamydiae in Free-Ranging and Captive Frogs in Switzerland. Vet Pathol 2007;44:144–50.
21. Berger L, Volp K, Mathews S, et al. *Chlamydia pneumoniae* in a free-ranging giant barred frog (*Mixophyes iteratus*) from Australia. J Clin Microbiol 1999;37: 2378–80.
22. Mühldorfer K, Wibbelt G, Szentiks CA, et al. The role of 'atypical' Brucella in amphibians: are we facing novel emerging pathogens? J Appl Microbiol 2017;122: 40–53.
23. Latheef S, Keyburn A, Broz I, et al. Atypical Brucella sp in captive Australian green tree frogs (*Litoria caerulea*): Clinical features, pathology, culture and molecular characterization. Austral Vet J 2020;98(5):216–21.
24. Helmick KE, Garner MM, Rhyan J, et al. Clinicopathologic features of infection with novel *Brucella* organisms in captive waxy tree frogs (*Phyllomedusa sauvagii*) and colorado river toads (*Incilius alvarius*). J Zoo Wildl Med 2018;49(1):153–61.
25. Bienentreu JF, Lesbarreres D. Amphibian Disease Ecology: Are We Just Scratching the Surface? Herpetologica 2020;76(2):153–66.
26. Duffus ALJ. Ranavirus ecology in common frogs (*Rana temporaria*) from the United Kingdom: transmission dynamics, alternate hosts and host-strain interactions. Ph.D. Thesis. UK: Queen Mary, University of London; 2010.
27. Miller D, Gray M, Storfer A. Ecopathology of ranaviruses infecting amphibians. Viruses 2011;3:2351–73.
28. Bennati R, Bonetti M, Lavazza A, et al. Skin lesions associated with herpesvirus-like particles in frogs (*Rana dalmatina*). Vet Rec 1994;135(26):625–6.
29. Origgi FC, Schmidt BR, Lohmann P, et al. Ranid Herpesvirus 3 and Proliferative Dermatitis in Free-Ranging Wild Common Frogs (*Rana Temporaria*). Vet Pathol 2017;54:686–94.
30. Origgi FC, Schmidt BR, Lohmann P, et al. Bufonid herpesvirus 1 (BfHV1) associated dermatitis and mortality in free ranging common toads (*Bufo bufo*) in Switzerland. Sci Rep 2018;8:14737.

31. Chai N, Whitaker BR. Amphibian chytridiomycosis. In: Divers SJ, Stahl SJ, editors. Mader's reptile and Amphibian. Medicine and surgery. 3rd editions. St Louis, Missouri: Elsevier Saunders; 2019. p. p1291–3.

32. Chowdry P, Eng C, Recchio I, et al. Saprolegniasis in a Chinese Giant Salamander (*Andrias davidianus*). J Herpetological Med Surg 2011;21(2):43–4.

33. Borteiro C, Verdes JM, Cruz JC, et al. *Ichthyophonus sp.* (Ichthyophonae, Ichthyophonida) Infection in a South American Amphibian, the Hylid frog *Hypsiboas pulchellus*. J Wildl Dis 2015;51(2):530–3.

34. Collymore C, White JR, Lieggi C. *Trichodina xenopodus*, a Ciliated Protozoan, in a Laboratory-Maintained *Xenopus laevis*. Comp Med 2013;63(4):310–2.

35. Pritchett KR, Sanders GE. Epistylididae ectoparasites in a colony of African clawed frog (*Xenopus laevis*). J Am Assoc Lab Anim 2007;46:86–91.

36. Graczyk TK, Cranfield MR, Bicknese EJ, et al. Progressive ulcerative dermatitits in a captive, wild-caught, South American giant tree frog (*Phyllomedusa bicolor)* with microsporidial septicemia. J Zoo Wildl Med 1996;27(4):522–7.

37. Keller S, Roderick CL, Caris C, et al. Acute mortality in California tiger salamander (*Ambystoma californiense*) and Santa Cruz long-toed salamander (*Ambystoma macrodactylum croceum*) caused by *Ribeiroia ondatrae* (Class: Trematoda). Int J Parasitol Parasites Wildl 2021;16:255–61.

38. Box EK, Cleveland CA, Garrett KB, et al. Copepod consumption by amphibians and fish with implications for transmission of Dracunculus species. Int J Parasitology:Parasites Wildl 2021;15:231–7.

39. Stanley J, MacHale J, Hedley J. Successful Treatment of Anchor Worm (*Lernaea cyprinacea*) Using Lufenuron in the Mexican Axolotl (*Ambystoma mexicanum*). J Herpetological Med Surg 2021;31(2):107–10.

40. Stacy BA, Parker JM. Amphibian oncology. Vet Clin North Am Exot Anim Pract 2004;7(3):673–95.

41. Brenner EE, Sanchez CR, Garner MM. Squamous Cell Carcinoma in a Group of Solomon Island Leaf Frogs (*Ceratobatrachus guntheri*). J Herpetological Med Surg 2020;30(4):242–7.

42. Cramp RL, Franklin CE. Exploring the link between ultraviolet B radiation and immune function in amphibians: Implications for emerging infectious diseases. Cons Physiol 2018;6:coy035.

Dermatologic Diseases of Four-Toed Hedgehogs

Grayson A. Doss, DVM, Dipl ACZM

KEYWORDS

- Acariasis • African pygmy hedgehog • *Caparinia* • Dermatology • Dermatophytosis
- Neoplasia • *Trichophyton* • Zoonosis

KEY POINTS

- Acariasis, dermatophytosis, and cutaneous neoplasia are the most common dermatologic abnormalities in four-toed hedgehogs.
- *C tripilis*, the hedgehog mite, is the most common mite affecting pet hedgehogs and is quickly identified by the 3 long setae present on the third pair of legs in both sexes.
- Transmission of *Trichophyton* infections from pet hedgehogs to humans is well-documented, so strict hygiene practices when working with hedgehogs with dermatologic disease are essential.
- Cutaneous neoplasia is commonly reported in pet hedgehogs, and the diagnostic approach typically starts with a fine-needle aspirate but often requires biopsy.

 Video content accompanies this article at http://www.vetexotic.theclinics.com.

INTRODUCTION

Dermatologic diseases are one of the most common groups of disorders affecting captive four-toed hedgehogs (*Atelerix albiventris*), also known as African pygmy hedgehogs. The four-toed hedgehog has a haired ventrum, and the dorsal portion of the body, known as the 'mantle', contains a dense network of thousands of keratinaceous spines. Beneath a thin epidermal layer, the mantle is composed of a fibrous dermal layer, abundant adipose tissue, and a complex network of muscles that control spine position and enable the hedgehog to roll into a defensive ball. This normal defensive behavior of curling into a tight ball makes evaluation of the ventral-haired skin near impossible in an awake animal, apart from a cursory view with the hedgehog positioned on a translucent surface (**Fig. 1**). For a complete physical examination, including inspection of the pinna, face, and ventrum for lesions,

Department of Surgical Sciences, School of Veterinary Medicine, University of Wisconsin-Madison, 2015 Linden Drive, Madison, WI 53706, USA
E-mail address: gdoss@wisc.edu

Vet Clin Exot Anim 26 (2023) 443–453
https://doi.org/10.1016/j.cvex.2022.12.007
1094-9194/23/© 2022 Elsevier Inc. All rights reserved.

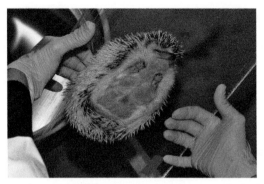

Fig. 1. The ventrum can be examined for abnormalities in an awake hedgehog by placing it on a translucent surface.

chemical immobilization is required. Disposable gloves should be worn due to the high frequency of zoonotic dermatophyte infections in this species.[1]

Common signs of dermatologic disease in hedgehogs include spine loss, scaling, pruritus, and crusting. Hedgehogs with chronic dermatologic disease may be presented for lethargy, anorexia, or weight loss. Spine loss can vary from mild, where the underlying skin is slightly more noticeable in a curled-up animal (**Fig. 2**), to severe, where most spines are missing. Hedgehog spines should not epilate easily, as they contain a basal bulb that firmly anchors them within the mantle (**Fig. 3**). Loss of multiple spines during an examination is abnormal (**Fig. 4**). However, for young hedgehogs, shedding of the smaller initial spines and simultaneous replacement with larger spines is normal, typically occurring around 8 to 12 weeks of age.[2] Also, four-toed hedgehogs normally lack spines in the skin over the midline of the head and neck (**Fig. 5**). The level of scale present in hedgehogs with dermatologic disease can vary, depending on the etiology and chronicity. Additionally, hedgehog owners may bathe or apply topical products to their pet hedgehogs before seeking veterinary care, making diagnosis more challenging. Like other species, pruritic hedgehogs extend their pelvic limbs forward to scratch rather than using their thoracic limbs (**Fig. 6**). Self-anointing, where a hedgehog turns its head caudolaterally and applies foamy saliva to its spines with its tongue, is normal behavior.

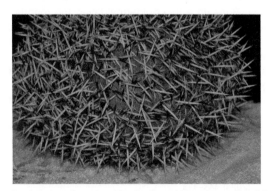

Fig. 2. Moderate spine loss in a four-toed hedgehog. Note the easily visible areas of underlying skin.

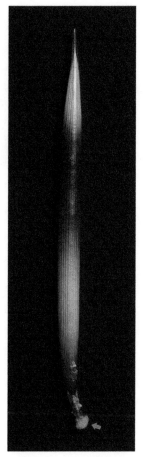

Fig. 3. Spine from a four-toed hedgehog. Note the pointed, translucent apex and disk-shaped protuberance at its base, known as the basal bulb (*arrow*).

Parasitic Diseases

Acariasis

Common clinical signs of acariasis include spine loss, scales, crusts, and pruritus. Powdery white deposits may be present around the eyes and nose.[3,4] Self-inflicted excoriations may occur secondary to chronic pruritus. Generalized erythema (see **Fig. 6**), lichenification, lethargy, and anorexia may also occur with infestations.[3,4]

Diagnosis of acariasis is through microscopic identification of mites or mite eggs collected from the skin, scales, or crusts.[5] Owing to the thin epidermis of the mantle, skin scrapes should be performed with caution. A toothbrush can be used to atraumatically collect mites from the skin and spines, even when the hedgehog is awake and balled up in its defensive posture.[4] In the author's experience, superficial mites can also be successfully collected by rubbing a cotton tip applicator coated with a small amount of mineral oil over the affected skin areas. Severe infestations may indicate underlying immunosuppression, necessitating a systemic workup.

The most common species affecting hedgehogs is the psoroptid mite *C tripilis*. *Caparinia* mites are grossly visible as motile, white-yellow powdery spots, and may be found in

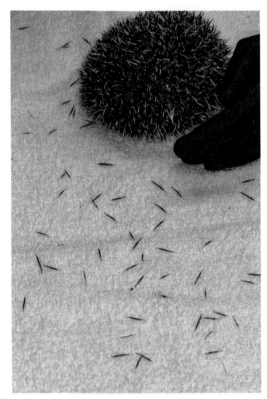

Fig. 4. Abnormal loss of a significant number of spines during a four-toed hedgehog examination.

large numbers (Video 1). The face and head, behind the ears, and around the eyes are common areas to find *Caparinia* mites.[4,6] *Caparinia* mites can be challenging to distinguish from other Psoroptidae mites like *Chorioptes*, *Otodectes*, and *Psoroptes*. However, both sexes of *Caparinia* mites can be quickly identified by the presence of three long setae (hairs) on the third pair of legs. The mnemonic 'three-on-three' can aid remembering this key feature (Video 2). Additionally, the pedicels (stalks) are unjointed, and the tarsal caruncles (suckers) are bell-shaped.[5,7] Tarsal caruncles are present on all legs of male *Caparinia* mites, but are absent on the third and fourth legs in females. Short, unsegmented pedicels in both sexes, the lack of caruncles on the fourth pair of legs in females, and the presence of three long setae on the third pair of legs in both sexes distinguishes *Caparinia* from *Psoroptes*, *Chorioptes,* and *Otodectes*, respectively.[5]

Infestations may seem to develop randomly in hedgehogs without a previous history of ectoparasites or an obvious source of transmission. Hedgehogs can have subclinical infestations with small numbers of mites.[6] It is possible that more severe infestations develop secondary to stress, underlying immunosuppression or systemic disease.

Treatment typically consists of topical selamectin (20 to 30 mg/kg, q21–28d for 2 to 3 doses; Revolution, Zoetis Inc, Kalamazoo, MI, USA). Other treatment options include ivermectin (0.2 to 0.4 mg/kg SC, PO, q10 to 14d for 3 to 5 doses) or a combination of imidacloprid (10%) and moxidectin (1%) (0.1 mL/kg topically; Advantage Multi for cats, Advocate for cats, Elanco Inc).[1,7] Isoxazolines also seem to be useful for *Caparinia* infestations in hedgehogs. Single oral doses of either fluralaner (15 mg/kg) or

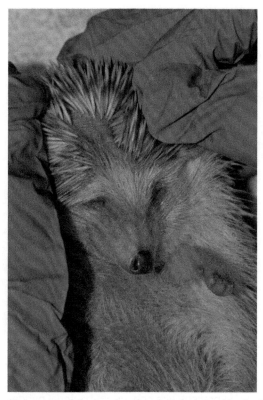

Fig. 5. The midline skin on top of the head and neck in four-toed hedgehogs, known as the "crown," normally lacks spines.

sarolaner (2 mg/kg) were reportedly successful in treating *Caparinia* in a small number of four-toed hedgehogs.[8,9]

As *C tripilis* is easily transmissible, all hedgehogs in the household should be treated simultaneously. Treatment can fail if environmental decontamination is not performed by the client and affected hedgehogs should be temporarily housed in enclosures that facilitate regular, complete cleaning.

Otodectes cynotis and *Notoedres cati* have been noted to cause otic disease in pet hedgehogs.[1,10] Clinical signs include waxy debris accumulation or crusting around the ears as well as aural pruritus. Treatment is similar to cats. *Demodex canis* was identified on light microscopy and molecular diagnostics in a hedgehog presented for generalized erythema and scaling and successfully treated with a combination of afoxolaner and milbemycin oxime.[11] Follow-up weekly skin scrapes were negative, the erythema resolved 14 days after treatment, and all lesions were completely healed by 30 days posttreatment.[11]

Fleas and lice
Although more commonly reported in wild hedgehogs, flea and lice infestations can occur in captive animals.[12] Treatment is similar to acariasis.

Dermatophytosis
Dermatophytosis is common in hedgehogs. Clinical signs include scaling and/or crusting around the base of the spines and face, facial alopecia, spine loss, and pinnal

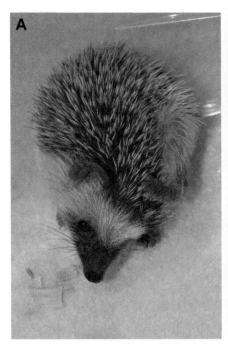 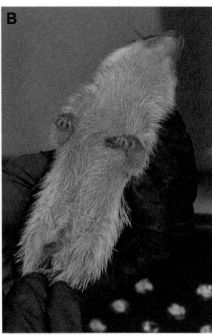

Fig. 6. Pruritic juvenile four-toed hedgehog with a *Caparinia* infestation. Note how the pelvic limb is extended to scratch at the dorsum (*A*) and the generalized erythema present (*B*).

dermatitis.[6,13–15] Dermatophyte infections are usually non-pruritic in hedgehogs, although pruritus may be present with concurrent bacterial pyoderma or acariasis.

T erinacei, part of the *Trichophyton mentagrophytes* complex,[16] is the most commonly reported dermatophyte isolated from captive four-toed hedgehogs.[12,17] There are several reports of zoonotic transmission of *T erinacei* from pet hedgehogs, and dermatophyte infections secondary to acariasis are common in pet hedgehogs.[18–23] *Microsporum* spp. have also been noted to cause infections in African pygmy hedgehogs.[10] Diagnosis is usually performed through fungal culture using dermatophyte test medium. The plate can be inoculated using a sterile toothbrush (MacKenzie brush technique) or with spines or hair plucked from affected areas (**Fig. 7**).[13,24] Treatment consists of topical antifungal agents like enilconazole, miconazole, clotrimazole, or lime sulfur in addition to oral systemic therapy, like terbinafine or itraconazole. A study in European hedgehogs (*Erinaceus europaeus*) infected with *T erinacei* showed a higher mycological cure rate with oral terbinafine (100 mg/kg, q12h) than itraconazole (10 mg/kg, q12h) after 28 days of therapy.[13] Routine monitoring of biochemistry panels during prolonged itraconazole use has been suggested.[14] Treatment should be continued until 2 negative fungal cultures (4 weeks apart) are obtained.[14] Strict environmental decontamination and treatment of all other hedgehogs in the household is indicated. Since transmission to humans is well-documented, clients should exercise proper hygiene practices when handling and cleaning enclosures of affected hedgehogs.

Pinnal dermatitis

Pinnal dermatitis is a common finding in captive hedgehogs and clinical findings consist of bilateral, ragged, hyperkeratotic ear margins (**Fig. 8**). Dermatophytosis and acariasis are major differentials, although inappropriate husbandry (eg, nutritional

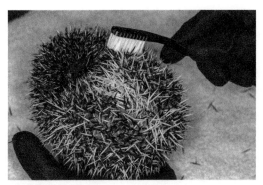

Fig. 7. Collecting a sample from a hedgehog with excessive spine loss. The MacKenzie brush technique was used to inoculate the dermatophyte test medium.

deficiencies, poor humidity) may play a role in development. Skin cytology and dermatophyte culture are recommended.

Otitis externa

Bacterial and yeast otitis have been reported in four-toed hedgehogs and may occur secondary to otic acariasis (**Fig. 9**).[1] Diagnosis is based on cytologic and culture findings and treatment consists of miticidal treatment in addition to antimicrobial or antifungal therapy. Owing to the small size of the external ear canal, visualization of the tympanic membrane is not possible with an otoscope.

Bacterial pyoderma

Bacterial infection has been reported secondary to acariasis in pet hedgehogs.[3] Lancefield Group A *Streptococcus* dermatitis was isolated from a pet hedgehog with bilateral dermatitis of the thoracic limbs. Crusting, ulceration, and purulent discharge was noted on examination.[25] Mycobacterial granulomatous dermatitis was reported in a hedgehog presented for a distal, nodular swelling on a thoracic limb.[26] Transcutaneous inoculation during a recent traumatic event was suspected to be the source of infection.[26]

Noninfectious Diseases

Neoplasia

Neoplastic skin diseases are common in pet hedgehogs (**Fig. 10**). The diagnostic approach for skin masses typically starts with a fine-needle aspirate, but a biopsy is frequently needed for a definitive diagnosis.

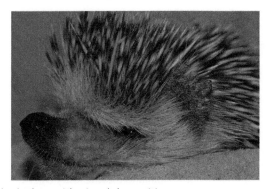

Fig. 8. Four-toed hedgehog with pinnal dermatitis.

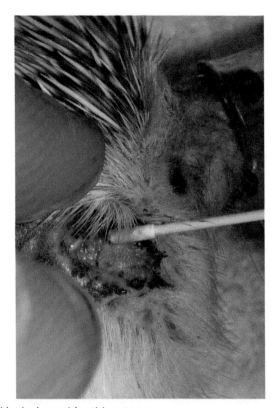

Fig. 9. Four-toed hedgehog with otitis externa.

Mammary gland tumors are one of the most common neoplasia types in the four-toed hedgehog, with the majority of reported cases being malignant.[27–30] Clinical signs include single or multiple subcutaneous masses along the ventrum.[27,28] Surgical excision and concurrent ovariohysterectomy are recommended, although the recurrence rate seems high.[27,28]

Oral squamous cell carcinomas are extremely common in pet hedgehogs.[1] However, there are a few descriptions of cutaneous squamous cell carcinomas in hedgehogs.[31,32] Reported clinical signs range from single masses to multifocal skin

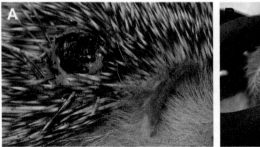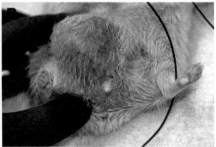

Fig. 10. Adult male four-toed hedgehog with an ulcerated round cell neoplasm, most consistent with a plasma cell tumor on immunohistochemistry (*A*). Adult female four-toed hedgehog with a subcutaneous fibrosarcoma in the inguinal area (*B*).

lesions. Ulcerated, exudative nodular lesions were present on the face, ears, and thoracic limbs in one case.[31] Diagnosis is through fine-needle aspirate or biopsy of affected areas.

Epitheliotropic T-cell lymphoma has been reported in four-toed hedgehogs.[33,34] Clinical signs in one case included generalized spine loss, alopecia and erythema as well as pruritus, and multifocal crust formation.[34] In another case, a nonhealing crusting lesion was noted on the pinna.[33]

Numerous other types of cutaneous neoplasia have been reported in hedgehogs, including fibrosarcoma,[29,30] sebaceous gland carcinoma,[35] mastocytoma,[29] hemangiosarcoma,[36] extraskeletal osteosarcoma,[37] and histiocytic sarcoma.[38]

CLINICS CARE POINTS

- Owing to their defensive behavior, a complete physical examination of pet hedgehogs requires chemical immobilization

- Acariasis and dermatophytosis are very common in pet hedgehogs, and often occur concurrently

- Skin cytology and dermatophyte culture should be prioritized in hedgehogs with spine loss and/or scale and crust build-up

- Various treatments exist for acariasis in hedgehogs, including topical and oral options

- Systemic antifungal treatment with terbinafine or an azole drug is recommended for dermatophyte infections

- Cutaneous neoplasia is common in four-toed hedgehogs and often requires biopsy for a definitive diagnosis

---

DISCLOSURE

The author has nothing to disclose.

SUPPLEMENTARY DATA

Supplementary data related to this article can be found online at https://doi.org/10.1016/j.cvex.2022.12.007.

REFERENCES

1. Doss G, Carpenter J. African pygmy hedgehogs. In: Quesenberry K, Orcutt C, Mans C, et al, editors. Ferrets, rabbits, and rodents: clinical medicine and surgery. 4th edition. St. Louis: Saunders; 2021. p. 401–15.

2. Greenacre C. Avian and exotic animal dermatology. In: Hnilica K, Patterson A, editors. Small animal dermatology. 4th edition. St. Louis: Elsevier; 2017. p. 508–74.

3. Fehr M, Koestlinger S. Ectoparasites in small exotic mammals. Vet Clin North Am Exot Anim Pract 2013;16:611–57.

4. d'Ovidio D, Santoro M, Santoro D. A clinical retrospective study of *Caparinia tripilis* (Psoroptidae) mite dermatitis in pet African pygmy hedgehogs (*Ateletrix albiventris*) in southern Italy. Vet Dermatol 2021;32:434, e115.

5. Kim DH, Oh DS, Ahn KS, et al. An outbreak of *Caparinia tripilis* in a colony of African pygmy hedgehogs (*Atelerix albiventris*) from Korea. Korean J Parasitol 2012;50:151–6.

6. Johnson D. African pygmy hedgehogs. In: Meredith A, Johnson-Delaney C, editors. BSAVA manual of exotic pets. 5th edition. Gloucester: British Small Animal Veterinary Association; 2010. p. 139–47.

7. Kim KR, Ahn KS, Oh DS, et al. Efficacy of a combination of 10% imidacloprid and 1% moxidectin against *Caparinia tripilis* in African pygmy hedgehog (*Atelerix albiventris*). Parasit Vectors 2012;5:158.

8. Romero C, Sheinberg Waisburd G, Pineda J, et al. Fluralaner as a single dose oral treatment for *Caparinia tripilis* in a pygmy African hedgehog. Vet Dermatol 2017;28:622, e152.

9. Antelo J, Núñez C, Contreras L, et al. Use of sarolaner in African hedgehogs (*Atelerix albiventris*) infested with *Caparinia tripilis*. J Exot Pet Med 2020;35:1–3.

10. Meredith A. Skin diseases and treatment of hedgehogs. In: Paterson S, editor. Skin diseases of exotic pets. Oxford: Blackwell Science Ltd; 2006. p. 264–74.

11. Núñez CR, Waisburd GS, Cordero AM, et al. First report of the use of afoxolaner/milbemycin oxime in an African pygmy hedgehog (*Atelerix albiventris*) with demodicosis caused by *Demodex canis* identified by molecular techniques. J Exot Pet Med 2019;29:128–30.

12. Gardhouse S, Eshar D. Retrospective study of disease occurrence in captive African pygmy hedgehogs (*Atelerix albiventris*). Isr J Vet Med 2015;70:32–6.

13. Bexton S, Nelson H. Comparison of two systemic antifungal agents, itraconazole and terbinafine, for the treatment of dermatophytosis in European hedgehogs (*Erinaceus europaeus*). Vet Dermatol 2016;27:500, e133.

14. Fehr M. Zoonotic potential of dermatophytosis in small mammals. J Exot Pet Med 2015;24:308–16.

15. Hedgehogs Heatley J. In: Mitchell MA, Tully T, editors. Manual of exotic pet practice. St. Louis: Saunders; 2009. p. 433–55.

16. Frías-De-león MG, Martínez-Herrera E, Atoche-Diéguez CE, et al. Molecular identification of isolates of the *Trichophyton mentagrophytes* complex. Int J Med Sci 2020;17:45.

17. Abarca ML, Castellá G, Martorell J, et al. *Trichophyton erinacei* in pet hedgehogs in Spain: occurrence and revision of its taxonomic status. Med Mycol 2016;55:164–72.

18. Riley PY, Chomel BB. Hedgehog zoonoses. Emerg Infect Dis 2005;11:1–5.

19. Frantz T, Rampton R, Wohltmann W. Bullous eruption caused by an exotic hedgehog purchased as a household pet. Cutis 2020;105:314–6.

20. Phaitoonwattanakij S, Leeyaphan C, Bunyaratavej S, et al. *Trichophyton erinacei* onychomycosis: The first to evidence a proximal subungual onychomycosis pattern. Case Rep Dermatol 2019;11:198–203.

21. Rhee DY, Kim MS, Chang SE, et al. A case of tinea manuum caused by *Trichophyton mentagrophytes* var. *erinacei*: the first isolation in Korea. Mycoses 2009;52:287–90.

22. Kromer C, Nenoff P, Uhrlaß S, et al. *Trichophyton erinacei* transmitted to a pregnant woman from her pet hedgehogs. JAMA Dermatol 2018;154:967–8.

23. Weishaupt J, Kolb-Mäurer A, Lempert S, et al. A different kind of hedgehog pathway: tinea manus due to *Trichophyton erinacei* transmitted by an African pygmy hedgehog (*Atelerix albiventris*). Mycoses 2014;57:125–7.

24. Moriello KA, Coyner K, Paterson S, et al. Diagnosis and treatment of dermatophytosis in dogs and cats: clinical consensus guidelines of the world association for veterinary dermatology. Vet Dermatol 2017;28:266, e68.

25. Rodenbaugh C, Ramachandran A, Brandão J. Lancefield group a Streptococcus-associated dermatitis in an African pygmy hedgehog (*Atelerix albiventris*). J Exot Pet Med 2020;33:27–30.
26. Blume GR, Eloi RSA, Oliveira LB, et al. Non-tuberculous mycobacterial granulomatous dermatitis in an African pygmy hedgehog (*Atelerix albiventris*). J Comp Pathol 2021;182:22–6.
27. Heatley J, Mauldin G, Cho D. A review of neoplasia in the captive African hedgehog (*Atelerix albiventris*). Semin Avian Exot Pet Med 2005;14:182–92.
28. Raymond J, Garner M. Mammary gland tumors in captive African hedgehogs. J Wildl Dis 2000;36:405–8.
29. Raymond J, Garner M. Spontaneous tumours in captive African hedgehogs (*Atelerix albiventris*): a retrospective study. J Comp Pathol 2001;124:128–33.
30. Okada K, Kondo H, Sumi A, et al. A retrospective study of disease incidence in African pygmy hedgehogs (*Atelerix albiventris*). J Vet Med Sci 2018;80:1504–10.
31. Huang J, Eshar D, Andrews G, et al. Diagnostic challenge. J Exot Pet Med 2014; 23:418–20.
32. Couture ÉL, Langlois I, Santamaria-Bouvier A, et al. Cutaneous squamous cell carcinoma in an African pygmy hedgehog (*Atelerix albiventris*). Can Vet J 2015;56:1275–8.
33. Spugnini EP, Pagotto A, Zazzera F, et al. Cutaneous T-cell lymphoma in an African hedgehog (*Atelerix albiventris*). In Vivo 2008;22:43–6.
34. Chung TH, Kim HJ, Choi US. Multicentric epitheliotropic T-cell lymphoma in an African hedgehog (*Atelerix albiventris*). Vet Clin Pathol 2014;43:601–4.
35. Matute AR, Bernal AM, Lezama JR, et al. Sebaceous gland carcinoma and mammary gland carcinoma in an African hedgehog (*Ateletrix albiventris*). J Zoo Wildl Med 2014;45:682–5.
36. Finkelstein A, Hoover JP, Caudell D, et al. Cutaneous epithelioid variant hemangiosarcoma in a captive African hedgehog (*Atelerix albiventris*). J Exot Pet Med 2008;17:49–53.
37. Phair K, Carpenter JW, Marrow J, et al. Management of an extraskeletal osteosarcoma in an African hedgehog (*Atelerix albiventris*). J Exot Pet Med 2011;20: 151–5.
38. Makishima R, Kondo H, Shibuya H. Clinical, histopathological, and immunohistochemical studies of histiocytic sarcoma in four-toed hedgehogs (*Atelerix albiventris*): a retrospective study. J Vet Med Sci 2021;83:419–26.

Dermatologic Aspects of Zoo Mammal Medicine

Endre Sós, DVM, PhD, DipECZM (ZHM)[a,b,*], Viktória Sós-Koroknai, DVM, PhD[a]

KEYWORDS

- Dermatologic examination • Zoo mammals • Diagnostic tools • Skin disorders

KEY POINTS

- Husbandry-related health problems occurring in a zoologic setting.
- The biological needs of the species and the careful evaluation of the husbandry must be part of the diagnostic plan.
- Medical training is a good general approach in many situations to achieve a definitive diagnosis and to implement treatment.
- Skin diseases must be differentiated whether they are primary ailments or part of a general disease, including zoonotic or notifiable ones.

INTRODUCTION

The concept of a modern zoo includes several elements, but the most important of these are species conservation, education/public awareness and research.[1] While implementing their mission, zoos are obliged to follow the highest standards of animal care and husbandry. These constantly change based on publications and evidence-based knowledge gained from both wildlife and animals under human care. This institutional role gives the zoo veterinarians an important responsibility for various reasons.

Zoo animals, in a broader sense, are ambassadors of their respective species in raising awareness, directly tackling conservation issues, and educating the general public about the individual biology of a species and their ecosystems, providing a more complex context of the role of a given species in its environment. On other occasions, zoo animals have a vital role in conservation breeding programs, which can have direct contact with reintroductions or major *in-situ* operations. Moreover, some of these programs can act as a "safety-net" (genetic insurance) for further conservation actions in the future when the reasons for the decline in the wild have been alleviated to a certain degree. Whichever is the case, it is obvious that all these objectives can be only served with both physically and mentally healthy animals. Specimens

[a] Budapest Zoo and Botanical Garden, Állatkerti krt. 6-12, Budapest, H-1146, Hungary;
[b] University of Veterinary Medicine, István u. 2. H-1078, Budapest, Hungary
* Corresponding author
E-mail address: drsos.endre@zoobudapest.com

Vet Clin Exot Anim 26 (2023) 455–474
https://doi.org/10.1016/j.cvex.2022.12.008
1094-9194/23/© 2023 Elsevier Inc. All rights reserved.
vetexotic.theclinics.com

destined to be part of such conservation breeding programs on the long run ought to meet general health requirements, and at the same time, the visitors of the institution where they are housed should see and learn about fit individuals with a normal behavioral repertoire.

It is well known that wild animals often hide the symptoms of general disease, meaning that it is not uncommon, that they only show signs of clinical disease by the time the process is profoundly advanced. However, dermatologic conditions are more difficult to hide and some signs can be rather obvious for veterinarians, anyone familiar with the species, and even the general public (eg, hair problems, alopecia, extensive pruritus, change of hair color). Some of these cases can even trigger a strong reaction from the general public and even call into question the keeping of animals in zoos. This phenomenon is especially impactful if it happens in a relatively large number of animals and the exact cause or contributing factors were not identified, such as in the case of the idiopathic alopecia in Andean bears (Tremarctos ornatus) in several zoos.[2,3]

Giving a detailed overview of the whole range of skin diseases in zoo mammals is well beyond the scope of this article, but general approaches through animal husbandry, diagnostic tools, and some very typical conditions are outlined below.

Dermatologic problems are often linked to and highlight inadequate husbandry or nutrition in captive-kept animals. The diagnosis can be challenging for various reasons, including, but not limited to the lack of cooperation from some species or animals, the risk of anesthesia, the limitations on multiple/consecutive sample collections, the limitations of treatment options, and the lack of "normal" values/descriptions. However, this is also a rapidly evolving field, in terms of both the amount of scientific information published and the information available from other sources, like extensive databases or expert forums. In addition, more updated handling techniques for wild animals, such as training based on operant conditioning techniques, do at least provide the ability to examine patients without the necessity of immediate anesthesia.[4] Medical training is achieved with the help of positive reinforcement, which allows the veterinarian to implement diagnostic techniques or treatments, in situations where the pain is lacking, or only minor pain is involved. Medical training gives us an option for consecutive treatments in dangerous or noncooperative species as the increased risk of multiple chemical restraint events does not exist, and more frequent handling is possible (even on a daily basis). This is especially relevant in slow healing processes (eg, a sole ulcer in a pachyderm) or in those treatment protocols when the medical treatment would require regular manipulation of the affected lesion (eg, a bitten, infected wound with pus accumulation and a regular need of debridement in a large carnivore).

Another important factor to consider in the case of zoos is the zoonotic potential of some dermatologic conditions, especially in immersion exhibits or in animals as part of an educational or demonstration program. In these settings, every precaution must be taken to avoid human infections.

Management-Related Disease and Prevention

Best practice guidelines are mostly made and distributed by specific zoo associations, such as EAZA (European Association of Zoos and Aquariums) in Europe or AZA (Association of Zoos and Aquariums) in North America. These documents serve as a guidance on how to keep the health of zoo animals at the highest standards but are not necessarily available for every species. Therefore, providing adequate husbandry is the sole responsibility of the institution housing the particular species.

Avoiding management-related ailments is a long-term concern in different taxa; if adequate husbandry is provided ailments will be eliminated. Reptiles and amphibians are prime examples for such concern, where potential banning from keeping these animals is under consideration in some countries because of animal welfare concerns and the lack of knowledge about the exact needs of many species. There are good, scientific arguments against such initiatives, but the problem exists and must be handled.[5] Inadequate husbandry as a source of disease is most likely prominent in reptiles and amphibians due to the fact that these species often originate from exotic conditions and are kept in fully artificial circumstances, where we must provide proper temperature, UV radiation, humidity, substrate, circadian/seasonal changes, and nutrition to meet their physiologic needs. As a comparison, zoo mammals can mostly be kept in less controlled environments, in terms of the difference in keeping conditions compared with their natural habitat or diet, even if they are considered to be an exotic species. However, careful planning and mimicking of the natural circumstances are required as much as possible to avoid husbandry-related health issues. The lack of provision of adequate conditions can lead to many diseases in mammals, including dermatologic disorders; among others, proper UV exposure has a paramount importance in many species, but the reference values are often unknown.

Animals housed only indoors are particularly an area of concern, where metabolic bone diseases are a very prominent risk. Vitamin D_3 is endogenously produced in mammalian skin when exposed to the appropriate wavelengths of UV-B. One study dealing with common marmosets (*Callithrix jacchus*) kept exclusively indoors revealed that this species requires dietary provision of vitamin D_3 due to the lack of sunlight exposure.[6] Their results show that marmosets tightly regulate their metabolism of dietary vitamin D_3 into the active metabolite $1,25(OH)_2 D_3$. This ability explains the tolerance of high levels of dietary vitamin D_3 and also suggests that the high dietary levels given in many institutions are not required. On the contrary, even UV supplementation is recommended and needed for callitrichids housed indoors; however, an excessive UV exposure can possibly lead to a skin neoplasia, as described in two Goeldi's monkeys (*Callimico goeldii*).[7] These animals developed multifocal alopecia with hyperkeratotic to ulcerative skin lesions on the lower abdomen and inner thighs, where hyperplastic dermatitis, carcinoma and intralesional *Demodex* mites were diagnosed. The cases took place 2.5 years apart under the same keeping conditions, demonstrating individual variances in such etiologies.

Apart from the vitamin D_3 metabolism, other nutrition-related problems have also been linked with dermatopathies. Some of these conditions are well-known in domestic species: adverse cutaneous reactions to food are common in small animals. Moreover, deficiencies of different compounds and their relationship with skin disease are also well described in certain species (eg, vitamins A and C, zinc and copper, fatty acids).[8,9]

Food-induced hypersensitivity (food allergy) is not a frequently occurring problem in zoo animals; however, even though the literature is devoid of reports, clinical cases have been anecdotally reported, with symptoms comparable to the ones observed in domestic species. As the caseload is small and diets are mostly extremely varied between institution, diagnostic challenges can occur. In our own experience at the Budapest Zoo and Botanic Garden a Brown bear (*Ursus arctos*) showed symptoms of food-induced hypersensitivity to chicken meat (in this case both the elimination trial and dietary rechallenge confirmed the suspicion). The clinical presentation included generalized partial alopecia (with altered quality hair growth) and severe pruritus with histopathological changes characterized by mild, mixed, perivascular infiltration of inflammatory cells with eosinophils, uneven epidermis hyperplasia and subcorneal pustule formation (unpublished data; **Fig. 1**).

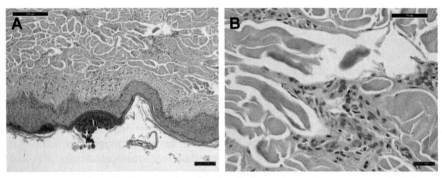

Fig. 1. Histopathological changes related to food allergy dermatitis in a Brown bear (*Ursus arctos*). Mild, mixed, perivascular infiltration of inflammatory cells with eosinophils are seen. The epidermis shows uneven hyperplasia and subcorneal pustule formation (HE staining, photo courtesy: Edina Perge, MATRIX).

Urticaria (or hives) is usually an acute immune response (most often seen as multifocal, dermal, swellings/called wheals/as a result of mast cell degranulation/histamine release/and subsequent edema), which is not uncommon and well-described in some domestic animal species (eg, horses and dogs).[10] In Asian elephants (*Elephas maximus*) anecdotal reports exists of urticaria being observed as one possible complication of tuberculosis treatment (https://www.aphis.usda.gov/animal_welfare/downloads/elephant/Challenges%20to%20Treatment.pdf). In our own records we encountered this problem on two occasions in June 2022 in our Asian elephant herd at the Budapest Zoo and Botanic Garden, when freshly cut grass was provided as part of their diet. We suspected a link between the fresh grass and this condition (manifested with intensive pruritus), which resolved rapidly after the diet was altered and this particular feedstuff was removed (**Fig. 2.**). Further studies are warranted to confirm the association between consumption of fresh grass and urticaria in elephants.

General descriptions are far scarcer regarding the link between zoo mammal skin disorders and animal husbandry; however, it is obvious that any form of unproper keeping conditions can have detrimental consequences on the general health of zoo

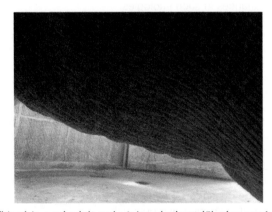

Fig. 2. Urticaria (hives) in a subadult male Asian elephant (*Elephas maximus*) at the ventral abdominal region. This condition was only observed when fresh grass was provided and resolved without treatment when this type of food was withdrawn. The dome shaped lesions were still visible after 1 week, even though the pruritic signs had resolved.

animals regardless of the species and can of course include dermatologic diseases. Black rhinoceroses (*Diceros bicornis*) can develop ulcerative dermatopathy with other, often life-threatening conditions (hemolytic anemia, hepatopathies) in certain circumstances, especially if a high-iron diet is provided for this browser species.[11,12] They are also prone to develop eosinophilic granulomas (2–10 cm diameter oral, nasal and cutaneous nodules/plaques, often with multifocal ulcerations), with unknown origin, but a possible link is suspected with an allergic process, based on histopathological features and a response to glucocorticoids and antihistamines.[13] Another case series (8 animals) also described the same type of oral, nasal, and cutaneous eosinophilic nodules/plaques in all rhinoceros included in the study.[14] The typical clinical presentation of the oral/nasal nodules included oral bleeding or epistaxis, with proliferative masses (with ulcerated areas). Two animals were treated with systemic corticosteroids but died later due to the consequence of a generalized fungal infection (*Aspergillus* spp. alone or in combination with *Mucor* spp.). Clinical experience indicates that corticosteroid usage should be done with great caution in Black rhinoceroses.[14,15]

Chronic stress and social problems were also found to be related to skin disorders in several taxa. Anecdotal reports do exist in some species: skin problems (hair loss, patchy alopecia, crusts on the affected area) are more frequent in Polar bears (*Ursus maritimus*) when a social problem (eg, the group composition does not follow the natural history of the species) persists (Kolter, L., personal communication). Other stressors (such as heat or high humidity) are also considered as highly stressful conditions for the species. However, systematic species-based evaluation for a particular species only exists in a few instances.[3,16] In the case of the Dorcas gazelles (*Gazella dorcas*) welfare assessment in a particular study indicated skin ailments induced by stress, as analogies were used from the farm animal industry. Those lesions (patchy alopecia and masses), which were a minimum of 2 cm in diameter were quantified as stress-induced findings; possibly secondary to rough handling, intra-specific aggression, or an inappropriate physical environment.[16] Moreover, stress-related skin problems can be self-inflicted as well and include but are not limited to excessive grooming, licking or even severe auto mutilation and may take place only as a manifestation of stress (**Fig. 3**).[17,18]

Moreover, stress dermatosis or dermatitis is a described clinical entity (syndrome) of South American rodent species (**Fig. 4.**). This condition is observed both in captivity

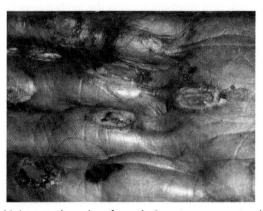

Fig. 3. Self-inflicted injury on the palm of a male Sumatran orangutan (*Pongo abelii*). This animal had severe difficulties during the integration into the group when the wounds developed. Moreover, as part of this condition, the animal developed paralytic ileus, which had to be treated surgically (Photo courtesy: Viktor Molnár).

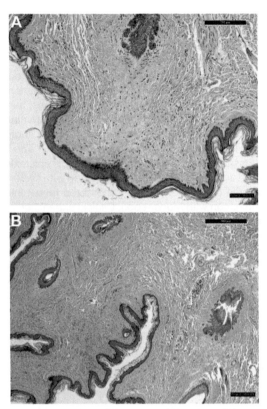

Fig. 4. Histopathological picture of the stress-dermatitis in a Capybara (*Hydrochoerus hydrochaeris*). Epidermal hyperplasia and mild hyperpigmentation; in the telogen follicles an abnormal trichilemmal keratinization is observed. (HE staining, M: 100x, photo courtesy: Edina Perge, MATRIX).

and the wild and is speculated to be related to high population density. The clinical presentation is alopecia and lacerations along the lumbosacral spine. Stress has a negative effect on skin fragility and overcrowding is related to intraspecific aggression (with possible secondary infections).[19]

It must be noted that the actual needs of a particular species are not always known even if zoo animal husbandry is rapidly evolving. This can especially be true, when a rare species is kept with a limited number of holders and also when minimal experience, or for example, a new conservation breeding program is set up, where previous husbandry-related knowledge is lacking in its entirely and only extrapolations can be made from similar species. The Hungarian birch mouse (*Sicista trizona*) is an endemic species with fragmented populations in Hungary and Transylvania, Romania. The uncertain status in the wild emphasized the need of bringing them under human care through a conservation breeding program recently established. However, skin ailments (eg, regional alopecia along the trunk and tail and biting) start to seem and they were most likely linked with the lack of deep understanding of the exact needs of the species (**Figs 5–7**).

As a final remark about husbandry and natural history that it is needless to say that both the keeping institution and the clinical veterinarians must know the species they care for. This is a basic condition to differentiate between a normal (physiologic) and

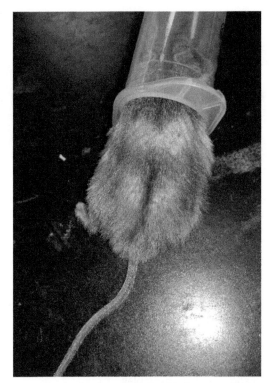

Fig. 5. Alopecic lesion on the back of a Hungarian birch mouse (*Sicista trizona*), caught in the wild cc. 6 months earlier to establish a conservation breeding program. Skin biopsy was collected during an anesthetic event to obtain a definitive diagnosis.

an abnormal (diseased) feature. This seems very obvious, but often it can be challenging to differentiate between a normal process (eg, seasonal moulting) or skin/hair problems due to nutritional or endocrine disorders (**Fig. 8**).

As a very relevant example of this topic, in some Old-World monkey species ischial callosities may be present and characterized by regional alopecia and hyperkeratotic skin. The sexual skin is also a physiologic characteristic in some primate genera

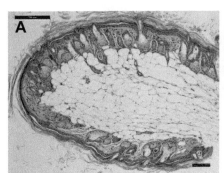
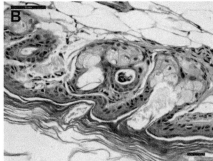

Fig. 6. Skin biopsy of the case in Hungarian birch mouse (*Sicista trizona*) (see **Fig. 5.**) revealed mild, nonspecific, chronic dermatitis with *Demodex* infestation (Photo courtesy: Edina Perge, MATRIX).

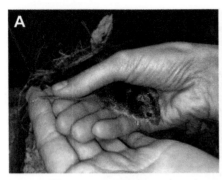 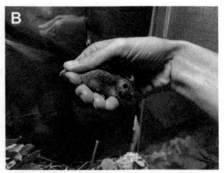

Fig. 7. Tail bites occurred in some cases among the Hungarian birch mice (*Sicista trizona*). At this stage it is unclear whether it was caused by intraspecific aggression or self-inflicted (stress-related) trauma. The picture on the left shows an intact-tailed animal, whereas the right one with a shorter tail, due to a bite injury.

(*Cercocebus, Macaca, Papio, Theropithecus, Miopithecus*, and Mandrillus).[20] In these taxonomic groups the sexual skin serves as a signalment for the conspecifics, as the perianal swelling and estrous-dependent reddening of the skin takes place according to hormonal cycles. All these characteristics are physiologic and do not indicate disease.[20,21]

Noninfectious Skin Disorders

Noninfectious skin disorders can arise for a fair number of reasons some of which will be listed below, with some relevant examples.

Physical aspects (such as extreme heat or cold), trauma arising from fights or other types of injuries (mainly caused by either fixture in the exhibit or self-inflicted, for various reasons, including chronic stress, obsessive behavior, fear, fight or flight response, etc.) can all occur. Chemicals can also cause severe skin conditions. Contact allergies (allergic contact dermatitis) are well-known in the companion animal medicine and theoretically could be seen in zoo mammals as well.[22] The improper

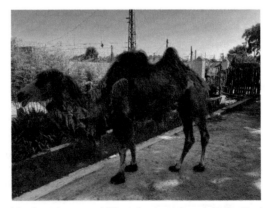

Fig 8. Perfectly healthy Bactrian camel (*Camelus bactrianus*) at the Budapest Zoo, showing signs of intensive, seasonal moulting while losing winter fur in June 2022. The patchy, scruffy appearance of the fur could suggest a hair growth problem for an unexperienced examiner.

use of disinfectants can cause severe skin problems, both irritant contact dermatitis or allergic contact dermatitis (the mode and type of disinfection in an enclosure can very clearly be a dangerous act, which must be implemented according to the instructions of the given substance).

Heat or cold traumas are in most cases husbandry-related issues; if the animals are kept under the required keeping conditions and shelters, places with appropriate temperature are available, these problems are rarely encountered. However, sometimes even animals that have the ability to choose where to stay within the exhibit can suffer heat/cold-related skin problems (eg, sunburn or frostbite). Heat/direct sunlight (especially with a high UV level) can be especially problematic in light-colored species or those, whose natural environment greatly differs from the keeping conditions (eg, pigs or cetaceans or species naturally living in the undergrowth of forests kept in enclosures where they are exposed to high UV radiation exposed).

Extreme cold will not only affect the skin per se but can result in severe tissue necrosis (frostbite); especially involving the extremities, tail, or ears (**Fig. 9.**). This is also called local cold injury; the elements of it are the direct freezing of the tissues, cold-induced vascular damage, and tissue anoxia at dry temperatures below 0 C°.[23]

Trauma is often encountered in a zoo environment and can be relevant in almost all taxonomic groups. In nonhuman primates, traumatic lesions are the second most common clinical problem after the diseases of the alimentary tract.[21] Skin injuries typically become infected with environmental bacteria. These wounds should be treated repeatedly, but the severity (depth, infection), the extent (how many lesions, the percentage of skin surface affected compared with the whole body surface), and the general health status of the individual (whether an immune-compromised status exists) will dictate the modality of treatment on an individual basis. In some species, fighting or predation is a normal physiologic behavior and even if we do not mimic these under human care the natural immune protection of the skin in these taxa should be considered when smaller-degree injuries are examined. This is particularly important due to the need of restricted antimicrobial use and the general battle against drug resistance. Compared with other veterinary fields, where even the narrow range of treated species shows how serious the problem is, a large-scale analysis has not been made yet in the zoologic medicine field, but discussions are ongoing on the legislative level.[24,25]

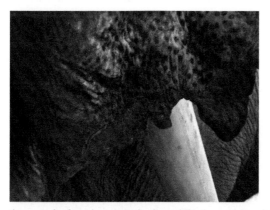

Fig. 9. Frostbite on the ear of a female Asian elephant (*Elephas maximus*). The animal spent too much time outside in dry, cold weather; this resulted a severe necrosis along the edge of the ear and erythema. The treatment included pain management and facilitation of the debridement of the necrotic tissue.

If trauma is caused by another animal, it can be of both inter- or intraspecific origin, and in some instances surgical intervention is inevitable (**Figs. 10** and **11**). Skin trauma can be caused by fences or other objects of the environment as well (**Fig. 12**).

Skin tumors are reported in different zoo mammal species. A study analyzed neoplasm cases in deceased animals revealed a 6.5% (7/108) incidence of cutaneous squamous cell carcinoma in zoo mammals in Taipei Zoo, Taiwan between 1994 and 2003.[26] In nonhuman primates primary and metastatic skin neoplasms were documented; benign tumors included papilloma, adnexal cell tumor, hemangioma, lipoma, neurofibroma, melanocytoma, fibroma, myxoid and basal cell tumor. In the same group malignant tumors consisted of squamous cell carcinoma, basal cell carcinoma, adnexal gland carcinoma, fibrosarcoma, liposarcoma, leiomyosarcoma, melanoma, lymphoma and mammary adenocarcinoma.[21] Though many types of neoplasms have been identified in zoo mammals, is not in the scope of this chapter to delve deeper into this subject.

Endocrine disorders can manifest in altered skin conditions as well, but our current knowledge on these conditions in zoo mammals is limited. Similar ailments that are well-documented in dogs, in which hypothyroidism, hyperadrenocorticism, hyperestrogenism, and hyperadrogenism are the most frequently occurring in relation to dermatologic disease. Hair loss, symmetric alopecia, seborrhea, and recurrent infections are often seen as clinical presentations of endocrinopathies.[27] These conditions pose challenges for the zoo veterinarian as in most of the species, hormonal reference values are not known.

As an example, Red pandas (*Ailurus fulgens*) often show seasonal alopecia, where the exact diagnosis is not always straightforward. Hair loss is most frequently seen on the tail and over the flanks (**Fig. 13**). If the condition is not a pronounced spring moult, then a full dermatologic examination should be performed, including ectoparasite control/investigation, histopathological evaluation of the affected skin, and an endocrinological panel, as hypothyroidism and hypoestrogenism are possible causes, but this commonly occurring problem is still not fully understood.[28]

DERMATOLOGIC PROBLEMS CAUSED BY INFECTIOUS AGENTS

Dermatologic disorders caused by infectious agents are well-documented in zoo mammals. Bacteria, viruses, fungi, and ectoparasites are all important causes of

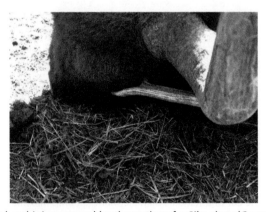

Fig. 10. Traumatic head injury caused by the antler of a Sika deer (*Cervus nippon*) in a European bison (*Bison bonasus*) (anesthetized individual). The wound was close to the eye, but only a relatively superficial skin injury was observed.

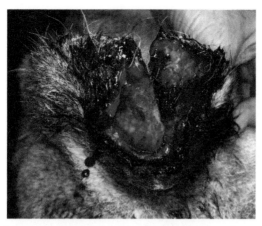

Fig. 11. Severe ear injury in an anesthetized Asiatic lion (*Panthera leo persica*), caused by its female conspecific (the lesion is shown after surgical debridement).

dermatopathies and their relevance differs according to the taxa, region, or environment in concern. Clinically manifested dermatitis can differ greatly on an individual level, ranging from isolated cutaneous signs (eg, alopecia or pustules or erythema) to severe generalized inflammation potentially leading to mortality.[29]

The zoonotic potential must be addressed in every case when handling such individuals, therefore protection measures must be taken regarding personnel safety, further infections, and biosecurity (depending on the agent in question).[30] Some of the diseases, which can infect certain zoo mammal species and also affect the skin are notifiable and the legal obligations must be followed. The 2001 foot and mouth disease outbreak in the United Kingdom showed the importance of the link between the domestic livestock and zoo mammal populations (with endangered taxa) and the

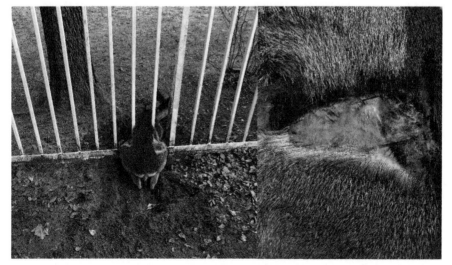

Fig. 12. When the objects of the environment cause the injury, the consequences can be very severe. In this case a wild Roe deer (*Capreolus capreolus*) was caught and stuck between the bars of a metal fence (left) and the animal had extensive skin lesions (right).

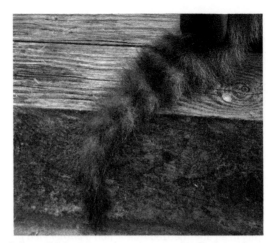

Fig. 13. Hair loss of the tail (above) or alopecia over the flank is often seen in Red pandas (*Ailurus fulgens*), but the exact diagnosis is not always straightforward. This clinical presentation was seen in May 2021 and was not considered a prolonged spring moult, but a definitive diagnosis was also not found, despite of the combined diagnostic effort and sample collection under anesthesia (including hormonal analysis and skin biopsy).

necessity of the One Health approach. In addition, it is important to mention that some zoo species are quite rare and very little information on potential zoonotic potential is known (eg, link between African swine fever and zoo-kept wild boar). More recently another notifiable disease, lumpy skin disease, originally endemic in Africa and parts of the Middle East, was observed and successfully halted in Southeast Europe, which could have had relevance in zoo animals as well.[29,31,32]

Some of the agents causing dermal disease (dermatitis) are significant not only in a captive setting, but can have a detrimental effect on wildlife populations too. The chytrid fungus in amphibians, *Ophidiomyces ophiodiicola* in snakes or White Nose Syndrome in bats are all extremely important examples with conservation relevance or even a direct link between keeping animals in captivity and the absolute need for biosecurity measures (eg, *Xenopus* frogs and chytridiomycosis in other frog species). The species-specific susceptibility/sensitivity is also known, in particular species like the Gray squirrel (*Sciurus carolinensis*), which is an invasive species in Europe and does not show clinical symptoms to the Parapox virus, contrarily to the native Red squirrel (*Sciurus vulgaris*) in which this virus manifests as exudative dermatologic lesions (ulcerations with crusts on the head, feet, and genitalia) and the dramatic decline of the species is attributed to a disease-mediated competition as well.[29,32,33]

The dermatologic condition observed by the clinician can be primarily a skin disease or can be a part of a general disease process where the integument is also affected. Moreover, it can be a localized condition, where the most obvious or first clinical signs are seen on the skin (**Fig. 14**).

One metanalysis study made a thorough literature survey and analysis of dermatitis cases in zoo and wildlife species (216 papers between 1925 and 2021) where findings indicated that 257 cases reported in 108 terrestrial and semi-aquatic wildlife mammal species were affected by skin problems. Seventeen definitive causes of dermatitis were identified in these reports, representing 76.4% of all cases. The highest single proportion of dermatitis cases were of an unknown origin (23.7%, *n* = 61), followed

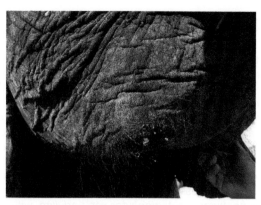

Fig. 14. Mandibular abscess and a consequent fistula in an African elephant (*Loxodonta africana*). The abscess leading to a fistula was a sign of an underlying (tooth) condition, but this can be the first symptom for detection.

closely by mites (21.4%, *n* = 55) and then both bacteria (16.3%, *n* = 42) and viruses (16.3%, *n* = 42).[29]

This statistical shows that even with a very long study period (96 years), a relatively low case load was found. This indicates several further points both for the clinicians and researchers. Firstly, the need of documentation (including photo documentation) to have a more comprehensive list of possible etiologies in all taxa. Second, the absolute necessity for metapopulation analysis to better understand species under human care based on collective data. This would be the role of the veterinary advisors of the relevant conservation breeding programs.

Bacterial agents are important causes of different skin diseases as well. It was found that among the reported cases *Dermatophilus congolensis* caused dermatitis most frequently and in the broadest taxonomic term (18 cases and 6 orders).[29] This disease is more common in young or immunosuppressed animals or among wet conditions, therefore the occurrence of it in polar bears could be linked with husbandry issues.[34,35] Apart from this pathogen several other bacteria are listed and recorded as causative agents in dermal disease, including *Staphylococcus* spp., including reports of MRSA, *Streptococcus* spp., *Pseudomonas aeruginosa*, *Pasteurella* spp., *Corynebacterium* spp., *Salmonella* spp., *Proteus mirabilis*, *Haemophilus influenzae*, *Erysipelothrix rhusiopathiae*, species of the Mycobacterium tuberculosis complex, *Mycobacterium leprae*, *Clostridium* spp., *Actinomyces* spp. to name a few.[21,36]

Viruses are well-known factors in several skin problems and in many species the skin symptoms are part of a systemic viral disease. In some groups taxonomically closely related to humans (eg, great apes and other primate species), the zoonotic nature of some of the diseases must also be considered and all precautions should be taken to avoid infections. The B virus (or Cercopithecine herpesvirus type 1) causes vesicles, pustules, and ulcers at the mucocutaneous junctions and in the skin[21] and though this disease is not considered to be a serious problem in its natural host (Asian macaque species), it can cause even a fatal illness in humans.[37]

Regarding viral infections, a general overview of the causes of dermatitis revealed that the Parapoxvirus genus was the causative agent in two orders (Rodentia and Artiodactyla) and 13 species.[29] Parapoxviruses are epitheliotropic viruses and in most cases have a narrow host range. There are several important viruses within this group; Orf virus has a special importance in petting zoos due to its zoonotic potential and can cause a proliferative dermatitis in several species.[18] Other Parapox-viruses must be considered as potential differential diagnoses as well (eg, bovine papular stomatitis virus and pseudocowpox virus).[38] Parapoxviruses were also identified from different seal and sea lion species (Sealpox), often in rehabilitation centers, where the zoonotic potential was an important factor.[39,40] Monkeypoxvirus was already a well-known pathogen, but more human cases are reported worldwide in 2022, including Europe and North America.[41]

Mycotic diseases are often linked with immunosuppression or husbandry-related matters. *Malassezia* spp. was reported in two orders and 6 species of dermatitis cases, whereas *Trichophyton* and *Microsporum* species do cause skin ailments in different taxa.[21,29,42,43]

A comprehensive questionnaire about mycotic skin disease in macropods revealed the first cases of dermatophytosis in several species in association with *Trichophyton verrucosum* and *Trichophyton mentagrophytes* var. *nodulare*, with young Red kangaroos (*Macropus rufus*) seemingly eliciting predisposition.[44]

Different ectoparasites are causing different clinical presentation in zoo mammals. *Demodex* spp., *Notoedres* spp., and *Sarcoptes scabiei* seem to be the most widespread ectoparasites in zoo mammals, but many other species are reported. Sarcoptic mange has the utmost importance in wildlife, though it has been reported in several zoo as well; New World camelids are very often affected by this condition and immunosuppressive conditions must be considered as well, whereas treatment requires a long duration with macrocyclic lactons.[45,46] Nevertheless, severely affected animals have often a grave prognosis, regardless of the species (**Fig. 15**).

Apart from different mite species lice, fleas, ticks, mosquitoes and flies are all can cause skin problems/disorders. These species can often transmit important, vector-borne diseases.

Diagnostic Challenges in Zoo Mammal Dermatology

Working with zoo mammal dermatologic problems in general can present many challenges to reach a definitive diagnosis. Even if this is accomplished, further difficulties may arise regarding adequate treatment, including the method, length and frequency of the therapy. These challenges include approaching our patients, anesthesia-related matters (where either the species is more difficult to anesthetize due to eg, anatomic

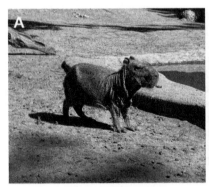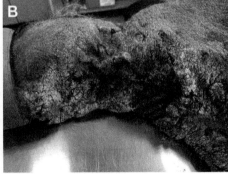

Fig. 15. Severe *Sarcoptes scabiei* infestation in a young Capybara (*Hydrochoerus hydrochaeris*). Despite of the intensive efforts the animal died during an intensive treatment course. Note the severe scaling and crusting with excoriations and wounds secondary to severe pruritus.

features or the condition of the patient defines a higher risk category), the need and relevance of medical training, and the lack of references of healthy individuals in many cases.

Altered skin or hair conditions are not always obvious, especially if these are mild or covered by hair/quills or other anatomic structures (eg, skin folds). There are certain taxonomic groups, where anesthesia if necessary to even perform a proper dermatologic examination and there are situations where even medical training is less practical due to time constraints or the traditional ways of how these animals are kept. As an example, hedgehogs, porcupines, and tree porcupines are rarely trained, thus their integument can only be properly visualized if the animals allow it, which is exceptional (**Fig. 16**).

It is always a difficult decision of how a zoo veterinarian approaches a clinical problem if the patient is noncooperative and the only way to collect samples or visualize a lesion from a close range under anesthesia. In a situation like this, many considerations must be evaluated including the risk of anesthesia regarding the species and the individual, the exhibit, the information to be gained through this procedure, the severity of the conditions, and many others. The other option is to treat the animal according to the clinical symptoms which are present and diagnosed, but it is often a great challenge to set up a definitive diagnosis, and is generally not possible without handling the patient.

The abovementioned practical aspects highlight the need for training (under operant conditioning) in a zoo setting, where noncooperative species can be examined,

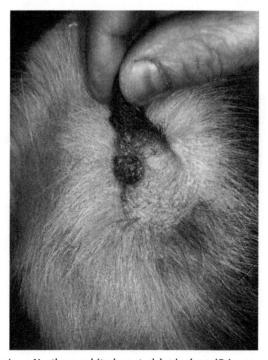

Fig. 16. Papilloma in a Northern white-breasted hedgehog (*Erinaceus roumanicus*). Any kind of skin lesion (due its location close to the elbow) would be difficult or sometimes impossible to see without proper chemical restraint. This fact is applicable to many other skin conditions, including wounds, maggots, ectoparasites, etc. in Erinaceidae.

sampled, and treated (with limitations) without chemical restraint, which eliminates anesthesia-related risk, cost and stress. It is species dependent whether special structures must be created for such activities, or if this can be implemented at the exhibit (**Figs. 17** and **18**). Medical training is not the "magic solution" for all problems in zoo mammals, it must be seen as a viable method and its limitations must be considered. It can easily be that an animal could be trained for a certain behavior and allow for a given diagnostic procedure to be implemented, but some ailments require a more urgent mode of action meaning time would be insufficient to achieve the behavior required through training. If a level of pain already exists, the anticipated pain inflicted through the diagnostic procedure, the physical characteristics of the exhibit and the urgency of the problem are all considerations that must be addressed and which must give a good basis for the clinician to decide how to proceed with the diagnostics/treatments in a particular case.

SAMPLE TYPES

A zoo mammal showing dermatologic symptoms requires a careful diagnostic plan, including many elements discussed above (cooperation level, feasibility of medical training, relevance of anesthesia, etc.). The different samples to be collected from the dermatologic lesions will have a conjunction with the type of lesion or the mode how we can collect these but will have an effect on the expected results as well.[47] Microbiological swabs or impression smears often only have limited diagnostic value, where contamination can be a relevant issue, but direct microscopic examination of the hair or other integumentary structures (eg, claws or nails) and coat brushing may also help in setting up a diagnosis. Skin scrapings (superficial and deep), tape strips, and using a Wood's lamp are all relevant, but skin biopsies (often with the highest diagnostic value if all layers are involved) can frequently provide us with the most complete information. Other examinations can be or must be (depending on the case)

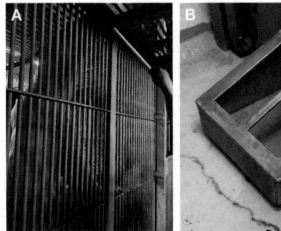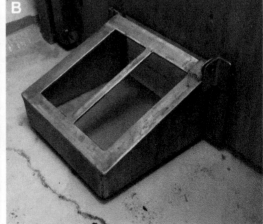

Fig. 17. Polar bears (*Ursus maritimus*) are among the most dangerous species in zoos. Nevertheless, they are good candidates for training and different body parts (including ventral abdomen and paws) can be presented for dermatologic examination if the technical circumstances are provided and a good training program exists. The ventral abdomen and paws are visualized in a standing position (left), whereas the paws are examined in a special device (right).

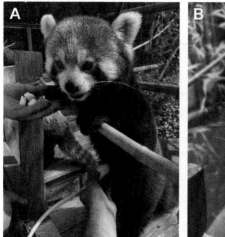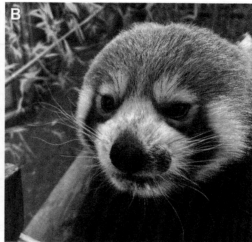

Fig. 18. Red pandas (*Ailurus fulgens*) require less technical modifications in their exhibit for an adequate training program. Dermatologic examination and even sampling is possible, whereas a general health status assessment can be implemented. In this case the lesion around the nose (picture on the right) was sampled and consequently treated long-term without the need for anesthesia.

part of our protocol. These may include for example, an ultrasonographic examination of the affected area and the surrounding/underlying tissues or different blood parameters (eg, hematology, biochemistry, endocrinology, serology, polymerase chain reaction, etc.). Blood collection is mandatory if the skin problem is suspected to be part of a generalized disease or process (eg, endocrine disorders, metabolic diseases, infectious processes, etc.).

It is also advised that sampling should be done only if a previous consultation was done with the laboratory carrying out the actual examination. This is helpful for both parties; the clinician, who will be thoroughly informed and will collect the exact type/material necessary and the lab will be prepared for the possible pathogens and will receive more background information about the course of the disease.

As a summary, zoo mammal dermatology requires a complex approach, where the natural history of the species, the keeping conditions, and the options for examination, diagnostics and treatment must be considered to successfully run a health program in a zoo setting.

CLINICS CARE POINTS

- The importance of understanding the biology of a given species and ensuring their husbandry and nutritional needs in order to prevent pathological conditions.
- If dermatological issues do occur, identification of the cause through diagnostic tests is key to understanding the ailment and how to establish a treatment protocol and potential prevention plan for the future.
- Identification of alterations differentiated along the lines of the following: infectious vs. non-infectious, primary vs. secondary, level of risk to conspecifics, other species (multi species group), staff.

- The importance of medical training in all stages of the management of dermatological disease (diagnosis, treatment and prevention).

REFERENCES

1. Barongi R, Fisken FA, Parker M, et al, editors. Committing to conservation: the World zoo and aquarium conservation strategy. Gland: WAZA Executive Office; 2015. p. 17–9.
2. Nicolau A, Lemberger K, Mosca M, et al. Clinical and histopathological aspects of an alopecia syndrome in captive Andean bears (*Tremarctos ornatus*). Vet Dermatol 2018;29(3):e34–85.
3. Van Horn RC, Sutherland-Smith M, Bracho Sarcos AE, et al. The Andean bear alopecia syndrome may be caused by social housing. Zoo Biol 2019;38(5): 434–41.
4. Mattison S. Training birds and small mammals for medical behaviours. Veterinary Clin North Am Exot Anim Pract 2012;15(3):487–99.
5. Pasmans F, Bogaerts S, Braeckman J, et al. Future of keeping pet reptiles and amphibians: towards integrating animal welfare, human health and environmental sustainability. Vet Rec 2017;181(7):450.
6. Goodroe AE, Fitz C, Power ML, et al. Evaluation of vitamin D3 metabolites in *Callithrix jacchus* (Common marmoset). Am J Primatol 2020;82(6):e23131.
7. Gruber-Dujardin E, Ludwig C, Bleyer M, et al. Cutaneous demodicosis and UV-induced skin neoplasia in two Goeldi's monkeys *(Callimico goeldii)*. J Zoo Wildl Med 2019;50(2):470–3.
8. Hensel P. Nutrition and skin diseases in veterinary medicine. Clin Dermatol 2010; 28(6):686–93.
9. Kearns K, Sleeman J, Frank L, et al. Zinc-responsive dermatosis in a red wolf (*Canis rufus*). J Zoo Wildl Med 2000;31:255–9.
10. Jensen-Jarolim E, Einhorn L, Herrmann I, et al. Pollen Allergies in Humans and their Dogs, Cats and Horses: Differences and Similarities. Clin Transl Allergy 2015;5:15.
11. Dennis PM, Funk JA, Rajala-Schultz PJ, et al. A review of some of the health issues of captive Black Rhinoceroses *(Diceros bicornis)*. J Zoo Wildl Med 2007; 38(4):509–17.
12. Munson L, Koehler JW, Wilkinson J, et al. Vesicular and ulcerative dermatopathy resembling superficial necrolytic dermatitis in captive black rhinoceroses (*Diceros bicornis*). Vet Pathol 1998;35:31–42.
13. Bishop GT, Zuba JR, Pessier PA, et al. Medical management of recurrent eosinophilic granuloma in two Black Rhinoceroses *(Diceros bicornis)*. J Zoo Wildl Med 2016;47(3):855–61.
14. Pessier PA, Munson L, Miller RE. Oral, nasal and cutaneous eosinophilic granulomas in the Black rhinoceros (*Diceros bicornis*): a lesion distinct from superficial necrolytic dermatitis. J Zoo Wildl Med 2004;35(1):1–7.
15. Weber M, Miller E. Fungal pneumonia in Black rhinoceros (*Diceros bicornis*). Yulee, FL: Proceedings American Association of Zoo Veterinarians; 1996. p. 34–6.
16. Salas M, Manteca X, Abáigar T, et al. Using farm animal welfare protocols as a base to assess the welfare of wild animals in captivity—Case study: Dorcas Gazelles (*Gazella dorcas*). Animals 2018;8:111.
17. Novak MA, Meyer JS. A Rhesus-monkey Model of Non-suicidal Self Injury. Front Behav Neurosci 2021;15:674127.

18. Titeux E, Gilbert C, Briand A, et al. From feline idiopathic ulcerative dermatitis to feline behavioral ulcerative dermatitis: Grooming repetitive behaviors indicators of poor welfare in cats. Front Vet Sci 2018;5:81.
19. Delaney MA, Treuting PM, Rothenburger JL. Rodentia, . Pathology of Wildlife and Zoo Animals. London, UK: Academic Press, Elsevier; 2018. p. 499–515.
20. Bernstein JA, Didier PJ. Nonhumane primate dermatology: a literature review. Vet Dermatol 2009;20(3):145–56.
21. Hubbard GB. Nonhuman Primate Dermatology. Veterinary Clin North Am Exot Anim Pract 2001;4(2):573–83.
22. Olivry T, Prélaud P, Héripret D, et al. Allergic contact dermatitis in the dog. Principles and diagnosis. Vet Clin North Am Small Anim Pract 1990;20(6):1443–56.
23. Wohlsein P, Peters M, Schulze C, et al. Thermal Injuries in Veterinary Forensic Pathology. Vet Pathol 2016;53(5):1001–17.
24. Hardefeldt LY, Gilkerson JR, Billman-Jacobe H, et al. Antimicrobial labelling in Australia: a threat to antimicrobial stewardship? Aust Vet J 2018;96(5):151–4.
25. Hur BA, Hardefeldt LY, Verspoor KM, et al. Describing the antimicrobial usage patterns of companion animal veterinary practices; free text analysis of more than 4.4 million consultation records. PLoS One 2020;15(3):e0230049.
26. Chang PH, Liu C-H, Jeng C-R, et al. Spontaneous neoplasms in zoo mammals, birds and reptiles in Taiwan – A 10-year survey. Anim Biol 2012;62(1):95–110.
27. Frank AL. Comparative dermatology – canine endocrine dermatoses. Clin Dermatol 2006;24(4):317–25.
28. Douay G, Ramsay EC. Captive red panda medicine. In: Glatson AR, editor. Red panda. Biology and conservation of the first panda. San Diego, USA: Academic Press, Elsevier Science Publishing Co Inc; 2022. p. 239–54.
29. Ringwaldt EM, Brook BW, Carver S, et al. The Patterns and Causes of Dermatitis in Terrestrial and Semi-Aquatic Mammalian Wildlife. Animals 2021;11(6):1691.
30. Parish LC, Schwartzman RM. Zoonoses of dermatological interest. Semin Dermatol 1993;12:57–64.
31. Namazi F, Tafti AK. Lumpy skin disease, an emerging, transboundary, viral disease: a review. Vet Med Sci 2021;7:888–96.
32. Bruemmer CM, Rushton SP, Gurnell J, et al. Epidemiology of squirrelpox virus in grey squirrels in the UK. Epidemiol Infect 2010;138(7):941–50.
33. Tompkins DM, Sainsbury AW, Nettleton P, et al. Parapoxvirus causes a deleterious disease in red squirrels associated with UK population declines. Proc R Soc Lond Ser B Biol Sci 2002;269:529–33.
34. Eo KY, Kwon OD. Dermatitis caused by *Dermatophilus congolensis* in a zoo polar bear (*Ursus maritimus*). Pak Vet J 2014;34:560–2.
35. Smith CF. Dermatitis caused by *Dermatophilus congolenesis* in Polar bears (*Thalarctos maritimus*). Vet Rec 1972;92(20):533–4.
36. Janssen D, Lamberski N, Dunne G, et al. Methicillin-resistant *Staphylococcus aureus* skin infections from an elephant calf – San Diego, California, 2008. Morbidity Mortality Weekly Rep 2009;58(8):194–8.
37. Elmore D, Eberle R. Monkey B Virus (*Cercopithecine herpesvirus 1*). Comp Med 2008;58(1):11–21.
38. Guo J, Rasmussen J, Wünschmann A, et al. Genetic characterization of orf viruses isolated from various ruminant species of a zoo. Vet Microbiol 2004; 99(2):81–92.
39. Clark C, McIntyre PG, Evans A, et al. Human sealpox resulting from a seal bite: confirmation that sealpox virus is zoonotic. Br J Dermatol 2005;152(4):791–3.

40. Nollens HH, Jacobson ER, Gulland FMD, et al. Pathology and preliminary characterization of a parapoxvirus isolated from a California sea lion (*Zalophus californianus*). J Wildl Dis 2006;42(1):23–32.
41. Kumar N, Acharya A, Gendelman HE, et al. The 2022 outbreak and the pathobiology of the monkeypox virus. J Autoimmun 2022;131:102855.
42. Kearns K, Pollock CG, Ramsay EC. Dermatophytosis in red pandas (*Ailurus fulgens fulgens*): a review of 14 cases. J Zoo Wildl Med 1999;30:561–3.
43. Sos E, Molnar V, Lajos Z, et al. Successfully treated dermatomycosis in California sea lions (*Zalophus californianus*). J Zoo Wildl Med 2013;44(2):462–5.
44. Boulton KA, Vogelnest LJ, Vogelnest L. Dermatophytosis in zoo macropods: a questionnaire study. J Zoo Wildl Med 2013;44(3):555–63.
45. Beck W. Treatment of sarcoptic mange in llamas (*Lama glama*) and alpacas (*Vicugna pacos*) with repeated subcutaneous moxidectin injections. Vet Parasitol 2020;283:109190.
46. Castilla-Castaño E, Herman N, Martinelli E, et al. Treatment of sarcoptic and chorioptic mange in an alpaca (*Vicugna pacos*) herd with a combination of topical amitraz and subcutaneous ivermectin. N Z Vet J 2021;69(2):121–6.
47. Neuber A, Nuttall T. Diagnostic Techniques in Veterinary Dermatology. In: Introduction to dermatological Tests. Hoboken, NJ: Wiley Blackwell; 2017. p. 1–20.

The Current State of Knowledge on Parasitic Copepods (Siphonostomatoida: Pandaridae) of Elasmobranchs

Marcia Raquel Pegoraro de Macedo, PhD[a],
Marialetizia Palomba, PhD[b], Mario Santoro, DVM, PhD[a],*

KEYWORDS

- Batoidea • Copepods • Ectoparasites • Elasmobranchs • Fish • Pandaridae
- Selachii • Sharks

KEY POINTS

- Parasitic copepods are commonly known to cause serious damage to their hosts.
- Pandarid copepods (Siphonostomatoida) are primarily ectoparasites of sharks.
- Taxonomic information on pandarid copepods remains conflicting, and data on their biology, ecology, and pathogenesis are poor known.
- The authors summarize and analyze the existing pandarid copepod literature as it relates to diversity, life cycles, host–parasite interactions, biogeography, pathology, and available treatments.

INTRODUCTION

Chondrichthyan is a term to group fishes with a cartilaginous skeleton consisting of about 1200 described species. This represents an evolutionarily conservative group that has persisted in marine and freshwater ecosystems for over 400 million years.[1] Within chondrichthyan, elasmobranch fishes (class Elasmobranchii) comprise sharks and sawfish (infraclass Selachii) and rays, skates, and stingrays (infraclass Batoidea).[2,3]

In spite of their evolutionary success, many elasmobranch species are threatened with overexploitation as a result of their life history traits and human activities.[4] On the other hand, elasmobranchs may serve as hosts for a great variety of parasites: Myxosporea, Monogenea, Cestoda, Trematoda, Nematoda, Hirudinea, Isopoda,

[a] Department of Integrative Marine Ecology, Stazione Zoologica Anton Dohrn, Villa Comunale n 1, Naples 80121, Italy; [b] Department of Ecological and Biological Sciences, University of Tuscia, Largo dell'Università snc, Viterbo 01100, Italy
* Corresponding author.
E-mail address: mario.santoro@szn.it

Vet Clin Exot Anim 26 (2023) 475–509
https://doi.org/10.1016/j.cvex.2022.12.006
1094-9194/23/© 2022 Elsevier Inc. All rights reserved.
vetexotic.theclinics.com

and Copepoda, to name a few examples.[5] Therefore, the decrease in the number or removal of elasmobranchs from their ecosystems can be driving a long-dated and worldwide decline in their parasites. The most interesting hypothesis about this is that fishing and, in general, anthropic pressures reducing the abundance of fish, in turn, reduces the transmission efficiency of their parasites.[6] Knowledge of parasite diversity, biology, taxonomy, geographic distribution, and host–parasite interactions are fundamental to understanding the impacts of abiotic and biotic factors on the host health and to promote appropriate intervention when it is needed.[7–11]

Many elasmobranch species are popular fishes exhibited in zoos and public aquariums. An excellent paper summarized the published data on metazoan parasites of chondrichthyans,[5] emphasizing on taxa that can promote disease in captive hosts. However, there is still a need to improve knowledge and to draw attention to particular issues of specific groups of parasites. In this article, the authors summarize and analyze the existing literature of the copepod parasites of the family Pandaridae (Milne Edwards, 1840) which are primarily ectoparasites of sharks, as it relates to their diversity, life cycles, biogeography, pathology, and available treatments.

HISTORICAL CONTEXT AND TAXONOMY

The copepods are small crustaceans (generally a few millimeters or less in length), ecologically very diverse, encompassing symbiotic, and free-living species.[12,13] Parasitic copepods display a great diversity of forms with marked structural modifications, having developed adaptations to attach to specific sites on the organism's host. For instance, siphonostomatoids have a tubular mouth containing stylet-like mandibular gnathobases. The mouthtube is formed by the labrum and the labium, which represents the fused paragnaths. The antennae and maxillipeds are typically subchelate in form and serve to attach these copepods to their hosts.[13] The overall morphology of copepods is maintained in many parasitic forms, but others undergo an extreme metamorphosis that their identity can only be determined by characteristics of the larval stages or by molecular diagnosis.[13] Furthermore, the same species can express different morphologic features when parasitizing on different host species possibly resulting in misidentifications.[14]

Historically, Aristotle is considered to have made the first record of the occurrence of parasitic copepods on fish.[15] Free-living copepods were easily recognized as crustaceans; however, the parasitic forms did not have an established classification until the nineteenth century. After establishing the copepod taxonomy, there are still gaps in knowledge about biology, parasite–host interaction, biogeography, and genetic information.

The Pandaridae (Siphonostomatoida Burmeister, 1835) comprises ectoparasites of fish, whose taxonomic information is conflicting, and data on biology, biogeography, phylogeny, and pathogenesis remain incomplete or poorly known. Taxonomy at the genus and species levels is not yet well resolved, leading to regular revisions and redescriptions of species.[16–23]

The more complete taxonomic revision of Pandaridae is that of Cressey.[17] He recognized 12 genera and 33 species and considered accidental infection if the report was on teleost fishes. Until the description of the genus *Kabataia* (Kazachenko, Korotaeva & Kurochkin, 1972) erected to place a species infecting the teleost fish *Opleg-nathus woodwardi*, this family was considered exclusive of copepods infecting only elasmobranchs. Finally, after transferring of the genera *Amaterasia* (Izawa, 2008), *Cecrops* (Leach, 1816), *Luetkenia* (Claus, 1864), *Philorthagoriscus* (Horst, 1897), and

Orthagoriscicola (Poche, 1902) to the Pandaridae, now this family comprises several species parasitizing also teleost fishes[18] (**Table 1**).

The most recent data on the taxonomic diversity of Pandaridae report 23 genera and 88 species parasitizing ray-finned fish and elasmobranchs.[13] However, Walter and Boxshall[24] consider only 64 of those as valid species (see **Table 1**). Many species are considered invalid or synonymies, making it difficult to gather information from the group. For example, for *Achtheinus pinguis* (Wilson, 1912) are considered 17 synonyms, whose descriptions occurred from 1912 to 1959, by different authors, from different geographic regions (ie, Cape of Good Hope[25] and Uruguay coast[26]) and hosts (ie, *Pliotrema warreni* and *Squalus mitsukurii*[27]). On the other hand, it is well established that elasmobranchs are the main hosts of Pandaridae, which harbor almost 90% of the known species. However, the precise number of valid species is still unclear due mainly to questions of the proposed synonymies and incomplete or conflicting descriptions. A summary of valid Pandaridae species, according to Walter and Boxshall[24] with hosts and geographic localities, is provided in **Table 1**. Representative examples of pandarid species are presented in **Figs. 1–5**.

LIFE CYCLES

Ectoparasite copepods of elasmobranchs use a wide spectrum of microhabitats in their hosts. They are found on body external surfaces and orifices with an exit route to the external environment.[17] The copepod permanence on the host can be for a short period or some stages of the parasite's life. In general, during the early part of their lives, these parasites increase stepwise in size, through a series of moults. On reaching sexual maturity and the definitive parasitic lifestyle, they stop to moult. At the same time, their growth becomes much more vigorous, accompanied by metamorphosis, as a result of which the adult female parasite becomes completely dissimilar from the early stages.[28] Most cycles can be divided into four segments: naupliar, postnaupliar, preadult, and adult. Except the adult, these segments commonly consist of more than one. Nauplii have been numbered I–V, and the postnaupliar stages numbered I–IV. The preadult is the stage that settles definitively on the host and begins a period of metamorphosis for the adult segment.[28,29] As in most parasitic copepods, the infective larva of Pandaridae is the first copepodid, and life cycles are direct, involving only a single host.

The specifics of Pandaridae life cycles are generally poorly understood, but it has been suggested that the life cycles of the members of this family are similar to those of Caligidae (Burmeister, 1835),[30] an issue supported by the monophyly of Pandaridae and Caligidae.[31] In general, the life cycle of caligids comprises two stages of free-living nauplii, followed by an infective copepodid stage and four stages of parasitic chalimus, two preadult parasitic stages and the parasitic adults.[28] Although there are small differences between the life cycles, the data can be useful to infer the cycles of other species, as was done for *Nesippus orientalis* (Heller, 1865).[32] Dippenar[32] inferred that *N orientalis* had a short free-living stage, whereas all other stages would be linked to a host. In the adult stage, males are likely to mate with several females, and females may be polyandrous, although it is unlikely that the parasites can move between different hosts.

Some species have particular life cycles. For instance, *Amaterasia amanoiwatoi* (Izawa, 2008) was described from a female developing inside encysted copepodid V, begin the copepodids I, III, IV, and V, all found in variable numbers, encysted in fin galls on *Xanthichthys lineopunctatus* from the eastern Pacific.[33] A similar life cycle was suggested for *Amaterasia lewisi* (Tang, Benz & Nagasawa, 2012) with females

Table 1
Valid species of Pandaridae (Siphonostomatoida) according to Walter and Boxshall,[24] and their respective hosts, geographic locations and sites of infection. Genera in bold are parasites of teleost fishes

Genus	Host	Location	Sites of Infection	References
Achtheinus (Wilson, 1908)	Carcharhiniformes Hexanchiformes Lamniformes Pristiophoriformes Squaliformes			
A dentatus (Wilson, 1911)	Carcharhinus leucas C limbatus C obscurus C sealei Carcharias taurus Carcharodon carcharias Galeorhinus galeus Haploblepharus edwardsii Mustelus canis M henlei M mosis Sphyrna mokarran S zygaena Squalus acanthias S blainville S megalops Triakis semifasciata	North Pacific Ocean (Japan); Mexico; South Pacific Ocean (Peru); North Atlantic (California, USA)	Body surface	20,37,59

A oblongus (Wilson, 1908)	C carcharias Galeorhinus galeus Haploblepharus edwardsii H pictus Hexanchus griseus Mustelus canis M henlei M manazo M mustelus M schmitti Notorynchus cepedianus Pliotrema warreni Poroderma africanum Prionace glauca Sphyrna zygaena Squalus acanthias S blainville S megalops S suckleyi Triakis semifasciata	South Pacific Ocean (Argentina); North Pacific Ocean (Japan); Peru; Southern Africa; North Atlantic (California, USA)	Body surface Claspers Fins Nostril Scar Skin	60–72
A pinguis (Wilson, 1912)	Carcharias taurus Carcharodon carcharias Galeorhinus galeus Mustelus mustelus M schmitti Pliotrema warreni Rhizoprionodon acutus Squalus acanthias S megalops S megalops	South Pacific Ocean (Argentina); North Pacific Ocean (Japan); Southern Africa	Claspers Fins	37,63,73,74
Amaterasia (Izawa, 2008) A amanoiwatoi (Izawa, 2008) A lewisi (Tang, Benz & Nagasawa, 2012)	Acanthuriformes Tetraodontiformes Eupercaria			24

(continued on next page)

Table 1
(continued)

Genus	Host	Location	Sites of Infection	References
Cecrops (Leach, 1816)	Pleuronectiformes Tetraodontiformes Scombriformes			24
C desmaresti (Risso, 1816)				
C fulgens (Telesius, 1819)				
C latreillii (Leach, 1816)				
C lutosus (Slabber, 1760)				
Demoleus (Heller, 1865)	Hexanchiformes Squatiniformes Squaliformes			
D heptapus (Otto, 1821)	Squatina squatina Hexanchus griseus	Hawaii; Mediterranean Sea; Slovenia	Body surface Skin of the chin	75–77
D latus (Shiino, 1954)	Squalus acanthias S megalops	Canada (Cape Trawler); New Zealand	Fins	17,78
Dinemoleus (Cressey & Boyle, 1978)	Lamniformes			
D indeprensus (Cressey & Boyle, 1978)	Megachasma pelagios	North Pacific Ocean (Japan)	Body surface	79–81
Dinemoura (Latreille, 1829)	Carcharhiniformes Lamniformes Squaliformes			
D discrepans (Cressey, 1967)	Alopias pelagicus A superciliosus A vulpinus Carcharinus limbatus C longimanus	Arabian Sea; Indian Ocean; Madagascar; North Atlantic; Taiwan	Body surface Fins	17,23,82,83

D ferox (Krøyer, 1838)	*Centrophorus squamosus* *Somniosus microcephalus* *S pacificus*	Taiwan	Body surface	84
D latifolia (Steenstrup & Lütken, 1861)	*Carcharodon carcharias* *Galeorhinus galeus* *Isurus oxyrinchus* *Lamna nasus* *Prionace glauca*	Hawaii; Indian Ocean North Pacific Ocean (Japan); Madagascar; Mediterranean Sea; Mexico; New Zealand South Africa; North Atlantic (California, USA)	Behind tooth Body surface Buccal cavity Fins Skin	20,38,40,45,68,75,77,78,85
D producta (Müller, 1785)	*Alopias vulpinus* *Carcharodon carcharias* *Cetorhinus maximus* *Isurus oxyrinchus* *Lamna nasus* *Prionace glauca* *Sphyrna zygaena*	Chile; Irish Sea; Mediterranean Sea;United States	Pelvic fin	17,44,77,86
Echthrogaleus (Steenstrup & Lütken, 1861)	Carcharhiniformes Lamniformes Myliobatiformes Squaliformes Torpediniformes			
E asiaticus (Ho, Liu & Lin, 2012)	*Alopias pelagicus* *A superciliosus*	Taiwan	Body surface	87
E coleoptratus (Guérin-Méneville, 1837)	*Carcharhinus brachyurus* *Carcharodon carcharias* *Centrophorus uyato* *Galeorhinus galeus* *Isurus oxyrinchus* *Lamna ditropis* *L nasus*	Australia; Canada (Bay of Fundy); Chile; Indian Ocean; Ireland (Dingle); North Pacific Ocean (Japan); Mediterranean	Body surface Buccal cavity Fins Gill arches Nares cavity Skin	17,20,38,44,45,68,70,77,78,87-92

(continued on next page)

Table 1
(continued)

Genus	Host	Location	Sites of Infection	References
	Mustelus henlei	Sea; New Zealand;		
	Prionace glauca	North Atlantic;		
	Rhizoprionodon acutus	North Pacific		
	Squalus acanthias	South Africa; Taiwan		
	S suckleyi	North Atlantic		
	T semifasciata	(California, USA)		
E denticulatus (Smith, 1873)	Alopias pelagicus	Arabian Sea; Indian	Body surface	17,20,38,68,82,83,93-95
	A superciliosus	Ocean; North Pacific	Branchial chamber	
	A vulpinus	Ocean (Japan);	Cloacal aperture	
	Carcharhinus falciformis	Madagascar; New	Fins	
	Carcharodon carcharias	Zealand; North		
	Isurus oxyrinchus	Atlantic; Pacific		
	Prionace glauca	Ocean; South		
	Sphyrna lewini	Africa; Thailand		
E disciarai (Benz & Deets, 1987)	Mobula thurstoni	North Atlantic (California, USA)	Fins	96
E mitsukurinae (Izawa, 2012)	Mitsukurina owstoni	North Pacific Ocean (Japan)	Body surface	97
E pellucidus (Shiino, 1963)	Carcharodon carcharias	North Pacific Ocean (Japan)		73
E spinulus (Morales-Serna, Crow, Montes & Gonzalez, 2019)	Tetronarce tokionis	Hawaii	Body surface	49
E torpedinis (Wilson, 1907)	Tetronarce nobiliana	South Africa;	Body surface	17,61
	T occidentalis	United States		
Entepherus (Bere, 1936)	Myliobatiformes			

	Host	Location	Site	
E laminipes (Bere, 1936)	*Mobula alfredi* *M birostris* *M hypostoma* *M kuhlii* *M tarapacana* *M thurstoni*	Mexico; Southern Africa	Branchial filters Tooth band	47,98
Gangliopus Gerstaecker, 1854	Carcharhiniformes Lamniformes			
G pyriformis (Gerstaecker, 1854)	*Alopias vulpinus* *Prionace glauca*	Indian Ocean; North Pacific Ocean (Japan); North Atlantic	Branchial lamellae Gill filaments	38,92,20,99
Kabataia (Kazachenko, Korotaeva & Kurochkin, 1972) *K ostorhynchi* (Kazachenko, Korotaeva & Kurochkin, 1972)	Centrarchiformes			24
Lepimacrus (Hesse, 1883)	Lamniformes			
L jourdaini (Hesse, 1883)	*Lamna nasus*			30
Luetkenia (Claus, 1864) *L asterodermi* (Claus, 1864) *L elongata* (Shiino, 1963)	Acanthuriformes			24

(continued on next page)

Table 1 (continued)				
Genus	**Host**	**Location**	**Sites of Infection**	**References**
Nesippus (Heller, 1865)	Carcharhiniformes Lamniformes Hexanchiformes Orectolobiformes Rhinopristiformes			
N crypturus (Heller, 1865)	*Carcharhinus brevipinna C galapagensis C leucas C limbatus C longimanus C plumbeus Carcharodoncarcharias Galeocerdo cuvier Rhizoprionodon acutus Scoliodon laticaudus Sphyrna lewini S mokarran S zygaena*	Australia; Hawaii; Indian Ocean; Madagascar; Mediterranean Sea; South Africa; North Atlantic (Florida, USA)	Body surface Gill arches Mouth Nasal cavity	17,32,38,75,77,100,102
N gonosaccus (Heegaard, 1943)	*Carcharhinus sorrah*	Gilbert Islands (Pacific Ocean)	Not stated	101
N nana (Cressey, 1970)	*Carcharhinus plumbeus*	North Atlantic (Florida, USA)	Gill arches	32,100
N orientalis (Heller, 1865)	*Alopias vulpinus Carcharhinus acronotus C brachyurus C brevipinna C leucas C limbatus*	Argentina; Chile; Indian Ocean; Japan; Madagascar; Mediterranean Sea; New Zealand; South Africa;		17,21,38,44,77,78,90,93,100 103,104

	Host	Locality	Site	References
	C obscurus C plumbeus Carcharias taurus Carcharodon carcharias Galeocerdo cuvier Ginglymostoma cirratum Isurus oxyrinchus Mustelus antarcticus M mustelus M punctulatus M schmitti Negaprion brevirostris Notorynchus cepedianus Rhizoprionodon acutus Scoliodon laticaudus Sphyrna lewini S mokarran S zygaena	Tunisia; North Atlantic (Florida, USA)		
N tigris (Cressey, 1967)	Carcharodon carcharias Galeocerdo cuvier	Madagascar; South Africa	Nasal cavities	17,32
N vespa (Kirtisinghe, 1964)	Rhina ancylostomus Rhynchobatus djiddensis	Madagascar; South Africa	Body surface Gill arches Mouth	17,32,105
Orthagoriscicola (Poche, 1902)	Carangiformes Tetraodontiformes			
O muricata (Krøyer, 1837)		North Atlantic (Woods Hole, USA); North Pacific (Japan)	Body surface Fins	30,106
Pagina (Cressey, 1963)	Carcharhiniformes Lamniformes			

(continued on next page)

Table 1
(continued)

Genus	Host	Location	Sites of Infection	References
P tunica (Cressey, 1964)	Alopias superciliosus, Carcharhinus longimanus, Prionace glauca, Sphyrna zygaena	Madagascar; North Atlantic; Taiwan; Thailand	Body surface, Fins	23,38,83,92,95,107
Pandarus (Leach, 1816)	Carcharhiniformes, Hexanchiformes, Lamniformes, Orectolobiformes, Rhinopristiformes, Squaliformes			
P ambiguus (Scott, 1907)	Alopias pelagicus			95
P bicolor (Leach, 1816)	Carcharhinus signatus, Carcharodon carcharias, Galeorhinus galeus, Hexanchus griseus, Isurus oxyrinchus, Mustelus henlei, M mustelus, Notorynchus cepedianus, Oxynotus centrina, Prionace glauca, Squalus acanthias, S suckleyi, Triakis semifasciata	Aegean Sea; Australia; Black Sea; Ireland (Dingle); Mediterranean Sea; New Zealand; North Sea; Sea of Azov; Sea of Marmara; South Africa; South Atlantic; Taiwan; Thailand; North Atlantic (California, USA)	Body surface, Branchial chamber, Fins	17,23,70,77,78,86,88,90,93,107–112
P brevicaudis (Dana, 1852–1853)	Unspecified shark	New Zealand		113

P carcharhini (Ho, 1963)	*Carcharhinus altimus* C *brevipinna* C *leucas* C *limbatus* C *plumbeus* C *sorrah* *Glyphis gangeticus*	Arabian Sea; Japan; Madagascar; Australia	Body surface Fins	38,17,82,102
P cranchii (Leach, 1819)	*Alopias pelagicus* A *vulpinus* *Carcharhinus amboinensis* C *brachyurus* C *falciformis* C *galapagensis* C *leucas* C *longimanus* C *obscurus* C *plumbeus* C *signatus* *Carcharodon carcharias* *Galeocerdo cuvier* *Galeorhinus galeus* *Isurus oxyrinchus* *Lamna nasus* *Poroderma africanum* *Prionace glauca* *Rhina ancylostomus* *Sphyrna lewini* S *mokarran* S *zygaena* *Stegostoma tigrinum*	Angola; Arabian Sea; Australia; Canary Islands; Hawaiian Islands; Indian Ocean; Japan; Mediterranean Sea; Mexico; New Zealand; North Atlantic; South Africa; Southern Africa; North Atlantic (Florida and North Carolina, USA); West Indies	Body surface Buccal cavity Cloacal aperture Fins Gills Jaws Skin	20,38,60,75,77,78,82,92,97,100,102,108,114–118

(continued on next page)

Table 1
(continued)

Genus	Host	Location	Sites of Infection	References
P floridanus (Cressey, 1967)	Carcharhinus amblyrhynchos Carcharias taurus Carcharodon carcharias Galeocerdo cuvier Isurus oxyrinchus Lamna nasus Prionace glauca Sphyrna zygaena Tetronarce nobiliana	Australia; Central Atlantic; North Atlantic; South Africa; North Atlantic (Dennis, USA)	Buccal cavity Fins Gills Jaws Snout	17,38,68,92,102,117
P katoi (Cressey, 1967)	Carcharhinus albimarginatus C falciformis C leucas	Cocos Islands; Central Pacific Ocean (Costa Rica); Pacific Ocean		17
P niger (Kirtisinghe, 1950)	Carcharhinus sorrah Sphyrna lewini	Arabian Sea; Australia		82,119
P rhincodonicus (Norman, Newbound & Knott, 2000)	Rhincodon typus	Australia; Mozambique	Body surface Fins Lips	19,120
P rouxii (Risso, 1826)	Not stated	Nice (Mediterranean Sea)	Body surface	121
P satyrus (Dana, 1849)	Alopias superciliosus Carcharhinus brevipinna Carcharodon carcharias Isurus oxyrinchus Prionace glauca Sphyrna zygaena	Central Pacific (Costa Rica); Hawaii; Indian Ocean; New Zealand; North Atlantic; Taiwan	Body surface Branchial chamber Fins Skin	38,45,75,83,92,93,122,123

P sinuatus (Say, 1818)	*Carcharhinus acronotus* *C leucas* *C plumbeus* *Carcharias taurus* *Carcharodon carcharias* *Ginglymostoma cirratum* *Mustelus canis* *M norrisi* *Negaprion brevirostris*	North Atlantic (Canada); North Atlantic (Massachusetts and Florida, USA)	Body surface Fins	17,100,124
P smithii (Rathbun, 1886)	*Alopias vulpinus* *Carcharhinus amboinensis* *C brevipinna* *C falciformis* *C galapagensis* *C leucas* *C limbatus* *C obscurus* *C plumbeus* *C signatus* *Carcharias taurus* *Carcharodon carcharias* *Galeocerdo cuvier* *Isurus oxyrinchus* *Prionace glauca* *Rhina ancylostomus* *Rhincodon typus* *Rhizoprionodon acutus* *Scoliodon laticaudus* *Sphyrna zygaena*	Arabian Sea; Australia; Central Atlantic Ocean; Hawaiian Islands; Indian Ocean; North Pacific (Japan); Mediterranean Sea; Mexico; North Atlantic; South Africa; South Atlantic (Brazil); North Atlantic (California, Massachusetts, and Florida, USA)	Body surface Buccal cavity Fins Gills	17,20,61,64,68,75,77,82,92,102,116,117
P zygaenae (Brady, 1883)	*Sphyrna zygaena*	Central Pacific (Mexico); South Atlantic (Brazil, São Paulo)	Fins	17

(continued on next page)

Table 1
(continued)

Genus	Host	Location	Sites of Infection	References
Pannosus (Cressey, 1967)	Carcharhiniformes			
P japonicus (Shiino, 1960)	*Sphyrna lewini*	North Pacific (Japan); South Africa	Body surface	105,125
Paranesippus (Shiino, 1955)	Squaliformes			
P incisus (Shiino, 1955)	*Deania calcea*	North Pacific (Japan)	Body surface	125
Perissopus (Steenstrup & Lütken, 1861)	Carcharhiniformes Lamniformes Rhinopristiformes Squaliformes			
P dentatus (Steenstrup & Lütken, 1861)	*Carcharhinus acronotus* C brevipinna Carcharhinus dussumieri Carcharhinus fitzroyensis C leucas C limbatus C obscurus C plumbeus C sealei C sorrah C tilstoni C tjutjot Carcharodon carcharias Galeocerdo cuvier Galeorhinus galeus Glaucostegus cemiculus Hemigaleus microstoma	Australia; Indian Ocean; Madagascar; Mediterranean Sea; South Africa; Tunisia; North Atlantic (Florida, USA)	Fins Clasper External nares Skin	17,38,61,77,82,90,100–105,119

	Mustelus asterias			
	M mosis			
	M mustelus			
	M norrisi			
	M punctulatus			
	Negaprion brevirostris			
	Rhizoprionodon acutus			
	R taylori			
	R terraenovae			
	Sphyrna lewini			
	S mokarran			
	S tiburo			
	S zygaena			
	Squalus megalops			
Philorthragoriscus (Horst, 1897)	Tetraodontiformes			24
P serratus (Krøyer, 1863)				
Phyllothyreus (Norman, 1903)	Carcharhiniformes Lamniformes			
P cornutus (Milne-Edwards, 1840)	Galeocerdo cuvier Isurus oxyrinchus Lamna nasus Prionace glauca Sphyrna zygaena	Hawaiian Islands; Indian Ocean; Ireland (Dingle); New Zealand; North Atlantic; South Africa	Body surface Gills Skin	38,45,75,78,89,92,105
Prosaetes (Wilson, 1907)	Orectolobiformes			
P rhinodontis (Wright, 1876)	Rhincodon typus	Madagascar; North Pacific (Japan)	Gills	18,59,126
Pseudopandarus (Kirtisinghe, 1950)	Carcharhiniformes Squaliformes			

(continued on next page)

Table 1
(continued)

Genus	Host	Location	Sites of Infection	References
P australis (Cressey & Simpfendorfer, 1988)	Carcharhinus dussumieri Hemigaleus microstoma Rhizoprionodon acutus R taylori Sphyrna lewini	South Africa; Australia; Arabian Sea	Females: pectoral, pelvic, and caudal regions; Male: flanks and nape	82,126,128
P cairae (Bernot & Boxshall, 2017)	Squalus bucephalus S melanurus	New Caledonia	Body surface	127
P gracilis (Kirtisinghe, 1950)	Mustelus griseus M mosis Rhizoprionodon acutus Sscoliodon laticaudus	Indian Ocean; North Pacific (Japan); Madagascar; South Africa	Body surface Fins	20,38,105,127
P longus (Gnanamuthu, 1951)	Carcharhinus dussumieri C obscurus C sealei C sorrah C tjutjot Mustelus mosis Rhizoprionodon acutus Triaenodon obesus	Arabian Sea; Indian Ocean; Madagascar; Mozambique; South Africa	Body surface Fins	38,82,104,127
P pelagicus (Rangnekar, 1977)	Unknown (collected in plankton)	India (Bombay)	-	129
P scyllii (Yamaguti & Yamasu, 1959)	Triakis scyllium	North Pacific (Japan)	-	130

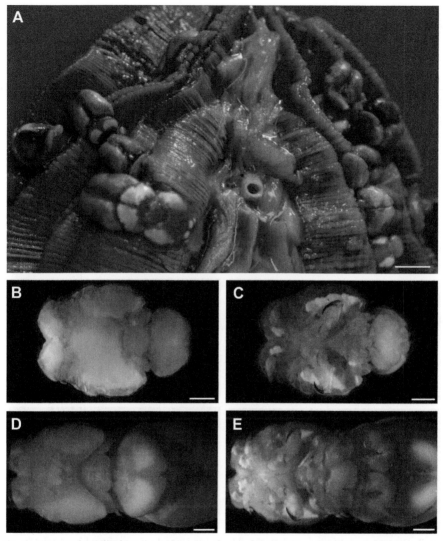

Fig. 1. *Cecrops latreillii* found on the gills of a sunfish (*Mola mola*), in the Mediterranean Sea (*A*). Male (*B*, dorsal view; *C*, ventral view) and female (*D*, dorsal view; *E*, ventral view). More information about *C latreillii* infection in this sunfish can be found in Santoro and colleagues.[131] Scale bars: A: 1 cm; B–E: 2 mm.

developing gall-forming juveniles.[33] *Amaterasia amanoiwatoi* and *A lewisi* are remarkable examples of the ecological diversity displayed by these parasitic copepods. They are the only pandarids known to fully encyst in fish fins during the post-naupliar phase of development.[18] This life cycle contrasts strongly with that of other pandarids, whose copepodids II–V anchor to the host's external surface by a frontal filament secreted by an anteriorly located gland on the cephalothorax.[20]

The knowledge of life cycles is important in understanding disease epidemiology and developing effective control strategies. However, there are many gaps about the life cycle of Pandaridae: routes of egg elimination, duration of each stage, lifetime

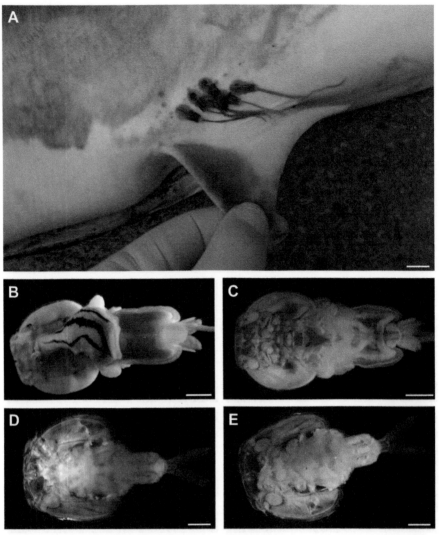

Fig. 2. *Dinemoura latifolia* found on the skin of the cloacal region of a white shark (*Carcharodon carcharias*) in the Mediterranean Sea (*A*, photo credit: Gianni Insacco). Female (*B*, dorsal view; *C*, ventral view) and male (*D*, dorsal view; *E*, ventral view); note an individual of *Conchoderma virgatum* attached to the anterior dorsal surface of *D latifolia* (*B*). Scale bars: A: 1 cm; B, C: 2 mm; D, E: 1 mm.

on the host and, environmental conditions that can interfere in stages or moults, to cite some issues.

HOST–PARASITE ASSOCIATIONS

The knowledge of the host–parasite associations is needed to increase the understanding of the dynamics between parasites and their hosts and their coevolutionary history. Except members of six genera (which are parasites of teleost fishes), all

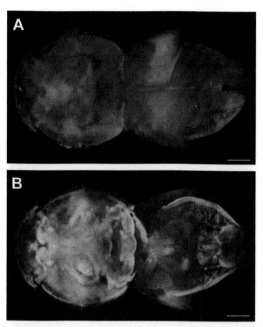

Fig. 3. *Echthrogaleus coleoptratus* found on the skin of a blue shark (*Prionace glauca*) in the Mediterranean Sea. Female (*A*, dorsal view; *B*, ventral view). Scale bars: A, B: 1 mm.

Pandaridae are parasites of elasmobranchs, usually, found on the skin, fins, and gills, and occasionally on mucosal surfaces of mouth and nasal passages (see **Table 1**). By analyzing literature and data available in public databases (ISI Web of Science, Google Scholar, and shark-references.com; accessed on July 2022) for the 64 pandarid species considered valid in Walter and Boxshall,[24] we found a total of 319 elasmobranch-pandarid associations (16 on Batoidea and 303 on Selachii). Of these, two were on sawfish (Pristiophoriformes), three on rays (Torpediniformes), thirteen on stingrays (eight in Myliobatiformes and five in Rhinopristiformes), and the remaining on various orders of sharks. The order of sharks with the higher number of associations was Carcharhiniformes (193 associations).

Most genera (12) infecting elasmobranchs are found only on Selachii and one genus with one species (ie, *Entepherus laminipes*; Bere, 1936) only on Batoidea (on six *Mobula* spp); four genera comprise most species that infect only Selachii and few species that infect only Batoidea or both. In particular, two species *Echthrogaleus spinulus* (Morales-Serna, Crow, Montes & González, 2019) and *Echthrogaleus torpedinis* (Wilson, 1907) are found only on *Tetronarce* spp (Torpediniformes), and *Echthrogaleus disciarai* (Benz & Deets, 1987) only on *Mobula thurstoni* (Myliobatiformes); *Nesippus vespa* (Kirtisinghe, 1964) only on *Rhynchobatus djiddensis* and *Rhina ancylostomus* (Rhinopristiformes), and *Pandarus cranchii* (Leach, 1819), *Pandarus sinuatus* (Say, 1818), and *Pandarus smithii* (Rathbun, 1886) are found on Selachii and Batoidea (see **Table 1**).

Almost all pandarids are generalist parasites with most species showing a wide range of hosts belonged to divergent orders and families. For instance, members of *Pandarus* (Leach, 1816) infect 48 elasmobranchs species in 10 orders and 19 families (see **Table 1**). The species infecting the highest number of host species is *Perissopus dentatus* (Steenstrup & Lütken, 1861), found on 31 Selachii species (almost all

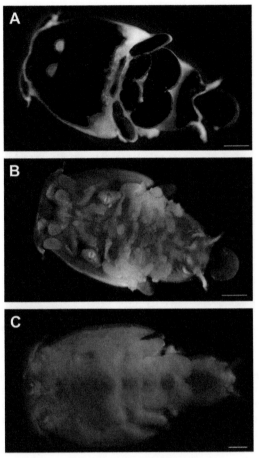

Fig. 4. *Pandarus satyrus* found on the skin of a blue shark (*Prionace glauca*) in the Mediterranean Sea. Female (*A*, dorsal view; *B*, ventral view) and male (*C*, dorsal view). Scale bars: A, B: 1 mm; C: 0.5 mm.

Carchariniformes). Conversely, few pandarid species are found only on one shark species. This is the case of *Dinemoleus indeprensus* (Cressey & Boyle, 1978), *Echthrogaleus pellucidus* (Shiino, 1963), *Echthrogaleus mitsukurinae* (Isaka, 2012), *Pandarus ambiguous* (Scott, 1907), *Pandarus rhincodonicus* (Norman, Newbound & Nott, 2000), *Pandarus zygaenae* (Brady, 1883), *Pannosus japonicus* (Shiino, 1960), *Paranesippus incisus* (Shiino, 1955), *Prosaetes rhinodontis* (Wright, 1876), and *Pseudopandarus scyllii* (Yamaguti & Yamasu, 1959) (see **Table 1**).

The attachment to the host occurs through copepod adaptations (ie, body dorsoventrally flattened, individuals inclined themselves over another and orientation of body axis to confront anteriorly into the flow and streamlining the body to the genital complex) which reduce the effects off drag and lift, which are caused by water flow over the host and have the potential to remove parasites.[17,34–36] In addition, Pandaridae has adhesion pads, organs to attachment (unique among the parasitic copepods[28]), which adhesive surface comprises a thick cushion of skin and transverse ridges.[30] The pads can be in one or more ventral locations; on the swimming legs 1

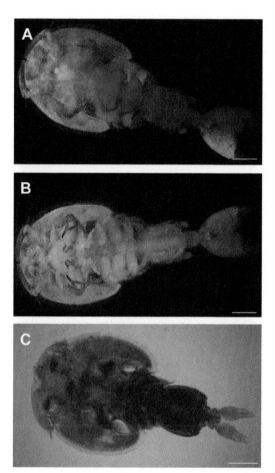

Fig. 5. *Phyllothyreus cornutus* found on the gills of a blue shark (*Prionace glauca*) in the Mediterranean Sea. Female (*A*, dorsal view; *B*, ventral view) and male (*C*, dorsal view). Scale bars: A, B: 2 mm; C: 1 mm.

to 4, at the base of the antennae, at the antennules, at the maxillipeds, at the distal corners of the dorsal shield or on the postero-lateral plates of the first free thoracic segment.[28] Usually, species that parasitize the skin surfaces have more pads than gill parasites, which in general have few pads or lack them fully.[17]

Despite of their low host specificity, pandarids are relatively site-specific and acquired particular adaptations to the hosts' surface where the parasite attaches. Pandarids of skin surface have the maxillipeds spatulate or sharply hooked, allowing clasping or hooking individual scale. *Achtheinus pinguis* inserts its antennae deep into the dermis of the shark's skin. The maxillipeds are used to attach to the placoid scales that cover the shark's skin and probably serve to keep the copepod and inserted antennae in position.[37] *Perissopus* (Steenstrup & Lütken, 1861) has maxillipeds distinct completely, even though species parasitize the skin surface of their hosts.[38] In this genus, the maxilliped possess a small claw and large adhesion pad, which is cemented to the host's placoid scales, probably to replace the reduced efficiency of the clasping attachment.[39] Conversely, pandarid parasites of the gills have sharply hooked maxillipeds to punch and anchor on the soft gill tissue.[17] However, *Gangliopus* (Gerstaecker, 1854) and *Phyllothyreus* (Edwards, 1840), which attach to the gills, have differenced antennae than others Pandaridae. Instead of only to hook the gill, they involve and punch the gill filaments.[17] In addition, the size of the ridges is variable among the genera, as in *Pandarus bicolor* (Leach, 1816) which the ridges are widest that in *Dinemoura latifolia* (Steenstrup & Lütken, 1861) and *Echthrogaleus coleoptratus* (Guérin-Méneville, 1837).[39]

GEOGRAPHIC RANGE

Pandarid species are cosmopolitan in their distribution, occurring especially in warm and temperate waters, mirroring the movements and distribution of their hosts.[40] For instance, *Pandarus bicolor* has its northern and southern limits of distribution in the North Sea (the Netherlands coast) and along the southern coast of New Zealand (Karitane), respectively (see **Table 1**). In general, pandarid species have been reported in the Mediterranean, North and South Atlantic, East and West Pacific, Indian Ocean, and West Indies.

Studies in areas such as the Western Pacific, the Atlantic coast of Central America, and the Indian Ocean report several species, conversely few reports exist from the coast of South America and most of the African coasts (see **Table 1**). The relative absence of data from some regions may reflect a relatively low local abundance of elasmobranchs, a low prevalence of pandarids, or the more restrictive reality, a low capacity, or a few opportunities for study and research, or poor interest on this group of parasites.

MOLECULAR AND PHYLOGENETIC STUDIES

In the last two decades, the advent of molecular technologies has accelerated the progress of the classical taxonomy, advancing our understanding of phylogeny and evolution and further the development of phylogenetically more accurate taxonomic classifications. The first genetic/molecular data on pandarids are those of Huys and colleagues,[41] when the small subunit ribosomal DNA (SSU rDNA, 18S−600 base pairs) gene sequences of *Pandarus smithii* and *Dinemoura latifolia* were deposited in a public database (National Center for Biotechnology Information). Huys and colleagues[41] highlighted by using a molecular approach, the phylogenetic position of caligiform families, formed by Pandaridae, Dissonidae (Kurtz, 1924), and Caligidae, within the Siphonostomatoida, placing the families as sister groups of the Monstrilloid taxa.[41] In subsequent years, Dippenaar and colleagues[22] generated SSU rDNA sequences of eight known pandarids (ie, *Nesippus vespa, Nesippus crypturus* [Heller, 1868], *Nesippus orientalis, Phyllothyreus cornutus* [Milne-Edwards, 1840], *Pannosus japonicus, Pseudopandarus longus* [Gnanamuthu, 1951], *Achtheinus oblongus, Perissopus dentatus* [Steenstrup & Lütken, 1861], and four unidentified *Pandarus* spp of sharks). The same species were also sequenced at two partial mitochondrial genes (16S rDNA− 508 base pairs and cytochrome oxidase 1 [*cox*1]−670 base pairs), in order to estimate the phylogenetic relationships among the six siphonostomatoid families found on elasmobranchs.[22] The same authors, by using a combined (18S, *cox*1, 16S) phylogeny reconstruction, established that Pandaridae is monophyletic and this family is the sister group of the Caligidae lineage. Two major clades within the family were identified: a first clade included the species of *Nesippus* (Heller, 1865) and a second clade included the species of *Phyllothyreus, Pannosus* (Cressey, 1967), *Pandarus, Pseudopandarus* (Kirtisinghe, 1950), and *Achtheinus* (Wilson, 1908).[22] The analysis of the partial *cox*1 sequences also permitted to reveal the presence of two cryptic species (ie, species morphologically similar, but reproductively isolated).[22] In particular, Dippenaar and colleagues[22] reported in *N orientalis* off the KwaZulu-Natal coast of South Africa, the existence of two divergent clades. The confirmation was detected by measuring the genetic divergence estimated from sequence analysis of the *cox*1 gene locus (17.44%) that was at a level expected for interspecific rather than intraspecific relationships in crustaceans.[42] Sequence divergence of 16% to 22% existed between defined *Nesippus* species which agrees with previous findings of 13% to 22% sequence divergence in congeneric species of copepods.[43] From here on out, little molecular and phylogenetic data have been generated for pandarids. Veliz and colleagues[44] identified, by using an integrative approach, pandarids of elasmobranchs collected from the central coast of Chile. Unfortunately, the obtained sequences are not available because not stored in a public database. Recently, in the Mediterranean Sea, Palomba and colleagues[45] obtained new additional DNA sequences for *D latifolia* and *P cornutus*. Furthermore, new molecular data for *Echthrogaleus coleoptratus* and *Pandarus satyrus* (Dana, 1849) were also added, based on, both the nuclear and mitochondrial (*cox*1) gene loci. The phylogenetic reconstruction revealed two major clades within the pandarids of elasmobranchs: the first included species of *Pandarus, Phyllothyreus, Pannosus,* and *Pseudopandarus* and the second included species of *Achtheinus, Perissopus, Echthrogaleus* (Steenstrup & Lütken, 1861)*, Nesippus,* and *Dinemoura.* The phylogenetic pattern for the species was congruent with the morphologic characters of the two species groups above mentioned, except for *A oblongus* and *P dentatus* which were placed into the second major clade with the genera *Echthrogaleus, Nesippus,* and *Dinemoura.* However, the scarcity of data regarding the host association and life cycle strategy of pandarid copepods does not help to resolve phylogenetic relationships among species. Indeed, to date, the phylogenetic analysis includes only a small subset of 12 of the 64 valid species of Pandaridae. Further new molecular data are needed to understand the true relationships within the family.

PANDARID COPEPODS OF VETERINARY IMPORTANCE

Parasitic copepods are commonly known to cause serious damage to their hosts by their attachment mechanisms and by their feeding activities.[5,46–48] Conversely, only few casual reports on pandarids causing pathologic changes have been published in elasmobranchs.[37,47,49,50] Pandarids comprise species which typically attach to the fins, gills, and skin of their hosts and occasionally to the mucosal surfaces of their buccal and nasal cavities (see **Table 1**).

Usually, they cause only minor mechanical injuries to their hosts when they attach to the skin. For instance, Dippenaar and Jordaan[37] reported that the attachment of females of *Achtheinus pinguis* on the skin and fins of shortnose spurdog (*Squalus cf megalops*), tope shark (*Galeorhinus galeus*), and sand tiger shark (*Carcharias taurus*) from the south and west coasts of South Africa caused adverse effects as seen by the erosion and disruption of the epidermal layers on their hosts. Lesions were associated to the copepod antennae embedded deeply into the middle reticular layer of the dermis.[37] The dorsal and ventral skin surfaces of a torpedo ray (*Tetronarce tokionis*) captured in the central Pacific Ocean (Hawaiian waters) with a severe infection by *Echthrogaleus spinulus* had diffuse white spot lesions associated to the copepod attachment sites.[49] *Pandarus rhincodonicus,* a specialist parasite on the skin of the whale shark (*Rhincodon typus*), occasionally caused excessive mucus production and localized epithelium erosions.[50]

A different scenario can occur when copepod species parasitize the gills. However, as for other pathogenic copepods, the possibility to cause pathologic changes increases in case of heavy infections. Grazing on the host tissues, these parasites can cause small hemorrhages and inflammatory processes. Pathologic changes caused by copepods may result in osmoregulation problems and expose the underlying tissues to opportunistic infectious agents as bacteria and fungi. In fish under stressful conditions, diseases can occur due to the development of severe secondary infections and in the case of the gill involvement the loss of respiratory efficiency. Moreover, when competing for substrate with other ectoparasites, pandarids can shift their usual substrate surface and displace on an unusual habitat. Cressey[51] observed that species of *Pandarus* (Leach, 1816) (ie, *P satyrus*, *P smithii*, and *P katoi* Cressey, 1967), which usually attach to the skin surfaces of sharks, were displaced by two additional pandarid species (*Dinemoura latifolia* and *Dinemoura producta* Müller, 1785) from their usual substrate to gills and buccal mucosa of mako sharks (*Isurus oxyrinchus*). When this occurs, the possibility that the parasites can cause pathologic changes increases because those parasites are not adapted to the new substrate as well as the host is not adapted to harbor those specialized skin parasites on its gills.

Borucinska and Benz[52] reported severe lesions caused by *Phyllothyreus cornutus* on the interbranchial septa of blue sharks (*Prionace glauca*) in coastal waters off Montauk Point, New York. The females of *P cornutus* were associated with grossly visible, soft, papillomatous lesions on the interbranchial septum in which their second antennae were embedded. Conversely, the males of *P cornutus* were occasionally associated with shallow gill epithelial ulcerations. Differences in features of lesions associated with female versus male of *P cornutus* were mostly explicated by the different behavior between the sexes of this species on the attachment site as well as by the size and morphology of the individuals of the two sexes (males are much smaller than females in body size and have different attachment appendices than females). Lesions associated to female copepods were suggestive of chronic infections in which parasites had been stationary for some appreciable period. Conversely, lesions associated with male copepods were compatible with acute infections suggesting that males are not stationary and systematically move to other attachment site to copulate with females.[52] Similar lesions were also observed by Benz and Deets[47] on the gill arch and adjoining branchial filters of a mobulid ray (*Mobula* sp), associated with the attachment of the female *Entepherus laminipes*. Finally, Cressey[17] reported *Dinemoura ferox* (Krøyer, 1838) as a common parasite attached to the eyes of the "Greenland shark." However, is likely that the copepod reported by Cressey[17] was *Ommatokoita elongata* (Grant, 1827) a member of the family Lernaeopodidae (Milne Edwards, 1840), a common parasite of the Greenland shark (*Somniosus microcephalus*) and the Pacific sleeper shark (*Somniosus pacificus*) which parasitize the eyes of its hosts being capable to cause corneal lesions and blindness leading to severe vision impairment.[48,53]

PREVENTIVE MEDICINE IN AQUARIUM COLLECTIONS

Quarantine is an essential management tool of preventive veterinary medicine to prevent or at least to reduce the risk of introducing infectious diseases into aquarium collections. Incoming fish, particularly from the wild, should be quarantined, observed, and carefully examined by veterinary specialists to minimize this risk. The most common infectious agents that can be introduced into the aquarium through the introduction of new individuals include parasites. Among these, many arthropod ectoparasites (copepods and isopods) are of veterinary importance because they are capable of causing significant morbidity and mortality, especially in wild caught fish restricted to captivity conditions. Indeed, when under stressful conditions due to captivity the host defense reduces its efficiency, the parasites may increase rapidly causing diseases that in the wild rarely occur. Because most copepods are visible with naked eye, they are considered an esthetic issue in exhibits. Moreover, most of these parasites have a direct life cycle (they do not need intermediate hosts to complete their life cycle) and when accidentally introduced into an aquarium collection, their subsequent elimination can be problematic. As many species are able to complete their life cycles and reproduce in captivity,[5] elimination involves emptying, washing, and disinfecting the aquarium tank and its filtering system.

Pandarid infections may be obvious when parasites attach to the skin and fins while not easily detected when they infect gills, mouth, and nasal cavities. Once the fish reaches the quarantine facility, clinical evaluation for ectoparasites should include the examination of gills, skin, fins, and mouth and nasal cavities. Fish can be restrained for physical examination either manually or chemically.[54] Manual restraint is possible for some elasmobranchs and is often adequate for physical examination and removal of skin and fins ectoparasites using forceps and tweezers. Conversely, the presence of ectoparasites into relatively inaccessible regions as gills and buccal and nasal cavities would be difficult to evaluate without the use of endoscopy equipment.[5,54]

TREATMENTS FOR COPEPOD INFECTIONS

There are several pharmacologic options available for treating of copepod infections in elasmobranchs, with much of the information relying on extrapolation from the effective treatments in the control of siphonostomatoids (caligids and lernaeopodids) in aquaculture-produced fish.[5] Nevertheless, before choosing the most appropriate treatment for each specific case, it is important to consider that the concentration of many chemicals required to kill the developmental stages or more resistant copepod taxa may be toxic for fish. For this latter reason, fish that are severely debilitated or stressed from concurrent disease or from capture should be treated for the life-threatening problems first before attempting to treat for copepods. Because several species of marine parasitic copepods may be sensitive and detach on freshwater, in case of moderate infections a bath in freshwater for 10 to 15 minutes can be attempted.

In many countries, organophosphates are the preferred drugs of treatment for copepod infections in farm fish. For instance, dichlorvos has been found to be effective against the species of *Caligus* (Müller, 1785) and *Ergasilus* (von Nordmann, 1832). Conversely, *Lernaea* spp may be difficult to control using this agent because different developmental stages show varied susceptibility to the chemical.[55–57] However, due to its high neurotoxicity in animals and humans, the use of dichlorvos is controversial. In the case of severe infections with resistant copepod species, the use of specific parasiticides such as diflubenzuron or lufenuron (benzoylphenyl urea derivatives) is recommended in elasmobranchs.[5] These drugs work as chitin synthesis inhibitors and have been shown to be effective against all larval and preadult stages of copepods. The main indication for the use of avermectins (ivermectin and emamectin) in fish is the infection with copepods. Both agents are well-documented as very effective on all developmental stages of *Lepeophtheirus* spp and *Caligus* spp in salmonid fish.[58]

CLINICS CARE POINTS

- Quarantine is an essential management tool to prevent the risk of introducing parasitic diseases into aquarium collections.
- When ectoparasites are accidentally introduced into an aquarium collection, their subsequent elimination can be problematic because many species are able to complete their life cycles and reproduce in captivity.

- Clinical evaluation for copepods should include the examination of gills, skin, fins, and mouth and nasal cavities.
- Manual restraint is possible for some elasmobranchs and is often adequate for physical examination and removal of copepods from the skin and fins. The presence of copepods into gills and buccal and nasal cavities would be difficult to evaluate without the use of endoscopy equipment.
- Drugs should be used with caution in elasmobranchs because the concentration of many chemicals required to kill the developmental stages or more resistant copepods may be toxic for fish.
- Fish that are severely debilitated or stressed from concurrent disease or from capture should be treated for life-threatening problems first before attempting to treat for ectoparasites.

DISCLOSURE

The authors have no conflicts of interest to disclose.

REFERENCES

1. Fowler SL, Cavanagh RD. Sharks, rays and chimaeras: the status of the Chondrichthyan fishes: status surveyvol. 63. Switzerland: IUCN; 2005.
2. Van Der Laan R, Eschmeyer WN, Fricke R. Family-group names of recent fishes. Zootaxa 2014;3882(1):1–230.
3. Horton T, Kroh A, Ahyong S, et al. World register of marine species (WoRMS). 2022. Available at: https://www.marinespecies.org. Accessed June 20, 2022.
4. IUCN. IUCN. SSC Shark Specialist Group. 2022. Available at: https://www.iucnssg.org/. Accessed June 20, 2022.
5. Benz GW, Bullard SA. Metazoan parasites and associates of chondrichthyans with emphasis on taxa harmful to captive hosts. In: Smith MFL, Thoney DA, Hueter RE, editors. The elamobranch husbandry manual: captive care of sharks, rays, and their relatives. Ohio biological survey. Columbus. USA: Ohio Biological Survey; 2004. p. 325–416.
6. Wood CL, Lafferty KD, Micheli F. Fishing out marine parasites? Impacts of fishing on rates of parasitism in the ocean. Ecol Lett 2010;13(6):761–75.
7. Marcogliese DJ, Cone DK. Food webs: a plea for parasites. Trends Ecol Evol 1997;12(8):320–5.
8. Lafferty KD, Allesina S, Arim M, et al. Parasites in food webs: the ultimate missing links. Ecol Lett 2008;11(6):533–46.
9. Santoro M, Iaccarino D, Bellisario B. Host biological factors and geographic locality influence predictors of parasite communities in sympatric sparid fishes off the southern Italian coast. Sci Rep 2020;10:13283.
10. Santoro M, Bellisario B, Tanduo V, et al. Drivers of parasite communities in three sympatric benthic sharks in the Gulf of Naples (central Mediterranean Sea). Sci Rep 2022;12:9969.
11. Timi JT, Poulin R. Why ignoring parasites in fish ecology is a mistake? Int J Parasitol 2020;50(10):755–61.
12. Hickman CP, Keen S, Eisenhour DJ, et al. Princípios integrados de zoologia. In: Koogan G, editor. Artrópodes. Rio de Janeiro: Grupo Gen; 2016. p. 367.
13. Boxshall G, Hayes P. Biodiversity and taxonomy of the parasitic Crustacea. In: Feldhaar H, Schmidt-Rhaesa A, editors. Parasitic Crustacea (Zoological Monogrvol 1. Switzerland: Springer; 2019. p. 73–134.

14. Hua CJ, Zhang D, Zou H, et al. Morphology is not a reliable taxonomic tool for the genus *Lernaea*: molecular data and experimental infection reveal that *L. cyprinacea* and *L. cruciata* are conspecific. Parasit Vectors 2019;12(1):579.

15. Damkaer DM. The copepodologist's cabinet: a biographical and bibliographical history, Volume One, Aristotle to Alexander Von Nordmann (330 B.C. to A.D. 1832). In: Mem Am Philosophical Socvol 240. Philadelphia: American Philosophical Society; 2002. p. 747–8.

16. Cressey RF. A revision of the family Pandaridae (Copepoda, Caligoida), parasites of marine fishes. Boston University; 1965.

17. Cressey RF. Revision of the family Pandaridae (Copepoda: Caligoida). Proc US Natl Mus 1967;121:1–133.

18. Tang D, Benz GW, Nagasawa K. Description of the male of *Prosaetes rhinodontis* (Wright, 1876) (Crustacea, Copepoda, Siphonostomatoida), with a proposal to synonymize Cecropidae Dana, 1849 and Amaterasidae Izawa, 2008 with Pandaridae Milne Edwards, 1840. Zoosymposia 2012;8(1):7–19.

19. Norman BM, Newbound DR, Knott B. A new species of Pandaridae (Copepoda), from the whale shark *Rhincodon typus* (Smith, 1828). J Nat Hist 2000;34(3):355–66.

20. Izawa K. Redescription of eight species of parasitic copepods (Siphonostomatoida, Pandaridae) infecting Japanese elasmobranchs. Crustaceana 2010;83(3):313–41.

21. Dippenaar SM, Jordaan BP. *Nesippus orientalis* Heller, 1868 (Pandaridae: Siphonostomatoida): descriptions of the adult, young and immature females, a first description of the male and aspects of their functional morphology. Syst Parasitol 2006;65(1):27–41.

22. Dippenaar SM, Mathibela RB, Bloomer P. Cytochrome oxidase I sequences reveal possible cryptic diversity in the cosmopolitan symbiotic copepod *Nesippus orientalis* Heller, 1868 (Pandaridae: Siphonostomatoida) on elasmobranch hosts from the KwaZulu-Natal coast of South Africa. Exp Parasitol 2010;125(1):42–50.

23. Ho JS, Lin CL. Redescription of *Dinemoura discrepans* Cressey, 1967 (Copepoda: Pandaridae) parasitic on four species of sharks off southeast coast of Taiwan. Folia Parasitol 2011;58(4):311.

24. Walter TC, Boxshall G. World of Copepods Database. Pandaridae Milne Edwards, 1840. In: World Register of marine species. 2022. Available at: https://www.marinespecies.org/aphia.php?p=taxdetails&id=135531. Accessed June 28, 2022.

25. Wilson CB. Descriptions of new species of parasitic copepods in the collections of the United States National Museum. Proc US Nat Mus 1912;42(1900):233–43.

26. Thomsen R. Copépodos parásitos de los peces marinos del Uruguay. Com Zool Mus Hist Nat Mont 1949;3:1–41.

27. Shen CJ, Wang KN. A new parasitic copepod, *Achtheinus impenderus*, from a shark taken at Peitaiho, Hopei Province? Acta Zool Sinica 1959;10(1):27–31.

28. Kabata Z. Copepoda (Crustacea) parasitic on fishes: problems and perspectives. In: Lumsden WHR, Muller R, Baker JR, editors. Adv Parasitolvol 19. Cambridge: Academic Press; 1982. p. 1–71.

29. Williams EH, Bunkley-Williams L. Life cycle and life history strategies of parasitic Crustacea. In: Parasitic Crustacea. Switzerland: Springer; 2019. p. 179–266.

30. Wilson CB. North American parasitic copepods belonging to the family Caligidae. Parts 3 and 4. A revision of the Pandarinae and the Cecropinae. Proc US Natl Mus 1907;33:323–40.

31. Dippenaar SM, van Tonder RC, Wintner SP. Is there evidence of niche restriction in the spatial distribution of *Kroyeria dispar* Wilson, 1935, *K. papillipes* Wilson, 1932 and *Eudactylina pusilla* Cressey, 1967 (Copepoda: Siphonostomatoida) on the gill filaments of tiger sharks *Galeocerdo cuvier* off KwaZulu-Natal, South Africa? Hydrobiologia 2009;619(1):89–101.

32. Dippenaar S, Jordaan B. Notes on the morphology and ecology of the adult females of *Nesippus* species (Siphonostomatoida: Pandaridae) with a key for identification. Zootaxa 2012;3170:18–30.

33. Izawa K. *Amaterasia amanoiwatoi* nov. gen., nov. sp. (Copepoda, Siphonostomatoida, Amaterasidae nov. fam.), with gall-forming juveniles parasitic on the fins of a balistid actinopterygian fish. Crustaceana 2008;81(11):1331–46.

34. Boxshall GA. Infections with parasitic copepods in North Sea marine fishes. J Mar Biol Assoc UK 1974;54(2):355–72.

35. Benz GW. Observations on the attachment scheme of the parasitic copepod *Pandarus satyrus* (Copepoda: Pandaridae). J Parasitol 1981;67:966–7.

36. Kabata Z. Parasitic copepoda of British fishes. In: Ray society monographs. London: Ray Society; 1979.

37. Dippenaar SM, Jordaan A. How females of *Achtheinus* spp. (Pandaridae: Siphonostomatoida) attach to their elasmobranch hosts with notes on their effects on the hosts' fins. Folia Parasitol (Praha) 2015;1:62.

38. Cressey RF. Caligoid copepods parasitic on sharks in the Indian Ocean. Proc US Natl Mus 1967;121:1–21.

39. Ingram AL, Parker AR. The functional morphology and attachment mechanism of pandarid adhesion pads (Crustacea: Copepoda: Pandaridae). Zool Anz 2006;244(3):209–21.

40. Alvarez F, Winfield I. New records of *Dinemoura latifolia* and *Pandarus smithii* (Copepoda, Siphonostomatoida, Pandaridae) parasitizing the shark *Isurus oxyrinchus* in the Gulf of Mexico. Crustaceana 2001;74(5):501–3.

41. Huys R, Llewellyn-Hughes J, Conroy-Dalton S, et al. Extraordinary host switching in siphonostomatoid copepods and the demise of the Monstrilloida: integrating molecular data, ontogeny and antennulary morphology. Mol Phylogenet Evol 2007;43(2):368–78.

42. Burton RS, Lee BN. Nuclear and mitochondrial gene genealogies and allozyme polymorphism across a major phylogeographic break in the copepod *Tigriopus californicus*. Proc Natl Acad Sci U S A 1994;91(11):5197–201.

43. Bucklin A, Guarnieri M, Hill R, et al. Taxonomic and systematic assessment of planktonic copepods using mitochondrial COI sequence variation and competitive, species-specific PCR. In: Zehr JP, Voytek MA, editors. Molecular ecology of aquatic communities. Switzerland: Springer; 1999. p. 239–54.

44. Véliz C, Lopez Z, González M, et al. Copépodos parásitos (Siphonostomatoida: Pandaridae) de *Prionace glauca* e *Isurus oxyrinchus*, capturados en la costa central de Chile. Rev Biol Mar Oceanogr 2018;53:51.

45. Palomba M, Insacco G, Zava B, et al. Occurrence and molecular characterization of some parasitic copepods (Siphonostomatoida: Pandaridae) on pelagic sharks in the Mediterranean Sea. Front Mar Sci 2022;8:778034.

46. Johnson PT, Calhoun DM, Riepe TB, et al. Chance or choice? Understanding parasite selection and infection in multi-host communities. Int J Parasitol 2019; 49(5):407–15.

47. Benz GW, Deets GB. Fifty-one years later: an update on *Entepherus*, with a phylogenetic analysis of Cecropidae Dana, 1849 (Copepoda: Siphonostomatoida). Can J Zool 1988;66(4):856–65.

48. Benz GW, Borucinska JD, Lowry LF, et al. Ocular lesions associated with attachment of the copepod *Ommatokoita elongata* (Lernaeopodidae: Siphonostomatoida) to corneas of pacific sleeper sharks *Somniosus pacificus* captured off Alaska in Prince William sound. J Parasitol 2002;88(3):474–81.

49. Morales-Serna FN, Crow GL, Montes MM, et al. Description of *Echthrogaleus spinulus* n. sp. (Copepoda: Pandaridae) parasitic on a torpedo ray from the central Pacific Ocean utilising a morphological and molecular approach. Syst Parasitol 2019;96(9):777–88.

50. Dove AD, Robinson DP. Parasites and other associates of whale sharks. In: Dove ADM, Pierce SJ, editors. Whale sharks: biology, ecology, and conservation. 1st edition. USA: CRC Press; 2021. p. 65.

51. Cressey RF. Caligoid copepods parasitic on *Isurus oxyrinchus* with an example of habitat shift. Proc US Natl Mus 1968;125(3653):1–26.

52. Borucinska JD, Benz GW. Lesions associated with attachment of the parasitic copepod *Phyllothyreus cornutus* (Pandaridae: Siphonostomatoida) to interbranchial septa of blue sharks. J Aquat Anim Health 1999;11(3):290–5.

53. Borucinska J, Benz G, Whiteley HE. Ocular lesions associated with attachment of the parasitic copepod *Ommatokoita elongata* (Grant) to corneas of Greenland sharks, *Somniosus microcephalus* (Bloch & Schneider). J Fish Dis 1998;21(6):415–22.

54. Francis-Floyd R. Clinical examination of fish in private collections. Vet Clin North Am Exot Anim Pract 1999;2(2):247–64.

55. Varó I, Navarro J, Amat F, et al. Effect of dichlorvos on cholinesterase activity of the European sea bass (*Dicentrarchus labrax*). Pestic Biochem Physiol 2003; 75(3):61–72.

56. Noga EJ. Fish disease: diagnosis and treatment. USA: John Wiley & Sons; 2010.

57. Wafer LN, Whitney JC, Jensen VB. Fish lice (*Argulus japonicus*) in goldfish (*Carassius auratus*). Com Med 2015;65(2):93–5.

58. Horsberg TE. Avermectin use in aquaculture. Curr Pharm Biotechnol 2012; 13(6):1095–102.

59. Wilson CB. Parasitic copepods in the United States National Museum. Proc US Natl Mus 1944;94:529–82.

60. Barnard KH. South African parasitic copepoda. Ann S Afr Mus 1955;41: 223–312.

61. Dippenaar S. Reported siphonostomatoid copepods parasitic on marine fishes of southern Africa. Crustaceana 2004;77(11):1281–328.

62. Etchegoin AJ, Ivanov AV. Parasitic copepods of the narrownose smooth-hound shark *Mustelus schmitti* (Chondrichthyes: Triakidae) from Argentina. Folia Parasitol 1999;46(2):149–53.

63. Izawa K. Resurrection of the parasitic copepod genus *Achtheinus* Wilson, 1908 (Siphonostomatoida, Pandaridae), with redescription of *A. oblongus* Wilson, 1908, *A. dentatus* Wilson, 1911, and *A. pinguis* Wilson, 1912 based on museum collections. Crustaceana 2010;83(8):971–95.

64. Kensley BF, Grindley JR. South African parasitic copepoda. Ann S Afr Mus 1973;62:69–130.

65. Luque JL, Farfán C. Some copepods parasitic on elasmobranch fishes from the Peruvian coast, with the description of two new species of *Eudactylina* van Beneden, 1853 (Eudactylinidae) and four new records. J Nat Hist 1991;25(5): 1233–46.

66. Nevatte RJ, Williamson JE. The sawshark redemption: current knowledge and future directions for sawsharks (Pristiophoridae). Fish Fish 2020;21(6):1213–37.

67. Oldewage W. Description of *Perissopus oblongus* (Wilson, 1908) (Copepoda, Pandaridae) from Southern African sharks with a first description of the male. Crustaceana 1992;63(1):44–50.

68. Oldewage WH, Smale MJ. Occurrence of piscine parasitic copepods (Crustacea) on sharks taken mainly off Cape Recife, South Africa. Afr J Mar Sci 1993;13(1):309–12.

69. Russo R. Notes on the external parasites of California inshore sharks. Calif Fish Game 1975;61:228–32.

70. Russo R. Observations on the ectoparasites of elasmobranchs in San Francisco Bay, California. Calif Fish Game 2013;99:233–6.

71. Yamaguchi A, Yokoyama H, Ogawa K, et al. Use of parasites as biological tags for separating stocks of the starspotted dogfish *Mustelus manazo* in Japan and Taiwan. Fish Sci 2003;69(2):337–42.

72. Yeld EM. Parasite assemblages of three endemic catshark species from the west and south coasts of South Africa. University of Cape Town, Faculty of Science, Department of Biological Sciences; 2009.

73. Dippenaar SM. Symbiotic Siphonostomatoida (Copepoda) collected from white sharks, *Carcharodon carcharias* (Lamniformes, Lamnidae), during the OCEARCH expedition along the coast of South Africa. Crustaceana 2018; 91(1):103–11.

74. Etchegoin JA, Ivanov VA, Timi JT. Resurrection of *Perissopus galeorhini* (Yamaguti, 1936), with notes on the genus *Perissopus* Steenstrup & Lütken, 1861 (Copepoda: Pandaridae) parasitic on sharks. Syst Parasitol 2001;50:31–9.

75. Lewis AG. Copepod crustaceans parasitic on elasmobranch fishes of the Hawaiian Islands. Proc US Natl Mus 1966;118(3524):57–154.

76. Lipej L, Acevedo I, Akel E, et al. New Mediterranean biodiversity records (March 2017). Mediterr Mar Sci 2017;18(1):179–201.

77. Raibaut A, Combes C, Benoit F. Analysis of the parasitic copepod species richness among Mediterranean fish. J Mar Syst 1998;15(1):185–206.

78. Hewitt G. Some New Zealand parasitic Copepoda of the family Pandaridae. NZJ Mar Freshw Res 1967;1(2):180–264.

79. Nagasawa K, Nakaya K. The parasitic copepod *Dinemoleus indeprensus* (Siphonostomatoida: Pandaridae) from the megamouth shark, *Megachasma pelagios*. In: Yano K, Morrissey JF, Yabumoto Y, et al, editors. Biology of the megamouth shark. Tokyo: Tokai University Press; 1997. p. 177–9.

80. Nagasawa K. A note on *Dinemoleus indeprensus*, a parasitic copepod of the megamouth shark. [In Japanese; English abstract. R Jpn Soc Elasm Stud 2009;45(45):39–43.

81. Nagasawa K, Senou H. Third record of *Dinemoleus indeprensus* (Copepoda: Pandaridae) from the megamouth shark, *Megachasma pelagios*. Biogeogr 2012;14:147–9.

82. Henderson AC, Reeve AJ, Tang D. Parasitic copepods from some northern Indian Ocean elasmobranchs. Mar Biodivers Rec 2013;6:e44.

83. Rokicki J, Borowicz A. Parasitic Copepoda on *Alopias superciliosus* (Lowe, 1839) from the Atlantic Ocean. VI Nutzfischkonferenz, Universität Rostock, Güstrow 1986;29(1.10):140–3.

84. Ho JS, Chang WB, Yang S, et al. New Records for *Dinemoura ferox* (Copepoda: Siphonostomatoida: Pandaridae) from pacific sleeper sharks captured in waters off Eastern Taiwan. J Parasitol 2003;89(5):1071–3.

85. Benz GW, Mollet HF, Ebert DA, et al. Five species of parasitic copepods (Siphonostomatoida: Pandaridae) from the body surface of a white shark captured in Morro Bay, California. Pac Sci 2003;57(1):39–43.

86. Henderson A, Flannery K, Dunne J. Biological observations on shark species taken in commercial fisheries to the West of Ireland. Proc R Ir Acad 2003; 103B:1–7.

87. Ho JS, Liu WC, Lin CL. Two species of *Echthrogaleus* (Copepoda: Siphonostomatoida: Pandaridae) parasitic on five species of sharks off the east coast of Taiwan. J Fish Soc Taiwan 2012;39(4):247–55.

88. Heegaard P. Parasitic Copepoda from Australian waters. Rec Aust Mus 1962; 25(9):149–233.

89. Henderson AC, Flannery K, Dunne J. Parasites of the blue shark (*Prionace glauca* L.), in the North-East Atlantic Ocean. J Nat Hist 2002;36(16):1995–2004.

90. Hewitt GC, Hine PM. Checklist of parasites of New Zealand fishes and of their hosts. NZJ Mar Freshw Res 1972;6(1–2):69–114.

91. Pratt J, Turnbull S, Emery P, et al. Prevalence, intensity, and site of infection of *Echthrogaleus coleoptratus* (Guérin-Méneville, 1837) (Siphonostomatoida, Pandaridae), ectoparasitic on the porbeagle shark (*Lamna nasus*) in the Bay of Fundy, Canada. Crustaceana 2010;83(3):375–9.

92. Rokicki J, Bychawska D. Parasitic copepods of Carcharhinidae and Sphyridae (Elasmobranchia) from the Atlantic Ocean. J Nat Hist 1991;25(6):1439–48.

93. Hewitt GC. Eight species of parasitic Copepoda on a white shark. NZJ Mar Freshw Res 1979;13(1):171.

94. Pradeep HMA, Shirke S. First report of *Echthrogaleus denticulatus* (Smith 1874) on the pelagic thresher shark (*Alopias pelagicus* Nakamura 1935) from Indian EEZ of Andaman Sea. Sains Malays 2017;46:1675–8.

95. Purivirojkul W, Chaidee P, Thapanand-Chaidee T. Parasites of deep-sea sharks from the Andaman Sea with six new records of parasites in Thailand. Agric Nat Resour 2009;43(5):93–9.

96. Benz GW, Deets GB. *Echthrogaleus disciarai* sp. nov. (Siphonostomatoida: Pandaridae), a parasitic copepod of the devil ray *Mobula lucasana* Beebe and Tee Van, 1938 from the Sea of Cortez. Can J Zool 1987;65(3):685–90.

97. Izawa K. *Echthrogaleus mitsukurinae* sp. nov. (Copepoda, Siphonostomatoida, Pandaridae) infesting the goblin shark *Mitsukurina owstoni* Jordan, 1898 in Japanese waters. Crustaceana 2012;85(1):81–7.

98. Lebepe MC, Dippenaar SM. A report of symbiotic Siphonostomatoida (Copepoda) infecting mobulids (Rajiformes: Mobulidae) off the KwaZulu-Natal coast, South Africa. Afr Zool 2013;48(2):326–32.

99. Izawa K. Free-living stages of the parasitic copepod, *Gangliopus pyriformis* Gerstaecker, 1854 (Siphonostomatoida, Pandaridae) reared from eggs. Crustaceana 2010;83(7):829–37.

100. Cressey RF. Copepods parasites on sharks from the west coast of Florida. Smithson Contrib Zool 1970;38:1–30.

101. Heegaard PE. Some new caligids from the Gilbert Islands. Arkiv for Zoologi 1943;34(16):1–12.

102. Newbound DR, Knott B. Parasitic copepods from pelagic sharks in western Australia. Bull Mar Sci 1999;65(3):715–24.

103. Benmansour B, Youssef F, Ali MB, et al. The survey of ectoparasites on two species of triakids (*Mustelus mustelus* and M. *punctulatus*) sharks from Tunisian coasts. Saudi J Biol Sci 2022;29(5):3610–6.

104. Youssef F, Tlig Zouari S, Benmansour B. New host–parasite records of siphon-ostomatoid copepods infesting elasmobranch fishes in Tunisian waters. J Mar Biol Assoc UK 2019;99(4):851–5.

105. Dippenaar SM, Jordaan BP. New host and geographical records of siphonosto-matoid copepods associated with elasmobranchs off the KwaZulu-Natal coast, South Africa. Onderstepoort J Vet 2007;74(2):169–75.

106. Nagasawa K. A note on *Dinemoleus indeprensus*, a parasitic copepod of the megamouth shark. R Jpn Soc Elasm Stud 2009;45(45):39–43.

107. Cressey R. A new genus of copepods (Caligoida, Pandaridae) from a thresher shark in Madagascar. Cah O.R.S.T.O.M Sér Océanogr; 1963. p. 285–97.

108. Barnard KH. XVIII—New records and descriptions of new species of parasitic Copepoda from South Africa. Ann Mag Nat Hist 1948;1(4):242–54.

109. Ebert D. Biological aspects of the sixgill shark, *Hexanchus griseus*. Copeia 1986;1986(1):131–5.

110. Gaevskaya A. Parasites and diseases of fishes in the Black Sea and the Sea of Azov. Sevastopol, Russia: EKOSI-Gidrofizika 2012.

111. Montú M. Records of parasitic copepods of sharks from the southwestern Atlantic. Nauplius 1996;4:179–80.

112. Öktener A, Ventura D, Şirin M. Occurrence of *Pandarus bicolor* (Siphonostoma-toida: Pandaridae) on vulnerable shark species: *Oxynotus centrina* and *Squalus acanthias* from Turkish marine waters. Vie Milieu 2020;70:19–32.

113. Dana JD. Crustacea: United States exploring expedition during the years 1838, 1839, 1840, 1841, 1842. Under the command of Charles Wilkes (vol 2). Philadel-phia: USNC Sherman; 1853. p. 1918.

114. Capart A. Copépodes parasites. (Expédition Océanographique Belge dans les Eaux Cotieres Africaines de l'Atlantique Sud - 1948-1949). Bruxelles: Institut Royal des Sciences Naturelles de Belgique; 1959.

115. Dippenaar SM, Narváez K, Osaer F, et al. Symbiotic Siphonostomatoida (Cope-poda) of the hammerhead shark species *Sphyrna zygaena* (Carcharhiniformes: Sphyrnidae) and stingray *Dasyatis pastinaca* (Myliobatiformes: Dasyatidae) off the Canary Islands, with a re-description of *Pseudocharopinus pillaii* Kabata, 1979. Parasitol Res 2021;120(11):3739–47.

116. Rodriguez Acosta E, Moya H, Fuentes J, et al. Copépodos parásitos asociados a tiburones capturados en pesquerías artesanales de la Isla Margarita, Venezuela. Mem Fund La Salle Cien Nat 2019;77(185):81–100.

117. Rokicki J, Morozinska J. Parasitic copepods from *Isurus oxyrinchus* Rafinesque, 1810, from the Central Atlantic Ocean. Crustaceana 1995;68(1):21–6.

118. Williams JE. *Conchoderma virgatum* Spengler, 1789 (Cirripedia Thoracica) in association with *Dinemoura latifolia* (Steenstrup & Lutken) (Copepoda, Caligi-dea), a parasite of the shortfin mako, *Isurus oxyrhynchus* Rafinesque, 1810 (Pisces, Chondrichthyes). Crustaceana 1978;34:109–10.

119. Simpfendorfer C. Pandarid copepods parasitic on sharks from North Queens-land waters. Mem Queensl Mus 1993;33:290.

120. Austin CM, Tan MH, Lee YP, et al. The complete mitogenome of the whale shark parasitic copepod *Pandarus rhincodonicus* Norman, Newbound & Knott (Crus-tacea; Siphonostomatoida; Pandaridae) – a new gene order for the copepoda. Mitochondrial DNA A 2016;27(1):694–5.

121. Brian A. Copepodi parassiti dei pesci d'Italia. Genova (Italy): Stabilimento Tipo-Litografico R. Istituto Sordomuti; 1906. p. 1–187.

122. Ho JS, Nagasawa K. New records of parasitic Copepoda from the offshore pelagic fishes of Japan. Bull Natl Res Inst Far Seas Fish 2001;38:1–5.

123. Rojas R, Solano O, Morales-Ramírez A. Size and distribution of *Pandarus satyrus* (Copepoda: Pandaridae) on the blue shark *Prionace glauca* (Carcharhiniformes: Carcharhinidae) in Costa Rica. Rev Biol Trop 2001;49:199–201.
124. Hogans WE, Dadswell MJ. Parasitic copepods of the white shark (*Carcharodon carcharius* L.) from the Bay of Fundy. Can J Zool 1985;63(3):740–1.
125. Nagasawa K, Uyeno D. A checklist of copepods of the family Pandaridae (Siphonostomatoida) from fishes in Japanese waters (1898-2017). J Grad Sch Biosp Sci 2017;56:87–104.
126. Tang D, Yanagisawa M, Nagasawa K. Redescription of *Prosaetes rhinodontis* (Wright, 1876) (Crustacea: Copepoda: Siphonostomatoida), an enigmatic parasite of the whale shark, *Rhincodon typus* Smith 1828 (Elasmobranchii: Orectolobiformes: Rhincodontidae). Zootaxa 2010;2493:1–15.
127. Bernot JP, Boxshall GA. A new species of *Pseudopandarus* Kirtisinghe, 1950 (Copepoda: Siphonostomatoida: Pandaridae) from sharks of the genus *Squalus* L. in New Caledonian waters. Vet Parasitol 2017;94(2):275–91.
128. Cressey R, Simpfendorfer C. *Pseudopandarus australis*, a new species of pandarid copepod from Australian sharks. Proc Biol Soc Wash 1988;101(2):340–5.
129. Rangnekar PG. Two species of copepods from the marine fishes of Bombay. J Univ Bombay 1977;44(71):26–34.
130. Yamaguti S. Parasitic copepods from fishes of Japan with descriptions of 26 new species and remarks on two known species. Biol J Okayama Univ 1959; 5:89–165.
131. Santoro M, Palomba M, Mattiucci S, et al. New parasite records for the sunfish *Mola mola* in the Mediterranean Sea and their potential use as biological tags for long-distance host migration. Front Vet Sci 2020;7:579728.

Zoonotic Dermatoses of Exotic Companion Mammals

Dario d'Ovidio[a],*, Domenico Santoro[b]

KEYWORDS

- Exotic companion mammals • Dermatology • Skin disease • Zoonoses • Rabbit
- Rodents • Ferrets

KEY POINTS

- Integumentary disorders caused by zoonotic agents are very common in exotic companion mammals.
- The prevalence of zoonotic dermatoses in people is unknown as those conditions are not reportable.
- An effective surveillance is crucial to understand pathogen epidemiology and prevent the spread of zoonotic diseases.

INTRODUCTION

Several exotic companion mammal species (eg, rabbits, rodents, ferrets, and hedgehogs) live in contact with humans as house pets. Similar to dogs and cats, they are a potential source of zoonoses with dermatologic manifestation transmissible to their owners.[1,2] Zoonotic dermatoses of exotic companion mammals (ECMs) include parasitic, fungal, bacterial, and viral infections. Parasitic dermatoses are very commonly diagnosed in these pets and include *Cheyletiella parasitovorax*, *Leporacarus gibbus*, *Trixacarus caviae*, *Sarcoptes scabiei*, *Notoedres cati*, and *Otodectes cynotis*. Similarly, fungal infections, caused by *Trichophyton mentagrophytes* and *Microsporum* spp, are among the most common zoonotic dermatoses affecting ECM. Bacterial (eg, *Staphylococcus aureus*, *Salmonella* spp, *Corynebacterium kutscheri*, and *Francisella tularensis*)[3–6] and viral infections (mpox virus [MPXV] and cowpox virus [CPXV]) may also occur, although they are rarely reported.[6,7]

Parasitic Disease

Superficial mites

Mite infestation occurs in a large number of ECM species and can be caused by burrowing and non-burrowing mites.

[a] Via C. Colombo 118, Arzano, Naples 80022, Italy; [b] Department of Small Animal Clinical Sciences, College of Veterinary Medicine, University of Florida, 2015 Southwest 16th Avenue, Gainesville, FL 32610, USA
* Corresponding author.
E-mail address: dariodovidio@yahoo.it

Vet Clin Exot Anim 26 (2023) 511–523
https://doi.org/10.1016/j.cvex.2023.01.002
1094-9194/23/© 2023 Elsevier Inc. All rights reserved.

Zoonotic fur mites such as *C. parasitovorax* and *L. gibbus* (formerly *Listrophorus gibbus*) live on the skin or hair of affected animals where they feed on sebaceous secretions and epithelial scales and do not borrow. Burrowing mites such as *T. caviae*, *S. scabiei*, *N. cati,* and *O. cynotis* live in the upper layers of the epidermis and create tunnels in which females lay their eggs.[8,9] The life cycle of such mites lasts approximately 21 to 28 days.[10] The use of antiparasitic drugs (eg, avermectines) as well as environmental disinfection is recommended in infested animals. These mites are not able to reproduce outside of their host; thus, they can only transiently cause papular dermatitis on the owner's arms, legs, or abdomen after close contact with infested pets.

Ear mites

O. cynotis is the ear mite of dogs, cats, and ferrets that live on the surface of the ear canal and can occasionally migrate in other regions of the body (eg, perineum).[11,12] This mite causes otitis externa characterized by the presence of a dry dark brown exudate (coffee ground-like) and eventually blood clots as well as intense pruritus and head shaking.[12] Diagnosis relies on mite identification on microscopic examination of the aural debris. As *O. cynotis* is not host specific, transmission from affected dogs, cats, and ferrets to other cohabitant pets may occur. Although rarely, people can be infested as well and develop a pruritic papular dermatitis on the skin or even true otic parasitic infestations.[2,10,13] The most common treatment options include avermectines (eg, ivermectin, selamectin, moxidectin/imidacloprid) or fipronil, possibly associated with otic topical preparations (eg, thiabendazole, dexamethasone, and neomycin).[12]

Scabies

S. scabiei is cutaneous, burrowing mites belonging to the family Sarcoptidae that have been isolated from all the domestic animals such as dogs, cats, rabbits, horses, ruminants, and pigs.[9] These mites live in the *stratum corneum* of the skin and complete their entire life cycle (larvae, protonymph, tritonymph, and adults) on the host in about 21 days.[14] *S. scabiei* causes delayed inflammatory and immune responses in its hosts.[15] Several genetic variants are associated with single mammalian species making *S. scabiei* infestation species-specific. This mite occurs commonly in rabbits, less frequently in ferrets (**Fig. 1**).[9,12] *S. scabiei* infestation causes severe pruritus, scales, crusts, erythema, alopecia, and lichenification mainly as a consequence of a hypersensitivity reaction to the mites' body, their excrement, and eggs.[9,12] Diagnosis, particularly in early stages, can be challenging due to the high number of false-negative results of skin scrapings.[9] In people, particularly in children, vesicles and papules associated with transient intense pruritus are the main clinical signs associated with *S. scabiei* var. *cuniculi* infestation.[16] As animal mites cannot complete their life cycle in human beings, animal scabies is self-limiting in people.[16,17] In these cases, a papular eruption and pruritus can be likely caused by a hypersensitivity reaction to the mites (**Fig. 2**). Treatment includes topical or injectable parasiticides such as avermectines (eg, ivermectin, selamectin, and moxidectin/imidacloprid), lime sulfur (in ferrets) or isoxazolines (eg, fluralaner).[9,12,18]

Fur mites

Cheyletiellosis. *Cheyletiella* spp is a not host-specific fur mite that can parasitize several mammalian species including rabbits, dogs, cats, and humans. This parasite feeds on dandruff and can be found on the skin or hair shafts and it is commonly associated to pruritus, erythema, alopecia, and scales, particularly on the dorsal neck and inter-scapular area, but it can be found everywhere in the haircoat (**Fig. 3**).[2]

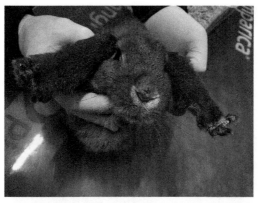

Fig. 1. Rabbit infected with *S. scabiei* var. *cuniculi* (rabbit scabies). Note the tick crusts on ear margins and bridge of the nose.

Asymptomatic forms are also reported in immunocompetent hosts, whereas symptomatic infestations are more common in animals affected by comorbidities (eg, dental disease) or in immunosuppressed animals.[2,19] The presence of compatible clinical signs as well as microscopic identification of mites is required for a definitive diagnosis. Pet owners can develop several clinical signs such as pruritus, erythema, papules, vesicles, vesiculobullous eruptions, and excoriations generally on the areas in contact with the infested animals (eg, forearms, chest, and abdomen) **(Fig. 4)**.[1,20,21] Persistent peripheral eosinophilia has also been rarely reported in affected people.[22] Owing to the ability to bite people and rapidly return to its animal host (bite and run behavior), diagnosis of human Cheyletiellosis is often challenging.[21] Several antiparasitic drugs such as ivermectin, selamectin, or moxidectin/imidacloprid along with concurrent environmental disinfestation with a miticide can be used in infested animals.[8,23,24]

Leporacarus gibbus infestation. *L. gibbus* (formerly *Listrophorus gibbus*) is a fur mite infesting both laboratory and pet rabbits belonging to the family *Listrophoridae*.[25]

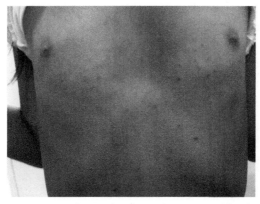

Fig. 2. Pruritic erythematous papules on the chest of an 8-year-old girl, after contact with a rabbit with scabies.

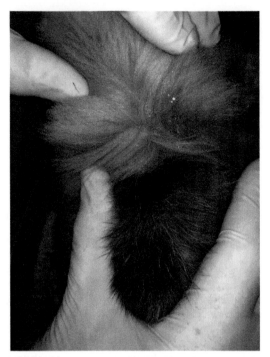

Fig. 3. Large non-adherent white scales on the dorsal neck and inter-scapular area of a rabbit affected by cheyletiellosis.

Rarely this mite can occur in other domestic species (eg, cats).[26] Its entire life cycle occurs on the host's coat, where the mites locate on the distal third of the hair shaft feeding on scales and sebaceous secretions. Transmission occurs with direct contact between infested and noninfested animals. Affected animals are generally asymptomatic. However, when rabbits are immunosuppressed or affected by other comorbidities, clinical signs such as non-well-demarcated alopecia, moist dermatitis,

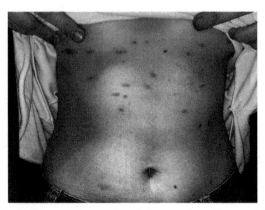

Fig. 4. Pruritic erythematous papules on the abdomen of an 11-year-old girl, after contact with a rabbit with cheyletiellosis.

erythema, scaling, and pruritus may occur.[25,27] Parasitologic examination on rabbit's hair after hair plucking, hair combing, skin scraping, and adhesive tape test, is essential to reveal *L. gibbus* mites. Cohabitant humans may develop small pruritic erythematous papules, tiny vesicles, and pustules generally on their arms and legs as well as intense pruritus after touching their rabbits likely caused by a hypersensitivity reaction to the biting of mites. Lesions may occur for a short time (days or weeks) after contact and disappear after treatment of infested animals.[10] Treatment is the same as for Cheyletiellosis.

Gamasids (Gamasid mites)

Ornithonyssus bacoti is not host-specific, obligate, blood-feeding ectoparasite belonging to the family Macronyssidae.[28] Previously considered specific of wild rats, this mite, which is found mostly in tropical and moderate climate zones, has been reported in several species of ECM in different European and North American regions.[3,28–31] The entire life cycle lasts 11 to 16 days at room temperature and at a relative humidity of 75% to 80%. Clinical signs in affected animals are generally not specific and include intense pruritus, anemia, weakness, alopecia, and erythema.[28,31] In people, *O. bacoti* infestation causes pruritic insect bite-like reactions with clusters of papules and vesicles localized on the forehead, limbs, and other regions of the body.[28] In addition, *O. bacoti* may serve as a vector for several arthropod borne diseases including *Coxiella burnetii* (Q fever), hantavirus, *Borrelia* spp., *Bartonella* spp., and *Rickettsia* spp.[28] Diagnosis is easily performed at light microscopy after ectoparasite collection on the affected animals. Owing to their large size *O. bacoti* can be visible with the naked eye (**Fig. 5**). Although uncommon *O. bacoti* infestation has been reported in pet owners in contact with affected animals as an erythematous-papular eruption on the contact areas (eg, arms) (**Fig. 6**A, B).[31] Treatment mainly consists of using avermectines (eg, ivermectin or moxidectin/imidacloprid) along with environmental disinfestation with environmental miticide products.[28,31]

Fleas

Fleas are small, hematophagous, wingless arthropods belonging to the order Siphonaptera that parasitize mammals and birds. They represent the most common cause of parasitic disease in dogs and cats, whereas they are generally rarely found in ECM.[10] The most common species found in rabbits, ferrets, and rodents include *Spilopsyllus cuniculi* (rabbit flea) and *Ctenocephalides felis* (cat flea) or *Ctenocephalides canis* (dog flea), *Echidnophaga gallinacea, Cediopsylla simplex, Odontopsyllus multispinosus, Hoplopsyllus* spp., *Paracaras meli* (the badger flea), *Ceratophyllus sciurorum* (the squirrel flea), and *Ceratophyllus vison* (the mink flea).[12,32,33] Flea infestation in ECM is characterized by moderate to severe pruritus leading to alopecia, erythema, excoriations, and crusts on the head, neck, and trunk.[34] Signs of flea-bite hypersensitivity (eg, pruritic papular-crusted dermatitis) have also been reported in ferrets.[12] In addition, fleas may act as carriers for several infectious diseases (eg, myxomatosis) some of which have a zoonotic potential (eg, *Bartonella* spp., *Yersinia pestis*).[35,36] Microscopic identification (at light microscopy) of the fleas or their excrements is required to achieve diagnosis. Molecular screening of fleas can help detect the zoonotic pathogens (eg, *Bartonella* spp.) for which they act as carriers. Both the infested animals and their environment should be treated with topical or systemic acaricidal drugs (eg, selamectin, imidacloprid, lufenuron).[32,34,37–39] Fipronil can be used in ferrets, but it should not be used in rabbits due to its high toxicity in this species.[12,34]

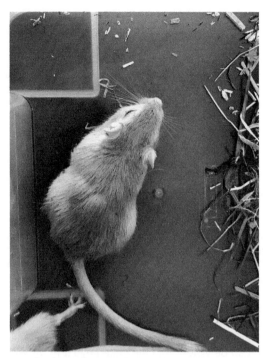

Fig. 5. Tropical rat mites (*O. bacoti*) on the haircoat and in the cage of two Mongolian gerbils (*Meriones unguiculatus*). The "big" mites are visible (as red spots) at naked eye.

Ticks

Ticks are not host-specific ectoparasites that can easily infest people cohabiting with pets causing irritation, pain, nodular reactions, and hypersensitivity reactions in both people and animals.[10,40] In addition, ticks serve as vectors of several vector-borne infectious diseases affecting animals (eg, myxomatosis) and humans (Lyme disease, Rocky Mountain spotted fever, and tularemia). Luckily, they are rarely found in ECM and have been reported mainly in wild rabbits as well as ferrets, rabbits, and hedgehogs housed outdoors or cohabiting with infested pets.[12,33,34,41] Both ixodid (namely

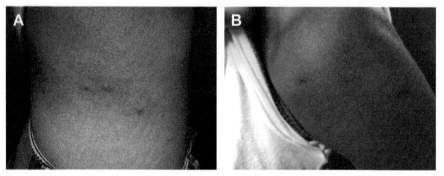

Fig. 6. Large erythematous papules on the abdomen (*A*) and arm (*B*) of a 16-year-old boy after contact with his Mongolian gerbils with *O. bacoti*.

hard) (eg, *Haemaphysalis leporispalustris*, *Amblyomma*, *Boophilus*, *Rhipicephalus*, and *Dermacentor*) and argasid (soft) ticks (eg, *Otobius lagophilus*, *Ornithodoros parkeri*, and *Ornithodoros turicata*) can be affect ECM.[42,43] Diagnosis is made similarly to dogs and cats, visualization and identification of the tick. Although there are no reported clinical cases of Lyme disease in rabbits, ferrets, or hedgehogs, and very few clinical cases of tularemia described in rabbits and rodents, these animals play in important role as carriers of the pathogen while arthropods (eg, ticks) act as vectors in the spread of the disease to humans or other companion animals (eg, cats and dogs).[44] Therefore, manual removal and use of antiparasitic preventative treatments (eg, avermectines) is recommended in tick-infested animals to reduce the risk of arthropod vector bites to cohabitant pets and humans.

Dirofilarioses
Dirofilaria immitis is the causative agent of canine heartworm disease, whereas *Dirofilaria repens* causes subcutaneous dirofilariosis. These nematodes are found mainly in wild carnivores (eg, foxes, wolves, coyotes, bears, muskrats, raccoons, and bobcats). However, they have been isolated in laboratory ferrets as well.[45] People can become accidental hosts with larvae or adult nematodes of *D. immitis* and *D. repens* localizing to the subcutaneous tissues as well as pulmonary vessels and central nervous system.[46–48] Human infestations are mainly asymptomatic; however, fatal symptoms may rarely occur. [46,49,50] The recommended treatment for ferret dirofilariasis consists of topical or injectable avermectines (eg, ivermectin, selamectin, imidacloprid/moxidectin) as well as oral milbemycin oxime.[51]

Fungal disease
Dermatophytes are pathogens of both animals and humans causing superficial fungal disease involving the skin (*stratum corneum*), hair, and nails.[2,10] Although several species of dermatophytes have been isolated from ECM, three species are more commonly isolated from dogs, cats, and ECM, namely *T. mentagrophytes*, *Microsporum canis*, and *M. gypseum*.[10] Of those, *T. mentagrophytes* is the most prevalent dermatophyte isolated in guinea pigs, rabbits, chinchillas, hedgehogs, and marsupials.[2,6] *Microsporum* spp occurs rarely and is mainly reported in rodents.[2,6] Several saprophytic fungi such as *Alternaria* spp., *Aspergillus* spp., *Cladosporium* spp., *Paecilomyces* spp., *Penicillium* spp., *Scolecobasidium* spp., and *Scopulariopsis* spp. have been isolated from ECM as well; however, they are rarely cause of human fungal infections.[52,53] As ECM can be asymptomatic carriers for both dermatophytic and nondermatophytic fungi, they represent a source of fungal infection in people.[2,5,52,54,55] Animals of all age can be infected; however, newly purchased ECMs have a higher potential to harbor such organisms.[2] Direct transmission occurs through contact with infective spores (on the animal or environment) to a susceptible host. Animals affected by dermatophytosis may be asymptomatic or show dermatologic sings such as alopecia, erythema, scaling, and crusting on the head (face, eyelids, and ears), nails, legs, and back (**Fig. 7**).[56,57] In people, areas of circular pruritic dermatitis may appear generally on arms and legs, but it can affect the entire body if left untreated (**Fig. 8A, B**).[10] Non-dermatophytic molds have also the potential to cause dermatitis in both animals and people.[2,53,58] Affected animals may show haircoat abnormalities (eg, hair opacity and fragmentation), hyperkeratosis, whereas onychomycosis, panophthalmia, granulomas and generalized infection may occur in humans.[53,58] Like for parasites, both the affected animals and their environment should be treated with systemic (eg, itraconazole, ketoconazole, terbinafine, griseofulvin) and topical (enilconazole or lime sulfur dips) drugs as well as fungicidal disinfectants (eg, bleach, enilconazole,

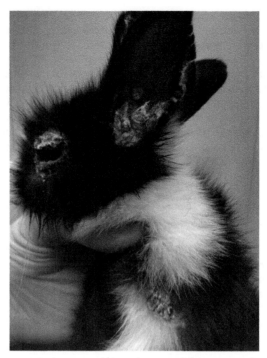

Fig. 7. Severe tick crusts, erythema, and alopecia around the eyes, on the ear margins and at the entrance of the ear canal, and thorax of a 3-month-old rabbit with *T. mentagrophytes*.

accelerated hydrogen peroxide, and over the counter general disinfectant with fungicidal activity).[12,41,59] Systemic therapy should be done until two negative fungal cultures are obtained 7 days apart.[41]

Bacterial Disease

Methicillin-resistant *S. aureus* (MRSA) is an emerging pathogen responsible for bacterial infections in animals and people. Isolation of MRSA has been documented in both pet and farm rabbits raised intensively for meat production as well as in wild lagomorphs.[60–64] Affected rabbits may show crusts and abscesses on head, neck, and lips.[60] A few cases of MRSA infections involving farm workers or their family members have been reported.[65] Affected people may show cutaneous, wound, and osteoarticular infections as well as endocarditis, pneumonia, and septicemia.[65] Diagnosis of MRSA infection is done mainly by bacteriologic culture of the lesions and/or molecular identification. Treatment relies on the results of the antimicrobial susceptibility test.

Viral Disease

MPXV is an emerging viral pathogen that has been reported in Africa and United States.[66,67] Outbreaks of MPXV disease have been reported in the staff of veterinary facilities and pet stores, pet owners, pet store visitors, and employees after contact with infected prairie dogs imported from Ghana and Gambian rats.[66,67] Affected people may show rash, fever, chills, sweats, headache, joint pain, or lymphadenopathy within 21 days of exposure to ill prairie dogs.[66,67]

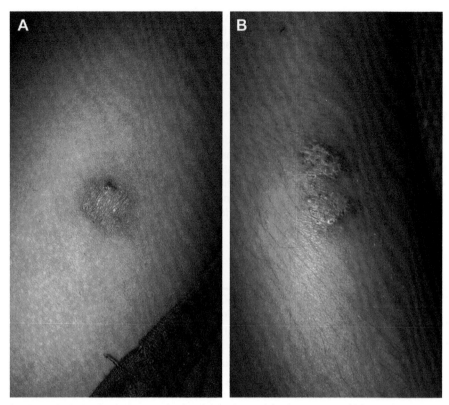

Fig. 8. Typical circular lesion on the leg (*A*) and arm (*B*) of a 14-year-old boy, after contact with his rabbit infected with *T. mentagrophytes*. Note the erythematous margin, alopecia, and scaling with some crusts.

Wild (eg, bank voles and wood mice) and occasionally pet (eg, pet rats) rodents are reservoirs of CPXV, family Poxviridae, genus *Orthopoxvirus*. Direct (through handling) or indirect (litter) contact with infected rats may occasionally cause human infection.[68,69] Infected people may present circumscribed nodules (up to 1.5 cm in diameter) with central necrosis and inflamed edges as well as pustules on the neck, chest, and abdomen potentially accompanied by fever and local lymphadenopathy.[68] Rarely cowpox infections can be associated with severe ocular signs such as necrosis of the upper eyelid, keratitis, leucomatous opacity, and corneal neovascularization.[70] Infections generally clear spontaneously without complications. Diagnosis is done by demonstration of causative agents by viral culture, polymerase chain reaction (PCR), immunohistochemistry, or electron microscopy. No treatment is reported for any viral disease.

Diagnostic Tests

Diagnosis of cutaneous or aural parasites can be done by skin scrapings, adhesive tape collection, coat brushing, and hair plucking followed by microscopic evaluation. To identify superficial fungal organisms, it is essential to perform a fungal culture (eg, dermatophyte test medium and Sabouraud's dextrose agar plates). Histopathologic examination (periodic cis-Schiff or Gomori methenamine-silver staining) and/or PCR have been used successfully.

Bacterial infections can be confirmed by bacterial culture associated to antibiotic susceptibility testing as well as molecular (PCR) analysis of the exudate. Finally, the diagnosis of viral agents is done through serologic or biomolecular laboratory testings (eg, enzyme-linked immunosorbent assay, or PCR) as well as histopathological and immunohistochemical examination of the skin lesions (See chapter on Diagnostic tests).

SUMMARY

Several ECM species (eg, lagomorphs, rodents, and carnivores) live in close contact with humans as house pets. Similar to dogs and cats, they may represent a potential source of cutaneous zoonotic infections/infestations. Specifically, in animals recently adopted or that live in overcrowded conditions. In most cases, the information about the prevalence and epidemiology of those conditions is lacking as many zoonotic dermatoses are not reportable in ECM. Therefore, an active surveillance is necessary to prevent the spread of zoonotic diseases.

CLINICS CARE POINTS

- Zoonotic parasites of exotic companion mammal (ECM) can cause papular dermatitis characterized by vesicles, papules, and transient intense pruritus in cohabiting people.
- Owing to their high potential of harbor fungi, newly purchased ECM should be screened for such pathogens even when asymptomatic.
- Fungal infection in ECM can cause areas of localized pruritic dermatitis in cohabiting people.
- Environmental disinfection should be always performed in combination with systemic and topical drugs to treat both parasitic and fungal dermatoses.

DISCLOSURE

The authors have nothing to disclose.

REFERENCES

1. Parish LC, Schwartzman RM. Zoonoses of dermatological interest. Semin Dermatol 1993;12:57–64.
2. d'Ovidio D, Santoro D. Survey of zoonotic dermatoses in client-owned exotic pet mammals in southern Italy. Zoonoses Public Health 2015;62:100–4.
3. Beck W, Pfister K. Occurrence of a house-infesting tropical rat mite (*Ornithonyssus bacoti*) on murides and human beings in Munich: 3 case reports. Wien Klin Wochenschr 2004;116(Suppl 4):65–8.
4. Pignon C, Mayer J. Zoonoses of ferrets, hedgehogs, and sugar gliders. Vet Clin North Am Exot Anim Pract 2011;14(3):533–49.
5. Rosen T, Jablon J. Infectious threats from exotic pets: dermatological implications. Dermatol Clin 2003;21:229–36.
6. Mitchell MA, Tully TN. Zoonotic diseases associated with small mammals. In: Quesenberry KE, Orcutt CJ, Mans C, et al, editors. Ferrets, rabbits and rodents clinical medicine and surgery. 4th edition. St Louis, MO: Elsevier Saunders; 2021. p. 609–19.
7. Souza MJ. One health: zoonoses in the exotic animal practice. Vet Clin North Am Exot Anim Pract 2011;14(3):421–6.

8. d'Ovidio D, Noviello. Diagnostic corner: Exotic pets. Veterinaria 2015;29(1):65–7.
9. d'Ovidio D, Santoro D. Efficacy of fluralaner in the treatment of sarcoptic mange (*Sarcoptes scabiei*) in 12 pet rabbits. Top Companion Anim Med 2021;43:100528.
10. Moriello KA. Zoonotic skin diseases of dogs and cats. Anim Health Res Rev 2003; 4(2):157–68.
11. Le Sueur C, Bour S, Schaper R. Efficacy and safety of the combination imidacloprid 10 %/moxidectin 1.0 % spot-on (Advocate(®) spot-on for small cats and ferrets) in the treatment of ear mite infection (*Otodectes cynotis*) in ferrets. Parasitol Res 2011;109(Suppl 1):S149–56.
12. d'Ovidio D, Santoro D. Dermatologic diseases of ferrets. In: Quesenberry KE, Orcutt CJ, Mans C, et al, editors. Ferrets, rabbits and rodents clinical medicine and surgery. 4th edition. St Louis, MO: Elsevier Saunders; 2021. p. 109–16.
13. Van de Heyning J, Thienpont D. Otitis externa in man caused by the mite *Otodectes cynotis*. Laryngoscope 1977;87:1938–41.
14. Arlian LG, Runyan RA, Vyszenski-Moher DL. Water balance and nutrient procurement of *Sarcoptes scabiei* var. *canis* (Acari: *Sarcoptidae*). J Med Entomol 1988; 25:64–8.
15. Morgan MS, Arlian LG, Markey MP. *Sarcoptes scabiei* mites modulate gene expression in human skin equivalents. PLoS One 2013;8:e71143.
16. Hengge U, Currie B, Jäger G, et al. Scabies: a ubiquitous neglected skin disease. Lancet Infect Dis 2006;6:769–79.
17. Menzano A, Rambozzi L, Rossi L. Outbreak of scabies in human beings, acquired from chamois (*Rupicapra rupicapra*). Vet Rec 2004;155:568.
18. d'Ovidio D, Santoro D. Efficacy of a spot-on combination of fluralaner plus moxidectin (Bravecto plus) against naturally acquired Sarcoptes scabiei infestation in 10 pet rabbits: Retrospective case series. Vet Dermatol 2022;34(1):3–6.
19. d'Ovidio D, Santoro D. Orodental diseases and dermatological disorders are highly associated in pet rabbits: a case-control study. Vet Dermatol 2013;24(5): 531, e125.
20. Cohen SR. *Cheyletiella* dermatitis. A mite infestation of rabbit, cat, dog, and man. Arch Dermatol 1980;116:435–7.
21. Wagner R, Stallmeister NS. *Cheyletiella* dermatitis in humans, dogs and cats. Br J Dermatol 2000;143:1097–131.
22. Dobrosavljevic DD, Popovic ND, Radovanovic SS. Systemic manifestations of *Cheyletiella* infestation in man. Int J Dermatol 2007;46:397–9.
23. Kim SH, Lee JY, Jun HK, et al. Efficacy of selamectin in the treatment of cheyletiellosis in pet rabbits. Vet Dermatol 2008;19:26–7.
24. Mellgren M, Bergvall K. Treatment of rabbit cheyletiellosis with selemectin or ivermectin: a retrospective case study. Acta Vet Scand 2008;50:1–6.
25. d'Ovidio D, Santoro D. *Leporacarus gibbus* infestation in client-owned rabbits and their owner. Vet Dermatol 2014;25:46, e17.
26. Dumitrache MO, Györke A, D'Amico G, et al. First case report of dermatitis associated with *Leporacarus gibbus* in cat. BMC Vet Res 2021;17:4.
27. Burns DA. Papular urticaria produced by the mite Listrophorus gibbus. Clin Exp Dermatol 1987;12:200–1.
28. d'Ovidio D, Noviello E, Santoro D. Prevalence and zoonotic risk of tropical rat mite (*Ornithonyssus bacoti*) in exotic companion mammals in southern Italy. Vet Dermatol 2018;29:522, e174.
29. Fox MT, Baker AS, Farquhar R, et al. First record of *Ornithonyssus bacoti* from a domestic pet in the United Kingdom. Vet Rec 2004;3:437–8.

30. Fiechter R, Grimm F, Müller G, et al. Cumulation of Ornithonyssus bacoti (tropical rat mite) infestations of pet rodents and their owners in the Canton of Zürich and Graubünden. Schweiz Arch Tierheilkd 2011;153:79–85.

31. d'Ovidio D, Noviello E, Santoro D. Tropical rat mite (*Ornithonyssus bacoti*) infestation in pet Syrian hamsters (*Mesocricetus auratus*) and their owner. Vet Dermatol 2017;28:256–7.

32. Jenkins JR. Skin disorders of the rabbit. Vet Clin Exot Anim 2001;4:543–63.

33. Patterson MM, Fox JG, Eberhard ML. Parasitic diseases. In: Fox JG, Marini RP, editors. Biology and diseases of the ferret. 3rd edition. Oxford, UK: Wiley-Blackwell; 2014. p. 553–72.

34. Fehr M, Koestlinger S. Ectoparasites in small exotic mammals. Vet Clin North Am Exot Anim Pract 2013;16:611–57.

35. Sobey WR, Conolly D. Myxomatosis: the introduction of the European rabbit flea *Spilopsyllus cuniculi* (Dale) into wild rabbit populations in Australia. J Hyg (Lond) 1971;69:331–46.

36. Sato S, Brinkerhoff RJ, Hollis E, et al. Detection of zoonotic Bartonella pathogens in rabbit fleas, Colorado, USA. Emerg Infect Dis 2020;26:778–81.

37. Hutchinson MJ, Jacobs DE, Bell GD, et al. Evaluation of imidacloprid for the treatment and prevention of cat flea (*Ctenocephalides felis felis*) infestations on rabbits. Vet Rec 2001;148:695–6.

38. Wenzel U, Heine J, Mengel H, et al. Efficacy of imidacloprid 10%/moxidectin 1% (Advocate/Advantage Multi) against fleas (*Ctenocephalides felis felis*) on ferrets (*Mustela putorius furo*). Parasitol Res 2008;103:231–4.

39. Carpenter JW, Dryden MW, Kukanich B. Pharmacokinetics, efficacy, and adverse effects of selamectin following topical administration in flea-infested rabbits. Am J Vet Res 2012;73:562–6.

40. Jones EH, Hinckley AF, Hook SA, et al. Pet ownership increases human risk of encountering ticks. Zoonoses Public Health 2018;65:74–9.

41. Varga M, Paterson S. Dermatologic diseases of rabbits. In: Quesenberry KE, Orcutt CJ, Mans C, et al, editors. Ferrets, rabbits and rodents clinical medicine and surgery. 4th edition. St Louis, MO: Elsevier Saunders; 2021. p. 220–32.

42. Cooney JC, Burgdorfer W, Painter MK, et al. Tick infestations of the eastern cottontail rabbit (*Sylvilagus floridanus*) and small rodentia in northwest Alabama and implications for disease transmission. J Vector Ecol 2005;30:171–80.

43. De Matos R, Kalivoda K. Dermatoses of exotic small mammals. In: Miller WH, Griffin CE, editors. Muller and Kirk's small animal dermatology. 7th edition. Philadelphia: Elsevier; 2013. p. 844–87.

44. Yeni DK, Büyük F, Ashraf A, et al. Tularemia: a re-emerging tick-borne infectious disease. Folia Microbiol (Praha) 2021;66:1–14.

45. Otranto D, Deplazes P. Zoonotic nematodes of wild carnivores. Int J Parasitol Parasites Wildl 2019;9:370–83.

46. Otranto D, Eberhard ML. Zoonotic helminths affecting the human eye. Parasites Vectors 2011;4:41.

47. Foissac M, Million M, Mary C, et al. Subcutaneous infection with *Dirofilaria immitis* nematode in human. France Emerg Infect Dis 2013;19:171–2.

48. Falidas E, Gourgiotis S, Ivopoulou O, et al. Human subcutaneous dirofilariasis caused by *Dirofilaria immitis* in a Greek adult. J Infect Public Health 2016;9:102–4.

49. McCall JW, Genchi C, Kramer LH, et al. Heartworm disease in animals and humans. Adv Parasitol 2008;66:193–285.

50. Genchi C, Kramer LH, Rivasi F. Dirofilarial infections in Europe. Vector Borne Zoonotic Dis 2011;11:1307–17.
51. Morrisey JK, Malakoff RL. Cardiovascular and Other Diseases of Ferrets. In: Quesenberry KE, Orcutt CJ, Mans C, et al, editors. Ferrets, rabbits and rodents clinical medicine and surgery. 4th edition. St Louis, MO: Elsevier Saunders; 2020. p. 55–70.
52. d'Ovidio D, Grable SL, Ferrara M, et al. Prevalence of dermatophytes and other superficial fungal organisms in asymptomatic guinea pigs in Southern Italy. J Small Anim Pract 2014;55:355–8.
53. Han J, Na KJ. Cutaneous paecilomycosis caused by *Paecilomyces variottii* in an African pygmy hedgehog (*Atelerix albiventris*). J Exot Pet Med 2010;19:309–12.
54. Chomel BB, Belotto A, Meslin FX. Wildlife, exotic pets, and emerging zoonoses. Emerg Infect Dis 2007;13:6–11.
55. Kraemer A, Mueller RS, Werckenthin C, et al. Dermatophytes in pet Guinea pigs and rabbits. Vet Microbiol 2012;157:208–13.
56. Moretti A, Agnetti F, Mancianti F, et al. Dermatophytosis in animals: epidemiological, clinical and zoonotic aspects. G Ital Dermatol Venereol 2013;148:563–72.
57. Overgaauw PAM, Avermaete KHAV, Mertens CARM, et al. Prevalence and zoonotic risks of *Trichophyton mentagrophytes* and *Cheyletiella* spp. in Guinea pigs and rabbits in Dutch pet shops. Vet Microbiol 2017;205:106–9.
58. Goncalves CAM, Tonin AA. Fungal dermatitis by *Scopulariopsis brevicaulis* in Guinea pig (*Cavia porcellus*). Acta Veterinaria Brasilica 2021;15:184–7.
59. Moriello KA, Coyner K, Paterson S, et al. Diagnosis and treatment of dermatophytosis in dogs and cats: Clinical Consensus Guidelines of the World Association for Veterinary Dermatology. Vet Dermatol 2017;28:266, e68.
60. Loncaric I, Kunzel F. Sequence type 398 meticillin-resistant *Staphylococcus aureus* infection in a pet rabbit. Vet Dermatol 2013;24:370, e84.
61. Agnoletti F, Mazzolini E, Bacchin C, et al. First reporting of methicillin-resistant Staphylococcus aureus (MRSA) ST398 in an industrial rabbit holding and in farm-related people. Vet Microbiol 2014;170:172–7.
62. Attili AR, Bellato A, Robino P, et al. Analysis of the antibiotic resistance profiles in methicillin-sensitive Staphylococcus aureus pathotypes isolated on a commercial rabbit farm in Italy. Antibiotics (Basel) 2020;9:673.
63. Moreno-Grúa E, Pérez-Fuentes S, Viana D, et al. Marked presence of methicillin-resistant Staphylococcus aureus in wild lagomorphs in Valencia, Spain. Animals (Basel) 2020;10:1109.
64. Chai MH, Sukiman MZ, Najib NM, et al. Molecular detection and antibiogram of Staphylococcus aureus in rabbits, rabbit handlers, and rabbitry in Terengganu, Malaysia. J Adv Vet Anim Res 2021;8:388–95.
65. Rankin S, Roberts S, O'Shea K, et al. Panton valentine leukocidin (PVL) toxin positive MRSA strains isolated from companion animals. Vet Microbiol 2005;108:145–8.
66. Croft DR, Sotir MJ, Williams CJ, et al. Occupational risks during a monkeypox outbreak, Wisconsin, 2003. Emerg Infect Dis 2007;13:1150–7.
67. Essbauer S, Pfeffer M, Meyer H. Zoonotic poxviruses. Vet Microbiol 2010;140:229–36.
68. Campe H, Zimmerman P, Glos K, et al. Cowpox virus transmission from pet rats to humans, Germany. Emerg Infect Dis 2009;15:777–80.
69. Ninove L, Domart Y, Vervel C, et al. Cowpox virus transmission from pet rats to humans, France. Emerg Infect Dis 2009;15:781–4.
70. Krankowska DC, Woźniak PA, Cybula A, et al. Cowpox: how dangerous could it be for humans? Case report. Int J Infect Dis 2021;104:239–41.

Moving?

Make sure your subscription moves with you!

To notify us of your new address, find your **Clinics Account Number** (located on your mailing label above your name), and contact customer service at:

Email: journalscustomerservice-usa@elsevier.com

800-654-2452 (subscribers in the U.S. & Canada)
314-447-8871 (subscribers outside of the U.S. & Canada)

Fax number: 314-447-8029

Elsevier Health Sciences Division
Subscription Customer Service
3251 Riverport Lane
Maryland Heights, MO 63043

*To ensure uninterrupted delivery of your subscription, please notify us at least 4 weeks in advance of move.

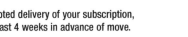

Printed and bound by CPI Group (UK) Ltd, Croydon, CR0 4YY

03/10/2024

01040473-0003